IMMUNOPATHOLOGY AND IMMUNOMODULATION

Edited by **Krassimir Metodiev**

Immunopathology and Immunomodulation
http://dx.doi.org/10.5772/59217
Edited by Krassimir Metodiev

Contributors

Krassimir Metodiev, Moosa Patel, Vinitha Philip, Atul Lakha, Sugeshnee Pather, Muhammed Faadil Waja, Lucille Singh, Mohamed Arbee, Yildiz Camcioglu, Tsvetan Sokolov, John N Giannios, Tatina Todorova, Gabriela Tsankova, Neli Lodozova, Tcvetelina Kostadinova, Assia Konsoulova, Kaloyan D. Georgiev, Marieta Georgieva, Peter Dobromirov, Liliya Ivanova, Denitza Tzaneva, Zhivka Stoykova, Ara Kaprelyan, Bogdanka Basekic Andric, Aleksandar Andric, Mileta Golubovic, Metodi Abadzhiev

Published by InTech

Janeza Trdine 9, 51000 Rijeka, Croatia

Publishing Process Manager Iva Lipovic

Technical Editor InTech DTP team

Cover InTech Design team

First published November, 2015

Printed in Croatia

Additional hard copies can be obtained from orders@intechopen.com

Immunopathology and Immunomodulation , Edited by Krassimir Metodiev

p. cm.

ISBN 978-953-51-2210-4

For EU product safety concerns:
IN TECH d.o.o., Prolaz Marije Krucifikse Kozulić 3, 51000 Rijeka, Croatia, info@intechopen.com or visit our website at intechopen.com.

Meet the editor

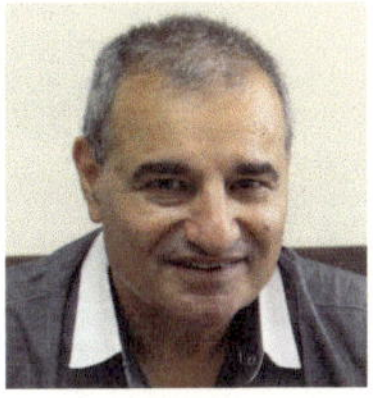

Professor Dr. Krassimir Metodiev, MD, PhD, DSc(Med), is Head of the Department of Preclinical and Clinical Sciences, Medical University, Varna, Bulgaria; President, IMAB; Vice-President, FESCI; Referent, UICC; and Director, ARW Bioterrorism, Scientific Affairs' Division, NATO. His specialties are immunology and clinical microbiology. He has published 240 papers, IF 174.00, 7 books on medicine, and 2 books on poetry. He is editor in chief of the *Journal of IMAB* and editorial board member of *IJIP*, *EJI*, *CEJM*, *JAA*, and JISAO. He has attended 120 congresses worldwide, is a plenary speaker, and has been the chairperson of several sessions and workshops. He has been guest professor in Germany (Institute for Immunology, Munich); Austria (Danube University, Krems); Norway (The Norwegian Radium Hospital, Institute for Cancer Research, Oslo); and Israel (Hadassah-Jerusalem, Rambam-Haifa, Sheba-Tel Hashomer). He has been assigned the following awards: Union Bulgarian Physicians (Doctor of the Year, twice); Honorary Medal IMAB; Annual Award ISC; Order Maimonides-Rambam (Haifa-Israel); Plate, Hellenic & International SMGM (Greece); Medal, Hadassah (Jerusalem-Israel); Medal, Sheba (Tel Aviv-Israel); Medal NKF (USA); and Plate, Israel Ministry of Foreign Affairs. He is also an honorary consul of Israel to Bulgaria.

Contents

Preface

Medicus curat, natura sanat!
(meaning, Doctor cures, nature saves!)

This book is a second attempt of a group of distinguished international authors to reveal out a number of disputable topics in regard to immunopathology, immunoregulation, immunosuppression, immunostimulation, immunotherapy, immune status, and clinical immunology as a whole.

Generally speaking, immunopathology (IP) is a branch of medicine that deals with immune responses associated with disease. It has various manifestations, both clinically expressed and latent processes, which, however, are also a high risk to the potential patient. IP includes the study of the pathology of an organism, organ system, or disease with respect to the immune system, immunity, and immune responses.

The main aim of the authors of the book is to take a deep look into serious immune disorders. The chapters reflect updated information of the current development and perspective of modern immunology in regard to immune diseases, and they tend to expand the present knowledge on the specific topics included in the content.

Defects or malfunctions in the immune response can provoke illness or disease. Such disorders are generally caused by an overactive immune response, manifested as hypersensitivity reactions, an inappropriate reaction to self, manifested as autoimmunity, or ineffective immune responses, known as immunodeficiency.

This book is a step forward to the positive discussion of proper diagnosis and appropriate therapeutic decisions, because *Bene diagnoscitur, bene curato*r (meaning, a disease known is half cured).

It is directed to all biomedical researchers and clinicians, from students to professionals, academic scientists, university professors, and specialists.

We, the authors, editors, and technical supervisors of the InTech Open Access Publisher, are fully aware that our product, the new book *Immunopathology and Immunomodulatio*n could be a useful tool in the hands of everybody who is keen and ambitious to know more about immunology.

Prof. Dr. Krassimir Metodiev, MD, PhD, DSc(Med),
Head, Dept. of Preclinical and Clinical Sciences,
Medical University of Varna, Bulgaria,
President of IMAB (www.imab-bg.org),
Vice-President of FESCI,
Referent and Fellow of UICC

Section 1

Original Papers

Chapter 1

Immunotherapy of Cancer — Some Up-To-Date Approaches

Krassimir Metodiev, Paula Lazarova, Jon Kyte, Gunnar Kvalheim and Jahn Nesland

Additional information is available at the end of the chapter

http://dx.doi.org/10.5772/61227

Abstract

Treatment of cancer is currently based on three main modalities: surgery, radiotherapy and chemotherapy. Most solid tumours can only be cured at an early stage, due to the lack of effective systemic treatment. Surgery and radiotherapy are highly effective for eradicating localized tumours, but unfortunately cannot target disseminated disease. Chemotherapy represents systemic treatment, but the clinical use of current drugs is to a large extent hampered by their limited specificity.

Over the last two decades, immunotherapy has emerged as an interesting novel approach. Contrary to the traditional treatment modalities, the immune system combines inherent specificity with a systemic range of action.

The term "vaccine" is traditionally used to describe substances that protect against the development of infectious diseases. In cancer therapy, this term refers to both therapeutic and prophylactic approaches for eliciting immunological and anti-tumour responses.

Prophylactic vaccines have only been developed in a few cancer forms, mainly cancers related to viral infection, such as cervical and hepatocellular carcinoma. Therapeutic vaccines, given to patients after the development of the disease, are however investigated in a number of cancer forms. Some of the therapeutic vaccines may also be used for prophylaxis, particularly in patients with increased risk of cancer process.

This paper throws light and depicts the international experience of a number of distinguished researchers in the field of development and testing of vaccines against some tumours, mainly malignant melanoma and prostate cancer.

Keywords: Immunotherapy, anti-tumour vaccine, malignant melanoma, prostate cancer

1. Introduction

The author analyzes the experience and the research projects worked out in the Dept. Cell Therapy of the University Hospital "Radium" (Inst. Cancer Research, Oslo, Norway) by the team of Prof. Gunnar Kvalheim, Prof. Jon Kyte, Prof. Jahn Nesland, the Bulgarian immunologist M.Sc. Biol. Paula Lazarova, and the author himself, for the last several years.

The colleagues from Radium have utilized gene-transfer technology for developing vaccine therapy with dendritic cells transfected with tumour-mRNA. These vaccines are designed to combine the immunostimulatory capacity of dendritic cells with the antigen repertoire of tumour cells.

There are two approaches to the project: preclinical/experimental evaluation and clinical trials on patients.

2. The first glance throws light on

2.1. Metastatic malignant melanoma – Prognosis and treatment

Malignant melanoma (MM) is among the most common cancers in the developed countries and the incidence has increased substantially over the last decades. Surgery is frequently curative at an early stage, but the prognosis for patients with disseminated disease is generally bleak, with a medium survival of 6-10 months and a 5-year survival of about 5% only.

Decarbazin is extensively used for treatment of metastatic melanoma and has been reported to induce objective tumour responses in 5-29% of all patients. A number of studies have compared other single agents or multi-drug regimes to Decarbazin, without demonstrating a superior effect. To date, no randomized controlled trials have demonstrated improved survival after treatment with Decarbazin or any other drug.

Furthermore, there have been numerous reports of spontaneous immune responses [1] in melanoma patients, to some extent associated with a favourable clinical development. This has prompted the development of various vaccines [1] to target defined or undefined melanoma antigens.

Immunological responses against vaccine antigens have been demonstrated in a number of studies [2, 3, 4, 5, 6, 7, 8]**, but there is limited evidence of clinical effect**

With regard to non-specific immunostimulation, high-dose interleukin-2 (IL-2) has been shown to induce complete remission in about 16% of melanoma patients, but is associated with considerable adverse effects. IL-2, Interferon-alpha (INF-alpha) and other cytokines are also investigated in combination with conventional chemotherapy. Adjuvant therapy with IFN-alpha is believed to prolong the disease-free period, but most studies do not indicate improved survival. Taken together, there is an urgent need for improved therapy of metastatic malignant melanoma.

2.2. The second glance throws light on: Metastatic prostate cancer – Prognosis and treatment

Prostate cancer is the most commonly diagnosed cancer in the male population of the developed countries world-wide. Though the majority of patients eventually die of other causes, prostate cancer is also among the most common cause of cancer death among males in Europe, North America and Japan.

Metastatic prostate cancer is usually treated with bilateral orchiectomy and/or androgen suppressive drugs. The resulting androgen deprivation frequently induces tumour regression and has a palliative effect. The treatment is also considered to give prolonged survival for subsets of patients. However, after a transient response period (median 12-24 months), virtually all patients develop progressive cancer refractory to hormone therapy.

In the RNA/DC-vaccine trial performed in Radium, all included patients had hormone refractory prostate cancer (HRPC).

At this advanced stage, the median survival is only 10-12 months. There has been no effective therapy for HRPC, and many physicians have thus recommended 'clinical observation'.

It is interesting that some separate trials, in other oncology centers, demonstrated prolonged survival after treatment with Doxetacel. This finding has been confirmed in subsequent studies, and Doxetacel is now considered as standard therapy for patients with HRPC.

It should be recalled, however, that the effect on mean survival is limited (2-3 months). Patients with HRPC may also to some extent benefit from different forms of palliative treatment, including certain cytotoxic drugs, bisphosphonates, second-line hormonal agents, glucocorticoids and radiation therapy.

There is, however, an evident need for improved systemic treatment, and immunotherapy may represent an attractive option. Several small-scale studies [2, 3, 5] have demonstrated promising immune responses after vaccine therapy, but there is limited evidence of clinical affect. Interestingly, a recent placebo-controlled phase III trial on HRPC patients has suggested a possible survival benefit from therapy with dendritic cells (DCs) pulsed with a fusion protein of prostatic acid phosphatase and granulocyte-macrophage colony-stimulating factor (GM-CSF).

3. General background for cancer immunotherapy

3.1. Immunosurveillance and immunoediting

A tumour-specific immune response will depend on the ability of immune cells to discriminate the tumour from normal host tissues. In contrast to infectious microbes and allogeneic human cells, the tumour cells are largely similar to normal host cells. According to the theory of immunosurveillance, as suggested by Burnet in 1970, the immune system is still able to recognize and eliminate tumour cells. This concept was severely challenged in the following years. However, there is now convincing evidence that the immune system may recognize tumour cells due to their expression of altered antigens. The early concept of tumour surveillance has highlighted the importance of the immune system in protecting against cancer.

Recent modifications of this theory, now named immunoediting, provide increased insight into the role of the immune system in sculpting the tumour into an immunologically selected cell population. The immunoediting perspective points to a major challenge in cancer immunotherapy: how to make the immune system destroy a tumour that has already escaped the immune attack.

A solution may be found in exploiting the difference between spontaneously occurring immune activation and optimally engineered immunization. This is the reason for the developing of immune-gene-therapy with tumour-mRNA transfected dendritic cells.

3.2. Activation of T cells that recognized tumour-associated antigens

T-lymphocytes express antigen-specific T-cell receptors (TCRs) that enable them to recognize target cells expressing a particular antigen. The antigens are presented as peptides on HLA-molecules on the target cell surface, and the recognition is mediated by binding of the T-cell receptor to the HLA/peptide complex. Proper T-cell stimulation, including TCR-binding, leads to activation and clonal expression of T cells with the relevant antigen specificity. During the development of a tumour, numerous mutations result in novel antigens and altered expression of normal antigens. The resulting tumour-associated antigens are presented as peptides on HLA-molecules.

Figure 1a shows how host T cells may recognize tumour cells by binding of the TCR to the HLA/peptide complex [7]. However, TCR-binding does not necessarily lead to T-cell activation. In general, the activation of previously unstimulated T cells ('naïve' T cells) requires additional stimulation through co-stimulatory molecules like CD80 and CD86. If stimulated only through the TCR, the naïve T cells enter a stage of anergy and permanently lose their ability to be properly activated. The expression of co-stimulatory molecules is largely restricted to professional antigen presenting cells (APCs), including dendritic cells (DCs), macrophages and B cells [7].

Two major subsets of T cells exist. CD4+ T cells recognize peptides bound to HLA class II, while CD8+ T cells recognize peptides presented on HLA class I (Figure 1b).

Most human cells, except erythrocytes and testicular cells, express HLA class I. In contrast, HLA class II is expressed mainly by professional APCs, activated T cells and the cortical epithelium in the thymus. Thus, CD8+ T cells may be stimulated by most cells, while CD4+ T cells depend on stimulation from APCs. As it will be discussed a bit later, the activation of both T-cell subsets is probably important for an effective anti-tumour response.

Effector T cells and the Th1/Th2 delineation [7]:

Proper T-cell activation results in differentiation into effector T cells. CD8+ effector T cells are cytotoxic, i.e. capable of killing cells that express the relevant antigen (Figure 1c).

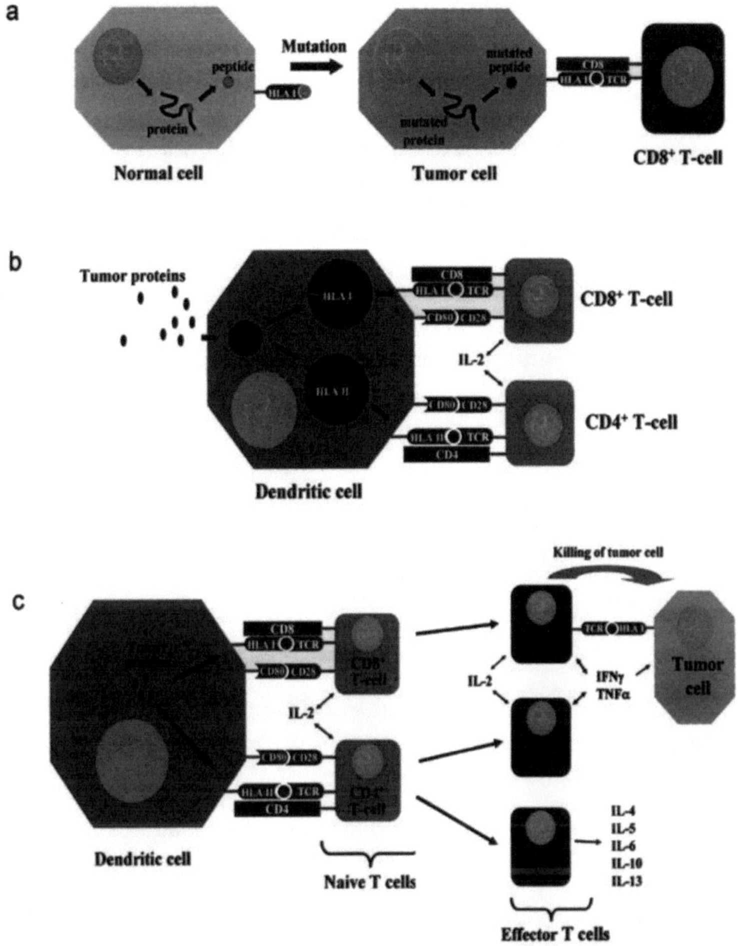

Figure 1. **a**) Mutations through the development of tumor lead to expression of mutated proteins. The mutated proteins are processed into peptides that are presented on HLA classI (HLA I) on the tumor cell surface. CD8+ T cells specific for mutated peptides may therefore recognize tumor cells by binding of their T cell receptor (TCR) to the HLA/peptide complex. **b**) Stimulation of tumor-specific T cells by dendritic cells (DCs). Tumor proteins are engulfed by DCs and processed into peptides. The tumor-associated peptides are presented by DCs on HLA class I and HLA class II, to CD8+ and CD4+ T cells respectively. For proper activation, previously unstimulated ("naive") T cells also requirestimulation from co-stimulatory molecules (e.g. CD80) and IL-2. Dendritic cells constitutively express HLA class II (and I) and co-stimulatory molecules, and the expression in up-regulated upon DC mutation. T cells start producing IL-2 when stimulated through TCR and co-stimulatory molecules. **c**) Activation of CD4+ and CD8+ T cells induce differentiation into effector T cells. CD8+ T cells differentiate into cytotoxic effector cells that specifically kill target cells expressing the relevant antigen. CD4+ T cells differentiate into T-helper cells secreting high levels of cytokines. Based on their cytokine profiles, the CD4+ effector cells are conventionally divided into Th1- and Th2-cells.

CD4+ effector T cells are conventionally divided into T-helper 1 (Th1) or T-helper 2 (Th2) cells, based on their cytokine secretion profiles (Figure 1c).

Interferon-γ (IFNγ), tumour-necrosis factor-α (TNFα) and IL-2 are usually designated as

Th1-cytokines, while the Th2-cytokines include IL-4, IL-5, IL-6, IL-10 and IL-13.

Th1 cells support cellular immunity, e.g. by secreting cytokines that induce up-regulation of HLA on target cells and stimulate macrophages and CD8+ T cells. Th2 cells promote antibody responses by interaction with B cells.

In cancer immunotherapy, Th1-type responses are generally believed to be desirable.

Antibody responses can only target surface antigens, whereas the CD8+ T cells are able to recognize intracellular antigens presented on HLA class I. Th1- and Th2-responses are mutually inhibitory. Th1-cytokines generally promote Th1-differentiation and inhibit Th2-differentiation, while Th2-cytokines have the opposite effects [5, 7].

Th2-cytokines may therefore suppress the development of cytotoxic anti-tumour responses.

There are considerable experimental data on the effects of individual Th1- or Th2-cytokines.

However, the validity of the Th1/Th2-delineation in humans may be questioned, which could be our next publication [8].

4. Dendritic cells – The most potent antigen presenting cells

Dendritic cells (DCs) are derived from CD34+ progenitor cells in the bone marrow, but otherwise constitute a heterogeneous cell type that is widely distributed in different tissues, including skin, mucosa, lymph nodes and spleen.

Resident DCs in the epidermis (Langerhans cells) and interstitial DCs found in other tissues [7] are believed to be derived from CD14+ myeloid precursor cells (Figure 2).

Recent studies in mice, however, have suggested that both subsets can be derived from fms-related tyrosine kinase 3 (Flt3)-expressing myeloid and lymphoid progenitors, and that plasmacytoid DCs may differentiate into myeloid DCs following viral infection.

Dendritic cells are considered to be the most potent antigen presenting cells and are instrumental in eliciting immune responses. DCs capture antigen in the tissues and then migrate to regional lymph nodes where they encounter T cells in the paracortal area.

Most DCs in the skin and other tissues have an immature phenotype. These cells are effective at engulfing antigen and constantly sample their environment, but have a limited ability to migrate and to stimulate T cells. If immature DCs reach the lymph nodes and present antigens to T cells, they are likely to induce anergy rather than activation, due to their low expression of co-stimulatory molecules. In the non-inflammatory setting, the immature DCs thus promote immunological tolerance by capturing and presenting endogenous antigens. Mature DCs, however, are potent inducers of immunity.

Maturation of DCs is commonly induced by inflammatory cytokines or by the capture of microbial ligands that stimulate Toll-like receptors (TLRs).

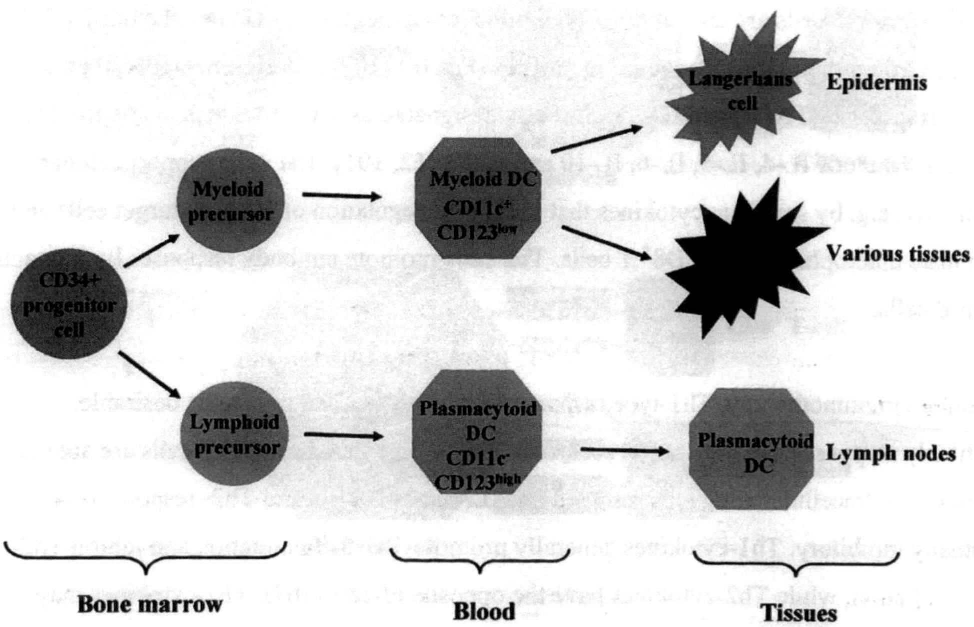

Figure 2. Subsets of dendritic cells (DCs). All DC-subsets are derived from $CD34^{+}$ haematopoietic profnitor cells in the bone marrow. Interstitial DCs and Langerhans cells are believed to be of myeloid origin. The plasmacytoid DCs are traditionally considered to be of lymphoid origin.

Contrary to immature DCs, the mature cells rapidly migrate to regional lymph nodes, as has been demonstrated in vivo in melanoma patients by Devries and his research group [7].

Moreover, mature DCs strongly up-regulate their expression of HLA class II and co-stimulatory molecules, and are highly effective at activating naïve CD4+.

DCs also present engulfed antigens on HLA class I and may thus directly stimulate CD8+ T cells.

Finally, the phenotype of mature DCs, including their cytokine secretion pattern, is believed to direct the differentiation of CD4+ T cells into Th1- or Th2-type cells.

5. Tumour-associated antigens

The tumour-associated antigens comprise tumour-specific antigens, overexpressed antigens, cancer-germline antigens, viral antigens and tissue-differentiation antigens. Antigens which are virtually tumour-specific may arise from genomic mutations, e.g. K-RAS or post-translational modifications, e.g. MUC-1. Other antigens used in cancer vaccines, like hTERT, survivin, and HER2/neu, are widely expressed in normal tissues, but overexpressed in tumour cells.

In contrast, the expression of cancer-germline antigens, e.g. the melanoma antigens MAGE-1 and MAGE-3, is restricted to tumour cells and normal germline cells (testis and placenta).

Viral antigens represent attractive vaccine targets for virus-induced cancers and are included in the prophylactic vaccines mentioned above for cervical carcinoma (Human papilloma virus) and hepatocellular carcinoma (Hepatitis B virus).

The differentiation antigens are tissue-specific, i.e. expressed only in normal and neoplastic cells from a particular lineage. These antigens may be utilized in cancer vaccines if an autoimmune reaction to the relevant tissue is tolerable.

For instance, prostatitis or vitiligo may represent acceptable adverse effects for patients with prostate cancer or malignant melanoma, respectively.

Several differentiation antigens are extensively used in cancer vaccines, including prostate-specific antigen (PSA) and the melanoma antigens Melan a/Mart-1, gp100 and tyrosinase [6, 7, 8].

6. Background for the present up-to-date tumour-RNA/DC vaccines

6.1. The use of dendritic cells in cancer immunotherapy

Most cancer vaccines have been based on peptides/proteins or tumour lysates that are injected intradermally. These approaches depend on uptake of vaccine antigen by immature DCs in the skin, and subsequent DC maturation and migration to lymph nodes. Alternatively, DCs may be loaded with tumour antigens ex vivo, and then injected into the patient. This strategy appears attractive, as it may result in enhanced antigen presentation and more effective T-cell stimulation. Moreover, DC-based vaccines may offer the opportunity of directing the immune response, by manipulating the DC phenotype.

The first DC-vaccine trials in cancer patients were reported by Hsu et al. in 1996 and Nestle et al. in 1998 [7]. Promising T-cell responses were obtained, and in recent years, various approaches to DC-vaccines have been explored.

Early studies applied immature DCs, but it is now generally believed that a mature phenotype is desirable.

Targeted loading of DCs in vivo represents another strategy.

Ralph Steinman's group has explored this option by use of antibodies targeting the receptor DEC-205 on the DC surface [7]. Their data from animal model indicate that potent T- and B-cell responses may be elicited.

Alternatively, vaccine antigens might be injected and subsequently transfected into tissue DCs by use of in vivo electropermeabilization.

6.2. Large-scale generation of dendritic cells

For clinical vaccine production, large quantities of autologous DCs are required. Most studies make use of monocyte-derived DCs (Mo-DCs).

http://dx.doi.org/10.5772/61227

On the other hand, DCs may be cultures from CD34+ cells obtained from bone marrow, umbilical cord blood or cytokine-mobilized peripheral blood progenitor cells.

DCs may also be purified from peripheral blood, e.g. after in vivo mobilization of DCs with Flt3-ligand.

At present, it is not clear which method results in the best DCs for cancer vaccination.

The only restriction of use of umbilical cord blood comes from the fact that the per cent of potentially active cells is rather limited and is not enough for bigger scales and clinical application.

In a study reported by Syme et al., Mo-DCs were compared to DCs generated from CD34+ cells 5, 6, 7). The results demonstrated higher expression of HLA class II and CD86 in the Mo-DCs, but no difference in the ability to elicit mixed lymphocyte reaction.

Immature DCs, with a phenotype resembling interstitial DCs, can be generated by stimulating monocytes from peripheral blood with IL-4 and GM-CSF.

The original methods made use of monocytes enriched by adherence.

However, the handling of large numbers of adherent cells is time consuming.

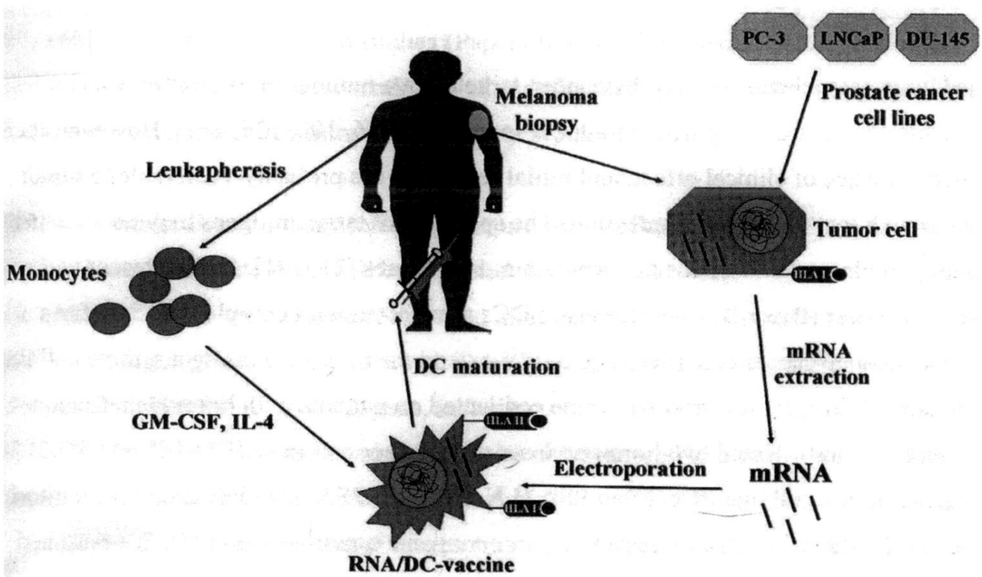

Figure 3. Production of the present RNA/DC-vaccines against malignant melanoma or prostate cancer. Tumor-mRNA was extracted from autologous melanoma biopsies (melanoma vaccine) or from three prostate cancer cell lines (PC-3, LNCaP, DU-145; prostate cancer vaccine). Autologus DCs were generated from monocytes obtained from leukapheresis products. The monocytes were cultured 5 days with IL-4 and GM CSF fro differentiation into immature DCs. Tumor mRNA was then transfected into DCs by electroporation. After transfection, the DCs were cultured for 2 days with cytokines promoting maturation and frozen in vaccine batches.

The production procedure used in the trials performed in Radium Hospital (Inst. Cancer Research, Oslo, Norway) by the group of Gunnar Kvalheim, Jon Kyte and Paula Lazarova [2, 6, 7] is outlined in Figure 3.

The research group did not make use of adherence, but isolated monocytes from leukapheresis products by immunomagnetic depletion of lymphocytes.

The monocytes were transferred to gas permeable Teflon bags that allowed the intrinsically adherent cells to stay in the suspension.

After five days' culture with IL-4 and GM-CSF, the cells were transfected with tumour-mRNA (Figure 3).

Finally, the transfected DCs were matured for 2 days ex vivo with TNFα, IL-6, IL-1β and PGE2.

Contrary to most previous studies, a serum-free culture medium was used. Thereby, unwanted antigens from bovine or human serum were excluded from the vaccine product.

The procedure for DC generation was first established at Radium Hospital by experiments on healthy donors, as reported by Mu et al. [3, 4] and Lazarova et al. [2, 6, 8], later on patients as well.

Subsequently, the generation of clinical grade DCs from patients was evaluated as part of the full-scale preclinical evaluation of the research group in Radium, namely Paula Lazarova et al. [2, 6, 8].

7. Choice of vaccine antigens

Defined tumour-associated antigens have been targeted in a number of interesting vaccine trials world-wide, resulting in antigen-specific immune responses. However, there is a limited evidence of clinical effect, and initial responses are probably vulnerable to tumour escape through loss of antigen expression. The spectrum of target antigens may be widened by use of peptide cocktails or allogeneic tumour cell lines. In the vaccine for prostate cancer, as proposed by the Radium group [2, 3, 4, 5, 6, 7, 8], the employed DCs are transfected with complete mRNA from allogeneic prostate cancer cell lines. To extend the number of antigens, three cell lines were combined.

The clinical trial was conducted on patients with hormone refractory cancer, and thus two hormone-insensitive tumour cell lines were selected (DU-145 and PC-3). A cell line expressing PSA (LN-CaP) was also included.

PSA is widely used for monitoring disease development and also represents an immunogenic tumour antigen.

It was considered that the allogeneic antigens included in the tumour cell lines may increase the risk of side effects, but may also be beneficial.

T-cell recognizing allogeneic antigens will be primed in the same lymph nodes as the tumour-specific T cells.

The allo-reaction may therefore result in an inflammatory milieu promoting the development of effective anti-tumour responses.

It is argued that the majority of tumour antigens are probably specific to each patient and not even expressed in allogeneic cancer cell lines. The individual tumour antigens are believed to arise from numerous incidental mutations occurring during the development of tumour.

The melanoma RNA/DC-vaccine, worked out by the Radium group [2, 3, 4, 5, 6, 7, 8], represents individualized immune-gene therapy. The autologous tumour material as source of mRNA is used in the procedure (Figure 3) and thereby targets the entire spectrum of tumour antigens in each individual. Moreover, non-expressed tumour antigens are excluded.

In general, it is believed that personalized vaccines, targeting the unique spectrum of tumour antigens in each patient, may emerge as a major principle in cancer immunotherapy

The tumour-mRNA strategy is in principle applicable to any cancer form and may prove particularly useful in rarer cancer forms, where common tumour antigens have not yet been defined. Contrary to peptide vaccines, the use of cell line/tumour-mRNA bypasses requirements for defined HLA alleles and for expression of identified antigens by tumours.

The mRNA can encode multiple epitopes and recruit a wide spectrum of T cell clones, including both CD4+helper and CD8+cytotoxic cells.

There is a number of cancer vaccine trials that have applied RNA-transfected DCs.

Certain parts of these studies include use of undefined antigens.

There are definite disadvantages related to the use of undefined antigens.

First, a wide array of possibly harmful autoantigens will be included, suggesting an increased risk of autoimmune side effects.

Second, the antigens recognized after vaccination will usually not be known.

If HLA-matching peptides can be obtained, T-cell responses to defined antigens may be demonstrated.

However, most antigens, including unique patient-specific targets, will remain unknown.

The T-cell responses can thus only be characterized to a limited extent.

Third, in a vaccine based on autologous tumour material, each individual will receive different vaccines.

This complicates the comparison of results from different patients. It should, however, be recalled, that in any trial on humans the inter-individual variability is immense, even though the vaccine itself may be fully standardized.

8. Loading of DCs with antigen

There are several strategies for loading DCs with antigen ex vivo. A number of important trials have applied simple co-incubation of DCs with peptides, proteins or tumour lysates. Other interesting vaccine studies have made use of tumour-DC hybrids, i.e. tumour cells that are fused with DCs. Similar to DCs loaded with tumour lysates or tumour-RNA, these hybrids may combine the antigen repertoire of tumour cells with the stimulatory capacity of DCs. However, sufficient numbers of living tumour cells are required. In most patients, clinical scale vaccine production may therefore only be feasible from allogeneic cell lines, not from autologous tumours.

DNA- or RNA-transfection represents other alternatives for DC-loading. It is accepted by the Radium group that mRNA has certain important advantages compared to DNA.

First, the use of mRNA bypasses the complex issues of transcriptional regulation.

Second, DNA requires entry into the nucleus, while mRNA has direct access to the translation machinery upon entry into cytoplasm.

In experiments with liposome-mediated loading of plasmid DNA, Saeboe-Larssen et al. found that only a minute fraction (10^{-4}) was detected in the nucleus.

Third, transfected DNA may persist in the cell and encode harmful proteins, while RNA will rapidly degrade.

The latter point is of particular relevance for the safety of using tumour-derived DNA/RNA, likely to encode proteins involved in tumour genesis.

The intrinsic instability of RNA, however, also carries a prominent obstacle to clinical use.

The tumour-mRNA may easily degrade if the tumour samples and RNA-preparations are not carefully handled right from the initial biopsy excision.

Contrary to tumour lysates or tumour/DC-hybrids, tumour–mRNA may be amplified from small tumour biopsies.

This may be of particular importance if the clinical trials are extended to patients with early-stage disease, where only small tumours will be available.

Moreover, mRNA-amplification may enable us to make vaccines from small biopsies of tumours located at difficult sites, e.g. in the brain or visceral organs.

The efficiency of RNA-transfection with conventional RNA/DC co-culture or liposome-mediated loading is limited, probably reflecting degradation of RNA both outside of the cell and in endocytic DC compartments.

The limited efficiency results in low intracellular concentrations of the transfected mRNA.

Though immune responses have still been obtained, it is believed that a higher transfection efficiency is desirable for recruiting a wider spectrum of T-cell clones.

While some T-cell clones will respond even to low peptide concentrations on the DC surface, the low affinity clones will require higher concentrations.

Viral vectors represent an effective alternative for both, DNA- and RNA-transfection, but there are considerable safety concerns and regulatory obstacles regarding their clinical application.

The Radium group [2, 3, 4, 5, 6, 7, 8] has developed an efficient method for mRNA-transfection by square-wave electroporation, compatible with clinical use.

The electroporation procedure has been optimized for full-scale vaccine production, as worked out by the group, and applied both, in the melanoma and the prostate cancer trials in Radium. The measured transfection efficiency is substantially higher than was expected to be obtained with other methods like liposome-mediated delivery.

In addition to dendritic cells, the research group works also on Epstein-Barr-Virus-transformed cell lines, monocytes and several cancer cell lines, and the initial results indicate efficient transfection.

9. Summary

The development and evaluation of immuno-gene therapy of cancer based on tumour-mRNA transfected dendritic cells, and focused on malignant melanoma and prostate cancer give certain optimism for future successful application of anti-cancer vaccines.

Acknowledgements

Warmest thanks to the research group of Radium Hospital in Oslo: J.A. Kyte, G. Kvalheim, J. Nesland, P. Lazarova, L.J. Mu et al. for their active support to provide materials and results for preparation of this paper.

Author details

Krassimir Metodiev[1*], Paula Lazarova[2,3], Jon Kyte[2], Gunnar Kvalheim[2] and Jahn Nesland[2]

*Address all correspondence to: kr.metod@yahoo.com

1 Dept. Preclinical and Clinical Sciences, Medical University, Varna, Bulgaria

2 Inst. Cancer Research, Univ. Hospital "Radium", Oslo, Norway

3 Clinical Laboratory, Univ. Hospital "St. Anna", Varna, Bulgaria

References

[1] Г. Капрелян, Кр. Методиев: Терминологичен речник по имунология, Медицина и физкултура, София, 1990, стр.120

[2] P. Lazarova, M. Lijun, H. Hammerstad, J. Nesland, G. Gaudernack, G. Kvalheim: Experimental attempt to introduce a vaccine therapy by using DC-developed from CD34+ cells. In: *Risk Infections and Possibilities for Biomedical Terrorism.* IOS Press, NATO Science Series I, vol. 361, 2004, 134

[3] L.J. Mu, P. Lazarova, G. Gaudernack, S. Saeboe-Larssen, G. Kvalheim: Development of a clinical grade procedure for generation of mRNA transfected dendritic cells from purified frozen CD34+ blood progenitor cells. *Intl J Immunopathol Pharmacol,* vol. 17, No. 3, 2004, 255-263

[4] L.J. Mu, J.A. Kyte, G. Kvalheim et al.: Immunotherapy with allotumour mRNA-transfected dendritic cells in androgen resistant prostate cancer patients. *Brit J Cancer*, 93, 2005, 749-756

[5] J.A. Kyte, L. Mu, S. Aamdal, G. Kvalheim et al.: Phase I/II trial of melanoma therapy with dendritic cells transfected with autologous tumour mRNA. *J Cancer Gene Ther*, I, 2006, 14

[6] P. Lazarova, Q. Wu, G. Kvalheim, Z. Suo, K.W. Haakenstad, K. Metodiev, J.M.Nesland: Growth factor receptors in hematopoietic stem cells: EPH family expression in CD34+ and CD133+ cell populations from mobilized peripheral blood. *Intl J Immunopathol Pharmacol*, vol. 19, No. 1, 2006, 49-56

[7] J.A. Kyte, Immuno-gene therapy of cancer with tumour-mRNA transfected dendritic cells, J Series of Dissertations, Faculty of Medicine, University of Oslo, Radium Hospital, SiO, 65, 2007

[8] P. Lazarova, G. Kvalheim, K. Metodiev: Is anticancer vaccine possible: Experimental application of produced mRNA transfected dendritic cells derived from enriched CD34+ blood progenitor cells. In: *Immunodeficiency*, InTech, Europe, Open Science, 2012, 77-88

Chapter 2

Immunoediting, Immunosurveillance, Tumor-induced Immunosuppression and Immunoresistance, Immunomodulation, Immunotherapy, and Immunonutrition in Personalized and Precision Cancer Medicine

John N. Giannios

Additional information is available at the end of the chapter

http://dx.doi.org/10.5772/61772

Abstract

Cancer immunoediting is composed of three phases: elimination, equilibrium, and escape. Tumor cells, which successfully navigate these phases, are capable of evading destruction by the immunity system of the host. Furthermore, there are different types of nonimmune surveillance against tumors, including genetic surveillance, which is based on DNA repair and checkpoint control, intracellular surveillance related to apoptosis or type I PCD, intercellular surveillance linked to the tumor microenvironment, and epigenetic surveillance related to the structure of chromatin, and specifically the stringency of imprinting. Circumventing immune destruction is one of the hallmarks of cancer pathogenesis, in addition to evading growth suppressors, deregulating cellular energetics, enabling replicative immortality, inducing angiogenesis, activating invasion and metastasis, sustaining proliferative signaling, and resisting cell death, which may lead to the uncontrollable promotion of tumor burden at the expense of the immune system. Although immunoediting may eliminate tumor cells with alterations in their antigenic epitope profile, many immunoresistant variants escape from the immune system of the host by various immunosuppressive molecular and cellular mechanisms. There are many immunomodulatory effects of targeted therapies that can circumvent tumor-mediated immunosuppression, improving the effector T-cell function, which enhances eradication of targeted tumors. Another even more efficient antitumor strategy consists of combining targeted therapies with immunotherapies, which exert many antitumor synergies. The subsequent complex interplay of targeted anticancer agents and immunotherapy may sensitize tumor cells to immune-mediated eradication with long-lasting immunotherapeutic effects, which may inhibit induction of tumor dormancy. These combinatorial immunotherapies with targeted therapies can be used as neoadjuvants and adjuvant treatments with conventional anticancer strategies, such as surgical debulking, radiation therapy, and chemotherapy. In conventional anticancer treatment, the chemotherapeutic-induced immunosuppression inhibits the anticancer efficiency of cell therapies, which are based on activated lymphocytes for eradication of tumor cells, enhancing susceptibility to infections. The majority of conventional chemotherapeutic agents interfere with hematopoiesis and subsequently with the immune system, affecting the surveillance of cancer cells leading to the promotion of tumor development and growth. Furthermore, cancer surgery causes tremendous alterations in the neuroendocrine, metabolic, and immune systems constituting the stress response, which may lead to infection and cancer recurrence. Generally by using an integrative medicine immunotherapeutic approach, where alternative medicine practice which follows a multitargeted and bidirectional regulation may compensate for deficiencies of conventional orthodox western medicine, which is characterized by specificity, we may achieve a synergistic effect concerning circumvention of tumor-induced immunosuppression and enhancement of antitumor immunomodulation followed by minimization or elimination of side effects, prolonging the survival rate of advanced stage and metastatic cancer patients promoting their quality of life. The key is to treat each cancer patient under a personalized evidence-based medicine approach, which must rely on clinomics, including transcriptomics, genomics, immunomics, lipidomics, glycomics, proteomics, metabolomics, nutrigenomics, and mainly epigenomics whose alterations in their noncoding RNA genes are reversible especially with immunonutrition. The precise immunotherapeutic approach against cancer may act synergistically with conventional anticancer therapies, such as surgery, chemotherapy, and radiotherapy combined with therapies based on molecular targeting, which are tailored for each patient on a pharmacogenomic basis, and they can be combined with nanomedicine for specific molecular targeting and circumvention of biological milieu interactions, which may enhance tremendously therapeutic efficacy with simultaneous reduction of systemic toxicity.

Keywords: Immunosurveillance, immunoediting, tumor-induced immunosuppression, immunoresistance, immunomodulation, immunotherapy, immunonutrition, personalized or precision cancer medicine, evidence-based medicine, omics

1. Introduction

The strategies to fight cancer are composed of mechanisms including surgery since 1600 BC, physics including radiotherapy since 1896, chemistry including chemotherapy since 1942, and biology including immunotherapy since 1976. Although immunotherapy has a long history that has been evaluated for more than a century, only recently has it entered a renaissance phase with anticancer biological agents, including the first monoclonal antibody approved in 1997, interleukin-2 (IL-2) cytokine approved in 1998, the first cellular immunotherapy as therapeutic vaccine approved in 2010, and the first checkpoint inhibitor approved in 2011, which has been succeeded by many more approved immunotherapeutic agents [1]. The cancer immunosurveillance hypothesis proposed by Ehrlich in 1909, modified by Burnet and Thomas in 1957, refers to the immunological resistance of the host against cancer development.

2. Immunoediting and immunosurveillance

The current term is cancer immunoediting, which is composed of three phases: elimination, equilibrium, and escape. Tumor cells, which successfully navigate these phases, are capable of evading destruction by the immunity system of the host [2]. Generally, the main component of the defensive army of the host's immune system for fighting tumors is composed of cytotoxic T cells (CTLs).

The elimination phase is a process, where the immune system components recognize transformed cells, eliminating them with the use of the innate and adaptive immune system [3]. Elimination consists of four phases, where the first phase of elimination initiates the antitumor immune response, after the cells of the innate immune system have detected a growing tumor mass, which has caused damage to the local tissue after it has been through stromal remodeling. This induces inflammatory signals, which recruit into the tumor-site cells of the innate immune system, such as macrophages, dendritic cells, and infiltrating lymphocytes such as natural killer cells and natural killer T cells that release interferon-gamma (IFN-γ). The second phase of elimination involving IFN-γ induces immunogenic tumor cell death (ITCD), and it activates the release of chemokines, such as CXCL9, CXCL10, and CXCL11, which inhibit angiogenesis inducing immunogenic necrotic tumor cell death, whose apoptotic bodies are phagocytosed by dendritic cells in the draining lymph nodes, as a bystander killing effect (BKE). The subsequent inflammation releases cytokines and chemokines, which attract additional immune cells. During the third phase of elimination, the reciprocal release of cytokines IL-12 and IFN-gamma transactivates macrophages and natural killer cells, expanding tumor cell death by apoptosis or PCD type I and releasing reactive oxygen and nitrogen intermediates. Tumor-specific dendritic cells in the draining lymph nodes activate the differentiation of Th1 cells, which mediate the production of killer T cells or CD8+ T cells. In the fourth phase of elimination, tumor-specific cytolytic T lymphocytes CD8+ and CD4+ T cells infiltrate the tumor site after recognition of tumor-specific or tumor-associated antigens, such as MHC class J and class II molecules, which in synergy with B cells that produce antibodies, such as IgG, IgA, IgM, IgD, and IgE, facilitate innate and adaptive immune mechanisms, which mediate release cytokines leading to immunogenic tumor cell death. The cancer cells that are not eradicated by the elimination phases of the immune system proceed to the equilibrium phase, where IFN-gamma and lymphocytes prevent expansion of tumor cells that are genetically unstable and mutate rapidly. All the tumor cell variants, which have evaded immune pressure due to acquired resistance to the elimination phases where the balance between the immune response and the tumor cells is driven toward tumor growth that expands in an uncontrolled manner with nonimmunogenic transformed cells, may lead to malignancies by entering the escape phase directly [4–9].

Furthermore, there are different types of nonimmune surveillance against tumors, including genetic surveillance, which is based on DNA repair and checkpoint control, intracellular surveillance related to apoptosis or type I PCD, intercellular surveillance linked to the tumor microenvironment, and epigenetic surveillance related to the structure of chromatin and specifically the stringency of imprinting [10–13].

Circumventing immune destruction is one of the hallmarks of cancer pathogenesis in addition to evading growth suppressors, deregulating cellular energetics, enabling replicative immortality, inducing angiogenesis, activating invasion and metastasis, sustaining proliferative signaling, and resisting cell death, which may lead to the uncontrollable promotion of tumor burden at the expense of the immune system [14].

3. Tumor-induced immunosuppression and immunoresistance

Although immunoediting may eliminate tumor cells with alterations in their antigenic epitope profile, many immunoresistant variants escape from the immune system of the host by the following immunosuppressive molecular and cellular mechanisms [15]. Not the immunoeffectors but only the immunosuppressive regulators are supported by the heterogeneous tumor microenvironment, which contains tumor cells, extracellular matrix (ECM) cells, local bone marrow-derived stromal progenitor cells, pericytes, endothelial cells, proteins, matrix degrading enzymes, chemokines, cellular factors, immune cells, tumor-associated fibroblasts, and angiogenic cells, which may cause desmoplasia after stromal cell infiltration and ECM deposition [16–18].

Tumors escape eradication from the immune system by mechanisms of the first category, which consists of the development of tumor immunoresistance, including the promotion of oncogenicity of tumor stem cells that causes resistance to conventional anticancer treatments and immune responses of the host due to tumor dormancy that cause tumor relapse by self-renewal, continuous ability of proliferation, incomplete differentiation, and production of immunosuppressive factors causing immunoresistance due to inhibition of apoptosis or type I PCD [19].

Another mechanism of tumor immunoresistance is the loss of abnormal surface antigens on the tumoral plasma membrane due to mutations and immunoescape of epitope loss tumor variants, which occurs due to the genetic instability of tumors, leading to continuous alterations of their surface molecules, hiding their antigenic profile by losing their epitope, especially after they sense the presence of cytotoxic T lymphocytes (CTL) in the tumor microenvironment. Thus, the immune system eradicates only the tumor cells that express the specific epitope, circumventing invisible epitope-negative tumor cells that become extremely resistant to CTL elimination [20].

One more immunoresistant mechanism exerted by the tumor cells is the lack of susceptibility to immune effector cells, such as natural killer cells (NK), cytotoxic T lymphocytes (CTL), macrophages, and dendritic cells (DC), which promote antibody-induced cytotoxicity, phagocytosis, or vaccine effects in cancer immunotherapy [21].

The second category of tumor immunoescape mechanisms consists of the interference with the antitumor-induced immune responses, such as reduced expression of costimulatory molecules on tumor cells or antigen presenting cells (APCs). This downregulation of costimulatory molecules on tumor cells or professional APC may inactivate or eliminate TAA-specific

http://dx.doi.org/10.5772/61772

CTLs, put in an immature state the dendritic cells conditioned by the tumor cells, and inactivate T cells leading to tumor tolerance by circumventing productive immune responses against the tumor cells [22]. Also, the tumor for escaping the immune system of the host alters the T-cell receptor (TCR) on the tumor infiltrating lymphocytes (TIL), especially in cases with advanced cancer, leading to reduced mediation of tumor cytotoxicity and decreased production of Th1-type cytokines [23–25].

The next tumor immunoescape mechanism of this category consists of death receptor/ligand signaling and tumor-induced counterattack on immune cells that induces apoptosis or type I PCD, in the majority of circulating CD8+ effector T cells in cancer patients, due to the overexpression of Fas (CD95) receptor on the plasma membrane of activated T cells cross-linked by FasL, which is overexpressed on tumor cells [26]. The tumor cells release immunosuppressive factors, such as PGE2, which downregulates Jak3, blocking the IL-2R downstream signaling pathway that downregulates the prosurvival members of the oncogenic bcl-2 family, leading to a defective signaling which inactivates T cells with subsequent circumvention of tumor cells [27].

Another immunosuppressive mechanism of this category consists of dendritic cell (DC) dysfunction in tumor-associated antigen (TAA) cross presentation to T cells, which leads to a deficient immune response against tumor cells, which may deplete dendritic cells (DCs) by inhibiting the induction of TAA-specific immunity that consists of cytokines and chemokines, such as interleukins (IL-1, IL-12, IL-15, IL-18, and IL-23), interferons, and costimulatory molecules, which are required as growth factors, and signals for T-cell proliferation, differentiation, and memory development [28–30]. The tumor cells may inhibit the maturation of dendritic cells (DCs) by utilizing VEGF and block their differentiation with exosomes. Also, tumor-associated gangliosides (TAG) may downregulate proteasomal constituents of antigen processing machinery (APM) of dendritic cells (DCs) [31–34]. Furthermore, there is another tumor-induced immunosuppressive mechanism consisting of induction of apoptosis or type I PCD of dendritic cells (DCs) in the tumor microenvironment (TME), leading to their elimination by the downregulation of antiapoptotic oncogene bcl-2, the production of nitric-oxide (NO), which downregulates cellular inhibitors of apoptotic proteins (cIAPs or cFLIP), the release of ceramide, which blocks PI3K-mediated survival signals, and alterations in intrinsic apoptotic pathways [35].

One more tumor-induced immunosuppressive category consists of insufficient function of effector cells in the tumor microenvironment (TEM). Its first mechanism consists of suppression of T-cell immune responses by regulatory T cells (Treg), such as CD4+CD25 highFOXP3+, which accumulate in tumors, and in the peripheral circulation of cancer patients [36]. They downregulate the immune response of the effector T cells by releasing TGF-b1 and IL-10 and involve the Fas/FasL and pathways linked to granzyme/perforin, and enzymatic ATP degradation to adenosine exerting immunosuppressive effects, which create tumor resistance [37,38]. The second mechanism of this immunosuppressive category consists of suppression of immune cells by bone marrow myeloid-derived immature suppressor cells (MDSC), such as CD13+, CD33+, and CD34+, which are located in the peripheral circulation of cancer patients, and they are recruited to the tumors after they release soluble immunosuppressive factors, such as PGE2, IL-6, GM-CSF, IL-10, VEGF, and TGF-b1, which produce the arginase-1 enzyme that metabolizes L-arginine, activate iNOS, and control the tumor release of indoleamine-2,2-dioxygenase (IDO), which catabolizes the essential for the differentiation of T-cell amino acid tryptophan, leading to the immunosuppression of T-cell responses that promotes the survival of tumor cells [39–41]. The third immunosuppressive mechanism of this third category consists of tumor-derived microvesicles (MV) or exosomes, which express TAA, HLA class I molecules, and death ligands, which exert their immunosuppressive action by the induction of apoptosis or type I PCD in activated CD8+ effector T cells, eradicating their antitumor action. Also, these tumor-derived exosomes exert an additional immunosuppressive action by blocking the differentiation of monocytes to dendritic cells. Subsequently, the monocytes are transformed by the tumor-induced exosomes (MV) into CD14-negative HLA-DR low TGF-b+ myeloid suppressor cells (MSC), blocking the differentiation of immune cells, which inactivates their antitumor properties by releasing TGF-b, downregulating HLA class II molecules, and inhibiting the proliferation of lymphocytes [42].

The fourth mechanism of this immunosuppressive mechanism consists of induction of apoptosis or type I PCD in effector T cells in the tumor and its periphery. Tumor cells may cause apoptotic DNA fragmentation in a proportion of activated CD8+ T lymphocytes and their effector subpopulations, such as CD8+CD28– and CD8+CD45RO+CD27–, in the tumor site, and the peripheral circulation of cancer patients may lead to tumor progression due to apoptotic death of effector T-cell functions, which compromises significantly the antitumor immune responses [43–46].

The last tumor-induced immunosuppressive category consists of insufficiency in tumor recognition signals consisting of four mechanisms. The first one consists of the downregulation of expression of HLA molecules on the surface of tumor cells. As the tumor progresses, it downregulates all HLA class I allospecificities, HLA-A, HLA-B, and HLA-C loci [47,48]. The tumor cells may cause alterations in the expression of the APM components and defects in the b2-microglobulin, and HLA class I heavy chain synthesis due to the deregulation of mechanisms involving the expression of HLA class I antigen and epigenetic alterations in the HLA class I heavy chain loci, creating resistance to adoptive T-cell-based immunotherapy due to defects into HLA class I which circumvents immune recognition, leading to tumor progression that reduces significantly survival rates of cancer patients [49]. The second mechanism consists of the downregulation of antigen processing machinery (APM) components in tumor cells or antigen presenting cells (APCs) that affect all the peptides, which are presented by HLA class I molecules to T cells enhancing tumor resistance to CTL lysis. The downregulation of total loss of expression of the HLA class I/peptide complexes circumvents the recognition and subsequent destruction of tumor cells by CTL, significantly reducing the disease-free interval and survival rate of cancer patients. The third mechanism consists of the suppression of natural killer cells (NK) in the tumor microenvironment (TME). The downregulation of the cytolytic activity against tumor cells is mediated by the action of inhibitory receptors, such as ILT2/LIRI, CD94/NKG2A, and KIR, which blocks lysis of cells expressing normal HLA class I [50]. The NK cells respond spontaneously to cytokines by expressing IL2R$\beta\gamma$, such as IFN-a, IFN-γ, IL-2, and IL-15. Upon activation, NK cells release TNF-a and IFN-γ for eradicating tumor cells. They also interact with dendritic cells (DCs) for exerting synergistic apoptotic cell death in tumor cells [51]. However, tumor cells release TGF-b1, which downregulates the expression of NKG2D on NK cells impairing their antitumor activity, especially in advanced stages [52]. Thus, tumors may escape the cytolytic activity of NK cells by the inhibition of interactions between receptors and ligands, the downregulation of tumoral ligands MICA or MICB, the eradication of activated NK cells mediated by overexpression of tumoral death-ligands, and the suppression of interactions between NKs and DCs in the tumor microenvironment (TME) promoting tumor growth and subsequent metastasis, which may kill the cancer patient [53]. The final mechanism of the last immunosuppressive category consists of loss or downregulation of surface antigens TAA by tumor cells, which evade the host's immune system by circumventing the cytolytic action of effector T cells (CTLs) due to genetic or epigenetic alterations, which may alter the tumoral protein expression, misleading recognition by the immune system, which promotes uncontrollable tumor growth. Thus, the loss or downregulation of epitopes, such as TAA, and differentiation antigens, such as TRP-1, tyrosinase, MART-1, gp100, and MUC-1, may promote tumoral growth due to escape from the host immune system [54,55]. Furthermore, mutations caused by the tumor in the TAA may circumvent the generation of epitopes, which are recognized immunogenically by cognate CTL regardless of the expression of TAA. These genetic alterations of tumor cells at the coding RNA level may affect posttranslational mechanisms at the protein level, including glycosylation, ubiquitination, and proteolytic enzymes, such as endopeptidases and metaloproteinases (MMPs), which degrade extracellular-matrix (ECM), leading to the downregulation or even total loss of TAA, which mediates tumor escape from the immune system of the host promoting tumor growth.

Thus, there is a continuous struggle between the tumor promoting and the antitumor immune components of the cancer patient where immune promoters of tumor growth and survival include Th17 cell, Cd4+Foxp3+ Treg cells, MDSC, TAM, and their associated chemokines/ cytokines, such as TGF-b, IL-23, IL-1b, TNF, and IL-6, while inhibitors of tumor development and growth consists mainly of CD8+ T, Th1, and CD4+ [56]. The inhibitory signaling pathways to the immune system must be suppressed by cancer immunotherapy [57]. Furthermore, the complexity of cancer involves a crosstalk between tumor microenvironment that interferes with the anticancer activities of the immune system, which in part is caused by the deregulation of the epigenetic machinery that involves methylation-mediated silencing, chromatin remodeling, and microRNA regulons, which may affect immune invasion, tumor–stromal interactions, and tumor angiogenesis [58]. Epigenetic silencing of coding RNA genes, such as retinoblastoma (Rb) gene mediated by histone deacetylase-2(HDAC-2), may regulate immune responses in cancer, which are facilitated by myeloid cells, such as myeloid-derived suppressor cells (MDSCs), polymorphonuclear MDSCs (PMN-MDSCs), and monocytic MDSCs (M-MDSCs), which are the normal counterparts of inflammatory monocytes that differentiate into macrophages, and dendritic cells whose dysfunction in cancer is a severe mechanism of immunosuppression [59,60]. Furthermore, tumor microenvironment (TME) may convert plasmacytoid dendritic cells by complex molecular pathways into tolerogenic immunosuppressive cells [61].

Other tumor microenvironment (TME)-induced immunosuppressive factors, which we must target with cancer immunotherapy not only in solid tumors but also in hematologic malignancies, include tumor intrinsic immunosuppressing ectoenzyme CD37, which is a disulfide-linked homodimer that regulates negatively the proinflammatory effects of extracellular ATP; activates P2X7R, which is a coactivator of the NLRP3 inflammasome-releasing proinflammatory cytokines such as IL-18 and IL-1b; and blocks antitumor T-cell immunity via upregulation of the adenosine receptor (AR) signaling, promoting tumor angiogenesis, growth, and metastasis [62–66].

4. Immunomodulation and immunotherapy

There are many potential therapeutic strategies for circumventing mechanisms of tumor immune evasion, including reversal of the inhibition of adaptive immunity, blocking the T-cell checkpoint pathways such as CTLA4, PD-1, TIM-3, adenosine A2A receptor and LAG-3 checkpoint molecule with agents such as IMP321, BMS-986016, pembrolizumab, nivolumab, pidilizumab, AMP-224, ipilimumab, tremelimumab, etc.

Another therapeutic strategy consists of improving the function of innate immune cells by manipulating the activation of natural killer (NK)-cell inhibitory receptors (KIP) and by stimulating dendritic cells and macrophages with therapeutic agents in clinical development, such as Lirilumab, and Toll-like receptors including TLR 2/4, TLR7, TLR 7/8, and TLR9 agonists, such as Hiltonol, Imiquimod, Resiquimod, CpG7909, and Bacillus Calmette–Guerin.

An additional mechanism consists of switching on adaptive immunity by promoting T-cell costimulatory receptor signaling, using agonist antibodies for the promotion of CD137 signaling with Urelumab, enhancement of CD27 signaling with CDX-1127, activation of CD40 with CP-870,893, and ChiLob 7/4 promotion of GITP signaling with TRX518, enhancement of OX-40 signaling with MEDI 6469, and administration of systemic recombinant IL-7, IL-15, IL-21 with Denenicokin, rhIL-7, and rhIL-15 for enhancing immune cell function including T-cell development.

The final therapeutic strategy consists of the activation of the immune system by potentiating immune-cell effector function with IDO inhibition with Indoximab or INCB024360, various vaccine-based therapeutic strategies, inhibition of TGF-b signaling with IMC-TRI, TEW-7197, LY2157299, or GC1008, and systemic IFN-a or IL-2 administration [67].

There are many immunomodulatory effects of targeted therapies, which can circumvent tumor-mediated immunosuppression, improving the effector T-cell function that enhances eradication of targeted tumors. Tumor and immune system effects of approved and experimental targeted agents include Sunitinib, which by inhibiting multiple tumor-associated tyrosine kinases, such as PDGFR and VEGFR, downregulates STAT3 and VEGF signaling pathways, reducing the population and effectiveness of T-reg cells and MDSCs. By blocking tumor-associated tyrosine kinases, such as KIT and ABL, imatinib inhibits IDO, reduces the population and effectiveness of T-reg cells, enhances the population of B-1 B cells and the concentration of natural antitumor carbohydrate antibodies, and promotes the crosstalk between NK and DC cells. By sensitizing tumor cells to the induction of apoptosis or type I PCD, IAP inhibitors stimulate responses of T cells, NKT cells, and NK cells. GSK3b inhibitors facilitate differentiation toward stem cell memory T-cell population by blocking GSK3b-mediated signaling of tumor cell growth, enhancing TLR4 signaling. By downregulating PI3K-AKT signaling in tumor cells, PI3K-AKT inhibitors enhance tumor susceptibility to perforin and granzyme-mediated lysis involving NK cells and CTLs, downregulating prosurvival signaling and reducing tumor promoting inflammation. By downregulating HSP-90, which enhances unfolded protein-associated stress in tumor cells, HSP-90 inhibitors exert immunostimulatory action by enhancing the expression of NKG2D ligands and by stimulating the CTL recognition of tumor cells. JAK2 inhibitors increase the maturation of DCs, enhance DC-mediated antigen presentation and T-cell priming, and downregulate immunosuppressive STAT3 signaling and expression of IAP and PDL1 of tumor cells by blocking JAK2 signaling in tumor cells. By downregulating BRAF-V600E, vemurafenib upregulates MART1, gp100, and other antigens, while it reduces tumor secretion of immunosuppressive cytokines. By inhibiting 26S subunit of the proteasome, bortezomib sensitizes tumor cells to lysis mediated by CTL and natural killer (NK) cells after the downregulation of the expression of MHC class I molecule, while it boosts antigen-specific T-cell response to vaccination. By inhibiting the mTOR pathway, rapamycin, temsirolimus, and other mTOR inhibitors exert immunostimulatory actions, increasing CD8+T-cell activation and production of IFN-γ, enhancing CD8+ T-cell differentiation into memory T cells, impairing the homeostasis of T-reg cells, and downregulating IDO. Cetuximab as a neutralizing antibody against EGFR inhibits tumoral growth signals and activates the immune system by complement fixation, antibody-dependent cellular cytotoxicity, MHC class I and class II upregulation, and enhancement of DC priming of tumor-specific CTLs. Trastuzumab inhibits tumor growth signaling by the downregulation of HER2, which activates antitumor CTL activity, activates NK cells to secrete IFN-γ, and induces antibody-dependent cell-mediated cytotoxicity (ADCC). Bevacizumab, which is a neutralizing antibody against VEGF, inhibits angiogenesis and subsequent metastasis, while it enhances the maturation of dendritic cells (DCs) and the DC priming of T cells and shifts differentiation of DC toward mature DCs instead of MDSCs [68]. Thus, by interfering with these targeted pathways that drive tumor maintenance and growth, we exert immune therapeutic action by modulating the differentiation, activation, function, and development of the immune cells, which are responsible for inhibiting tumor growth and development, while tumor-induced immunosuppressive mechanisms are circumvented. These immunomodulatory properties that activate the antitumor response include antagonism of tumor-mediated immunosuppressive mechanisms; increase of T-cell activation, differentiation, and effector function; and enhancement of T-cell priming and bolstering of presentation of tumor antigens, indicating a synergistic antitumor action between targeted therapies, which inhibit genomic pathways and anticancer immunomodulatory effects. These synergistic anticancer effects may become even much more effective with the use of combinatorial immunotherapies, which can be used in combination with other conventional anticancer treatment modalities, such as chemotherapy, radiotherapy, and surgery whose inflammatory and immunosuppressive actions may be circumvented with immunonutrition which can improve metabolomics, while it may circumvent the deadly risk of infection to cancer patients. More analytically, combinatorial immunotherapy may act synergistically by combining two different immunotherapeutic agents, such as inhibitors of immune checkpoints for preventing T-cell energy, and cancer vaccines for producing antitumor T cells. For instance, PD1 inhibitors or CTLA4 vaccines, such as autologous granulocyte macrophage colony-stimulating factor (GM-CSF) secreting tumor vaccine, may exert a significant synergistic antitumor action associated with higher overall survival rates by targeting multiple immunosuppressive pathways. Another combinatorial immune therapeutic approach consists of combining costimulatory receptors, which are overexpressed on activated T cells with agonistic antibodies, leading to enhancement of antitumor T-cell function, which eradicates tumors. Promising combinatorial immunotherapies target synergistically the dual T-cell checkpoints, downregulating CTLA-4, PD-1, PD-L1, and LAG-3 with ipilimumab, tremelimumab, nivolumab, pembrolizumab, MEDI4736, and BMS-986016 against NSCLC, colon Ca, gastric Ca, SCLC, pancreatic Ca, melanoma, RCC, triple (-) breast Ca, and other solid tumors. Combinatorial immunotherapeutic regimens include T-cell inhibitors with costimulatory receptor agonists targeting CTLA-4 and CD40 with administration of tremelimumab and CP-870,893 against metastatic melanoma. Another combinatorial regimen consists of T-cell inhibitors, and function enhancers of innate immune cells targeting CTLA-4, PD-1, and KIR with administration of lirilumab, ipilimumab, and nivolumab against solid tumors. Finally, T-cell inhibitors are combined with other activators of the immune system, such as vaccines and passive immunotherapeutics targeting CTLA-4, IL-21, PD-1, IDO with administration of denenicokin, ipilimumab, Nivolumab, INCB024360, indoximod, sipuleucel-T, nivolumab, gp100, NY-ESO-1, TriMix-DC, and adoptive cell transfer against melanoma, prostate Ca, and other solid tumors [67]. Currently, combinatorial therapeutics may combine more than two agents, such as, immunotoxins, Fc-fusion proteins, and bispecific T-cell engagers (BiTEs) [69–72].

Another even more efficient antitumor strategy consists of combining targeted therapies with immunotherapies which exert many antitumor synergies. As we have observed previously antitumor targeted therapies by breaking oncogene addiction, they may optimize the action of immunotherapies by enhancing their sensitivity after circumvention of resistant immunosuppressive mechanisms, leading to elimination of tumorigenic inflammation, enhancing long lived memory T-cell priming, activation, differentiation, function, and effective dendritic cell (DC) maturation, which trigger tumor cell senescence and eradication of tumor cells by induction of apoptosis or type I PCD leading to a bystander killing effect [73]. The derived apoptotic bodies release large quantities of multiple cancer-associated antigenic debris, which activate dendritic cell (DC) functioning as a vaccination in situ, leading to long-lasting remissions by combining the inhibition of oncogenic downstream signaling pathways, enhancing immunosensitivity after elimination of tumor-induced immunosuppressive mechanisms, which may lead to immunomodulatory effects, such as attenuation of the function of specific immunocomponents that block the action of cytotoxic T lymphocytes (CTLs), including myeloid-derived suppressor cells (MDSCs) and FOXP3+ regulatory T (Treg) cells. Other targeted antitumor agents may enhance the priming of tumor-specific CTLs and increase tumor antigen presentation by dendritic cells [74–76].

Thus, this complex interplay of targeted anticancer agents, and immunotherapy may sensitize tumor cells to immune-mediated eradication with long-lasting immunotherapeutic effects, which may inhibit induction of tumor dormancy [77–79].

Thus, we can combine targeted therapies with combinatorial immunotherapies, which consist of conventional immunotherapy, including administration of cytokines and/or chemokines, such as IL-7, IL-15, IL-21, adoptive T-cell transfusion with effector T cells, APC vaccination with dendritic cells (DCs), and tumor-associated antigens with tumor peptides combined with novel tumor immunotherapies, which target tumor-induced immunosuppressive molecules, circumventing tumor immunoresistance by inhibition of soluble suppressive molecules, such as TGFb, COX2, VEGF, and IL-10; suppressive molecules, such as PD1, and CTLA4 on T cells; and suppressive molecules, such as arginase, B7-H1, B7-H4, and IDO on APCs. They also target immunoresistant regulatory T cells by inhibition of trafficking with CCL22-specific antibody differentiation and signaling, such as FOXP3 signal, and depletion of T-reg cells with denileukin diftitox, cyclophosphamide, and CD25-specific antibody [80].

These combinatorial immunotherapies with targeted therapies can be used as neoadjuvants and adjuvant treatments with conventional anticancer strategies, such as surgical debulking, radiation therapy, and chemotherapy. For instance, immunotherapies such as indoximod, Denecikocin, CP-870,893, PF-05082566, urelumab, IMP321, pidilizumab, MEDI14763, MPDL3280A, pembrolizumab, tremelimumab, and nivolumab [67], which target CTLA-4, PD-1, PD-L1, LAG-3, CD137, CD40, IL-21, and IDO, have been combined with chemotherapeutic regimens or agents, such as FOLFOX, paclitaxel, cyclophosphamide, carboplatin, docetaxel, gemcitabine, etc., and molecular targeting agents, such as gefitinib, dasatinib, bevacizumab, erlotinib, sunitinib, pazopanid, lenalidomide, vemurafenib, trametinib, rituximab, sorafenib, etc., against liquid tumors, such as CML, NHL, etc., and solid tumors including NSCLC, RCC, multiple myeloma, melanoma, pancreatic Ca, CRC, prostate Ca, breast Ca, etc.

In conventional anticancer treatment, the chemotherapeutic-induced immunosuppression inhibits the anticancer efficiency of cell therapies, which are based on activated lymphocytes for eradication of tumor cells enhancing susceptibility to infections [81].The majority of conventional chemotherapeutic agents interfere with hematopoiesis and subsequently with the immune system affecting the surveillance of cancer cells promoting tumor development and growth [82].

Generally, cancer surgery causes tremendous alterations in the neuroendocrine, metabolic, and immune systems constituting the stress response, which may lead to infection, and cancer recurrence due to release of catecholamines, cortisol, and cytokines that interfere with the adaptive or specific immunity, which is composed of humoral immunity that consists of B cells, and cellular immunity containing T-cytotoxic cells, T-suppressor cells, and T-helper cells, and the innate or nonspecific immunity. During the postoperative stage, there is balance between pro-inflammatory and anti-inflammatory cytokines. Deficient responses may cause immunosuppression leading to infections. Excessive responses may cause the systemic inflammatory response syndrome (SIRS), which has been associated with the clinical syndrome of sepsis and multiorgan failure (MOF) or multiple organ dysfunction syndrome (MODS) [83].

The postoperative immune response is multifactorial with the release of inflammatory Th1 cytokines, such as IL-6 and TNF-a, and corticosteroids immediately after cancer surgery. Subsequently, even after 2 h from the surgical procedure, there is a reduction of the Th1 cytokines, while the Th2 cytokines, such as TGF-b, and IL-10 rise rapidly increasing the accumulation of immunosuppressive myeloid-derived suppressor cells, and immune-inhibitory cytokines [84]. This shift toward the Th2 immune response deregulates the cellular immunity, enhancing susceptibility of the cancer patient to infection, sepsis, and MOF [85–87]. Furthermore, there is a quantitative reduction of T lymphocytes, which depends on the volume of blood loss during surgery. Also, there is a reduction in the number of white blood cells (WBCs) called leucopenia, which causes immunosuppression that combined with reduced cytokine secretion and suppression of T-lymphocyte responses, and reduced levels of macrophages may cause postoperative sepsis that may lead to morbidity. However, sepsis may be inhibited by postoperative release of anti-inflammatory cytokines, prostaglandins, and nitric oxide, which requires arginine as a substrate for its production by nitric oxide synthase [88]. Since plasma levels of arginine are reduced in septic patients, we need to establish a positive nitrogen balance by supplementation of arginine as an immunonutrition approach. This amino acid regulates blood flow by producing nitric oxide (NO), and it functions as an immunomodulator by enhancing the antitumor cytotoxicity of neutrophils and macrophages [89–92]. Furthermore, the proper antitumor function of T cells requires arginine. The tumor microenvironment contains nitric oxide synthase (NOS) and arginase I, which are upregulated by tumor-induced MDSC, acting as an immunosuppressive mechanism that leads to a deficiency of arginine, which subsequently suppresses the antigen-specific T-cell responses by downregulating the T-cell receptor [93,94]. Within a few hours after cancer surgery, there is an evident reduction of arginine in the circulation of the cancer patient [95,96] because arginine is metabolized by arginase-I, which may be downregulated by omega-3 fatty acids that are metabolized to PGE3, inhibiting production of immunosuppressive Th2 cytokine, and increasing the production of protectins and resolvins, which promote tissue repair [97]. Immunonutrition in the surgical cancer patient with arginine may improve trauma healing, enhance macrophage function, and lymphocyte immune responses enhancing resistance to infection at the postoperative stage [98]. A functional immune system is required for protecting the surgical cancer patient from the high risk of postoperative infections, which can be achieved by perioperative immunomodulating formulations that can circumvent postoperative immunoparesis and prevent sepsis by activating the immune cell responses, and modulating inflammation.

Other protective perioperative practices include minimally invasive surgical procedures, circumvention of immunosuppressive drugs, and reduction of blood transfusions [99]. Radical surgery combined with old-age neuroendocrine response and administration of analgesics may suppress the activity of the innate immunity and specifically NK cells, which leads to tumor progression since tumor cells circumvent tumor immunosurveillance and subsequent cytolysis [100–104]. In addition, operative anesthetics, such as halothane, thiopental, and ketamine, may suppress even further the activity of NK cells promoting metastasis. Thus, immunonutrition may stimulate the immunity, while other factors such as hypothermia, alcohol, and mainly stress may enhance tumor progression [105].

Supplementation with polysaccharides or glutamine may increase natural killer (NK) cell activity [106]. A requirement for a functional anticancer immunity includes a balanced Th1/Th2 ratio because after surgery, a dominant Th2-type immune response, especially in tumors of the gastrointestinal (GI) tract, may suppress tumor surveillance and cellular immunity [107]. Other immunosuppressive and inflammatory factors such as IL-6 and immunosuppressive acidic protein (IAP) may reduce the antitumor activity of cellular immunity leading to tumor progression.

Other immunosuppressive factors include IL-10, TGF-b, and angiogenic VEGF, which is regulated by CD47 signaling that suppresses activity of T cells promoting tumor growth [108]. Thus, after oncological surgery, we must help the patient to maintain homeostasis against the consequences of cancer, tissular attrition, hormonal and metabolic changes, and mainly inflammatory reaction, which induces metastases by a cascade of genomic signaling pathways that may lead to angiogenesis, which is associated to a potent immunosuppression [109,110]. In addition to surgery, other conventional cancer treatments, such as chemotherapy and radiation therapy, may suppress the immune system of the cancer patient by causing a tremendous reduction in the production of all the cells of the bone marrow leading to leucopenia and anemia, which may lead to severe infections. Specifically, if a neutrophil count is below 1000, the risk of infection by bacteria, germs, and fungi is increased, which becomes worse if the count is below 500 where we have neutropenia. This may be treated with administration of colony stimulating factors (CSF) or white blood cell (Leukocyte) growth factors. With bone radiation for metastatic tumors, leucopenia and even neutropenia may be caused by chemotherapy. Furthermore, local radiation therapy can irritate the skin causing small breaks from which germs and bacteria may enter causing infections. Also when lymph nodes are irradiated, infection may occur, which leads to lymphedema. Moreover, there are many tumor-induced immunosuppressive mechanisms, which have been described previously that act synergistically.

5. Immunonutrition

It is very important that more than one third of all cancer deaths are related to nutritional complications, which have been caused by side effects of the major treatments for cancer even the targeted ones. With the administration of nutritional therapy, we can reduce or even inhibit the nutritional complications of cancer, improving nutritional status and healing, maintain normal weight by preventing muscle wasting, and mainly reduce side effects and mortality or morbidity by enhancing the overall effectiveness of anticancer treatments and their combinations while we may preserve and even enhance quality of life. Furthermore, with immunonutrition, we may boost the immune system of cancer patients, especially those who are hospitalized and malnourished. The immune system of cancer patients can be modulated with immunonutritional formulations, which may contain immunostimulant and anti-inflammatory nutrients such as protein, carbohydrate, amino acids, lipids, mineral, trace elements, and vitamins including glutamine, which may enhance immune cell activity, improve nutritional status, and reduce hospitalization time reducing risk of infections. Other nutraceuticals include arginine, which boosts immune function, prevents infection, and repairs tissue after surgery; omega-3 fatty acids, which have anti-inflammatory properties minimizing the risk for cancer cachexia; ribonucleic acid (RNA), which may stimulate immune cell division and activity; taurine, which reduces inflammation; vitamin C or ascorbic acid, which supports immune function and promotes wound healing; selenium, which supports immune function preventing infection; turmeric, which has anti-inflammatory effects especially at the post-operative stage; vitamins B12, B6, and B1, which may prevent post-operative immunosuppression; zinc, which is important for normal immune system function; and wound healing after surgery [111]. Also, natural products of alternative medicines, such as botanical or herbal plant derivatives, and mind–body practices under an integrative medicine approach may enhance the anticancer effects of conventional anticancer treatments, reducing their systemic toxicity; alleviate clinical symptoms including pain, which are induced by cancer; and prolong survival rates of cancer patients mainly by enhancing tumor immune responses via overexpression of classic MHC molecules, induction of apoptosis in tumor cells via the Fas/FasL pathway, and elimination of oncogenic cancer stem cells by inhibiting tumor immunoresistance [112–115]. Further, alternative medicine therapeutic strategies may reverse the tumor-induced immunosuppressive phenotype regulating the antitumor properties of the immune cells of the cancer patients by enhancing the antitumor abilities of T lymphocytes, regulating the M1/M2 phenotypes of tumor-associated macrophages (TAM), eliminating myeloid-derived suppressor cells (MDSC), enhancing antigen-presenting capacity of dendritic cells (DCs), and regulating the secretion of Th1/Th2 immune factors.

Generally, by using an integrative medicine immunotherapeutic approach where alternative medicine practice which follows a multitargeted and bidirectional regulation may compensate for deficiencies of conventional orthodox western medicine, which is characterized by specificity, we may achieve a synergistic effect concerning circumvention of tumor-induced immunosuppression and enhancement of antitumor immunomodulation followed by minimization or elimination of side effects prolonging the survival rate of advanced stage and metastatic cancer patients promoting their quality of life [116–121].

6. Conclusion

The key is to treat each cancer patient under a precision or personalized evidence-based medicine approach, which must rely on clinomics, including transcriptomics, genomics, immunomics, lipidomics, glycomics, proteomics, metabolomics, nutrigenomics, and mainly epigenomics, whose alterations in their noncoding RNA genes are reversible especially with immunonutrition. The precise immunotherapeutic approach against cancer may act synergistically with conventional anticancer therapies, such as surgery, chemotherapy, and radiotherapy combined with therapies based on molecular targeting, which are tailored for each patient on a pharmacogenomic basis. Also, they can be combined with nanomedicine for specific molecular targeting and circumvention of biological milieu interactions, which may tremendously enhance therapeutic efficacy with simultaneous reduction of systemic toxicity.

Author details

John N. Giannios*

Address all correspondence to: prdrjng@gmail.com

Translational Cancer Medicine, London, UK

References

[1] Kyi C,Postow M.Checkpoint blocking antibodies in cancer immunotherapy.FEBS Letters.2014 Jan;588(2):368-376.

[2] Prendergast GC.Immune escape as a fundamental trait of cancer:focus on IDO.Oncogene.2008;27:3889-3900.

[3] Vajdic CM,van Leeuwen MT.Cancer incidence and risk factors after solid organ transplantation.Int J Cancer.2009 Oct;125(8):1747-1754.

[4] Dunn GP,Bruce AT,Ikeda H,Old LJ,Schreiber RD.Cancer Immunoediting:from immunosurveillance to tumor escape.Nat Immunology.2002 Nov;3(11):991-998.

[5] Steinman RM,Mellman I.Immunotherapy:bewitched,bothered,and bewildered no more.Science.2004 Jul;305(5681):197-200.

[6] Lake RA,der Most RG.A better way for a cancer cell to die.N Engl J Med. 2006;354(23):2503-2504.

[7] Zitrogel L,Tesniere A,Kroemer G.Cancer despite immunosurveillance: immunoselection and immunosubversion.Nat Rev Immunol.2006 Oct; 6(10):715-727.

[8] Zitrogel L,Casares N,Pequignot MO,Chapul N,Albert ML,Kroemer G. al.Immune response against dying tumor cells.Adv Immunol. 2004; 84:131-179.

[9] Dunn G,Koebel C,Schreiber R.Interferons,immunity and cancer immunoediting.Nature Reviews Immunology.2006 Nov;6:836-848.

[10] Glick AB,Yuspa SH.Tissue homeostasis and the control of the neoplastic phenotype in epithelial cancers.Semin Cancer Biol.2005 Apr;15(2):75-83.

[11] Klein G.Cancer,apoptosis,and nonimmune surveillance.Cell Death & Differentiation. 2004;11(1):13-17.

[12] Cui H,Cruz-Correa M,Giardiello FM,Hutcheon DF,Kafonek DR,Brandenburg S,Wu Y,He X,Powe NR,Feinberg AP. Loss of IGF2 imprinting:a potential marker of colorectal cancer risk.Science.2003 Mar;299(5613):1753-1755.

[13] Paz MF,Avila S,Fraga MF,Pollan M,Capella G,Peinado MA,Sanchez-Cespedes M,Herman JG,Esteller M.Germ-line variants in methyl-group metabolism genes and

susceptibility to DNA methylation in normal tissues and human primary tumours. Cancer Res.2002 Aug;62(15):4519-4524.

[14] Hanahan D,Weinberg RA.Hallmarks of cancer:the next generation. Cell.2011 Mar; 144(5):646-674.

[15] Tsuda H,Gene and chromosomal alterations in sporadic breast cancer:correlation with histopathological features and implications for genesis and progression.Breast Cancer.2009;16:186-201.

[16] Hanahan D,Weinberg RA.Hallmarks of cancer:the next generation. Cell.2011 Mar; 144(5):646-674.

[17] Junttila M,de Sauvage FJ,Influence of tumour micro-environment heterogeneity on therapeutic response.Nature.2013 Sep;501(7467):346-354.

[18] Heldin CH,Rubin K,Pietras K,Ostman A.High interstitial fluid pressure-an obstacle in cancer therapy.Nat Rev Cancer.2004 Oct;4(10):806-813.

[19] Zhou BB,Zhang H,Damelin M,Geles KG,Grindley JC,Dirks PB.Tumour-initiating cells:challenges and opportunities for anticancer drug discovery.Nat Rev Drug Discov.2009 Oct;8(10):806-823.

[20] Khong HT,Wang QJ,Rosenberg SA.Identification of multiple antigens recognized by tumour-infiltrating lymphocytes from a single patient:tumor escape by antigen loss and loss of MHC expression. J Immunother.2004 May;27(3):184-190.

[21] Houot R,Kohrt H,Marabelle A,Levy R.Targeting immune effector cells to promote antibody-induced cytotoxicity in cancer immunotherapy. Trends in Immunology. 2011 Nov;32(11):510-516.

[22] Lang S,Atarashi Y,Nishioka Y,Stanson J,Meidenbauer N,Whiteside TL.B7.1 on human carcinomas:costimulation of T-cells and enhanced tumour-induced T-cell death.Cell Immunol.2000;201:132-143.

[23] Mihm MC,Jr,Clemente CG,Cascinelli N.Tumor infiltrating lymphocytes in lymph node melanoma metastases:a histopathologic prognostic indicator and an expression of local immune response.Lab Invest.1996;74:43-47.

[24] Kiesslinger R,Kono K,Petersson M,Wasserman K. Immunosuppression in human tumor-host interaction:role of cytokines and alterations in signal-transducing molecules.Springer Sem Immunopathol.1996;18(2):227-242.

[25] Uzzo RG,Clark PE,Rayman P,Bloom T,Rybicki L,Novick AC,Bukowski RM,Finke JH. Alterations in NFkappaB activation in T lymphocytes of patients with renal cell carcinoma. J Nat Cancer Inst.1999 Apr; 91(8):718-721.

[26] Whiteside TL.Immune response to malignancies.J Allergy Clin Immunol.2010 Feb; 125(2 Suppl 2):S272-283.

[27] Sheng H,Shao J,Morrow J,Beauchamp RD,DuBois R.Modulation of Apoptosis and Bcl-2 Expression by Prostaglandin E2 in Human Colon Cancer Cells. Cancer Res.1998 Jan; 58:362-366.

[28] WhitesideTL, Odoux X.Dendritic cell biology and cancer therapy. Cancer Immunol Immunother.2004;53: 240-248.

[29] Gabrilovich DI,Chen H,Girgis K,Cunningham TH,Meny G,Nadaf S,Kavanaugh D,Carbone D.Production of vascular endothelial growth factor by human tumours inhibits the functional maturation of dendritic cells.Nature Medicine. 1996;2:1096-1103.

[30] Aalamian M,Pirtskhalaishvili G,Nunez A,Esche C,Shurin GV,Huland E,Huland H,Shurin MR.Human prostate cancer regulates generation and maturation of monocyte-derived dendritic cells.Prostate.2001 Jan; 46(1):68-75.

[31] Katsenelson NS,Shurin GV,Bykovskaia SN,Shogan J,Shurin MR.Human small cell lung carcinoma and carcinoid tumor regulate dendritic cell maturation and function.Modern Path.2001;14:40-45.

[32] Shurin GV,Shurin MR,Bykovskaia S,Shogan J,Lotze MT,Barksdale Jr EM.Neuroblastoma-derived gangliosides inhibit dendritic cell generation and function. Cancer Res. 2001;61:363-369.

[33] Gabrilovich D,Ishida T,Oyama T,Ran S,Kravtsov V,Nadaf S,Carbone DP.Vascular endothelial growth factor inhibits the development of dendritic cells and dramatically affects the differentiation of multiple hematopoietic lineages in vivo.Blood. 1998;92:4150-4166.

[34] Tourkova IL,Shurin G,Chatta G,Perez L,finke J,Whiteside T,ferrone S,Shurin M.Restoration by IL-15 of MHC Class I antigen-Processing Machinery in Human dendritic Cells Inhibited by Tumor-Derived gangliosides.The Journal of Immunology. 2005;175:3045-3052.

[35] Esche C,Shurin GV,Kirkwood JM,Wang GQ,Rabinowich H,Pirtskhalaishvilli G,Shurin MR.Tumour necrosis factor-alpha-promoted expression of Bcl-2 and inhibition of mitochondrial cytochrome c release mediate resistance of mature dendritic cells to melanoma induced apoptosis.Clin Cancer Res.2001;7(3):974S-979S.

[36] Curiel TJ,Coukos G,Zou L,Alvarez X,Cheng P,Mottram P,Evdemon-Hogan M,Conejo-Garcia JR,Zhang L,Burow M,Zhu Y,Wei S,Kryczek I,Daniel B,Gordon A,Myers L,Lackner A,Disis ML,Knutson KL,Chen L,Zou W.Specific recruitment of regulatory T cells in ovarian carcinoma fosters immune privilege and predicts reduced survival.Nat Med.2004 Sep;10(9):942-949.

[37] Strauss L,Bergmann C,Szczepanski M,Gooding W,Johnson TJ,Whiteside TL.A unique subset of CD4+ CD25high FOXP3+Tcells secreting IL-10 and TGF-b1 mediates suppression in the tumour microenvironment.Clin Cancer Res.2007;13:4345-4354.

[38] Strauss L,Bergmann C,whiteside TL.Human circulating CD4+CD25highFox3+ regulatory T-cells kill autologous CD8+ but not CD4+ responder cells by fas-mediated apoptosis. J Immunol.2009; 182:1469-1480.

[39] Nagaraj S,Schrum AG,Cho HI,Celis E,Gabrilovich DI.Mechanism of T cell tolerance induced by myeloid-derived suppressor cells.J Immunol. 2010;184:3106-3116.

[40] Cabrilovich DI,Nagaraj S.Myeloid-derived suppressor cells as regulators of the immune system.Nat Rev Immunol.2009 Mar;9(3):162-174.

[41] Muller AJ,Prendergast GC.Indoleamine 2,3-dioxygenase in immune suppression and cancer.Curr Cancer Drug Targets.2007;7:31-40.

[42] Valenti R,Huber V,Filipazzi P,Pilla L,Sovena G,Villa A,Corbelli A,Fais S,Parmiani G,Rivoltini L.Human tumour released microvesicles promote the differentiation of myeloid cells with TGF-beta mediated suppressive activity on T-lymphocytes.Cancer Res.2006;66:9290-9298.

[43] Lybarger L,Wang X,Harris M,Hansen HT.Viral immune evasion molecules attack the ER peptide-loading complex and exploit ER-associated degradation pathways.Curr Opin Immunol.2005;17:71-78.

[44] Tsukishiro T,Donnenberg AD,Whiteside TL. Rapid turnover of the CD8+CD28– T-cell subset of effector cells in the circulation of patients with head and neck cancer. Cancer Immunol Immunother.2003;52:599-607.

[45] Kuss I, Hathaway B, Ferris RL, Gooding W, Whiteside TL. Decreased absolute counts of T lymphocyte subsets and their relation to disease in squamous cell carcinoma of the head and neck. Clin Cancer Res.2004a;10:3755-3762.

[46] Kuss I, Schaefer C, Godfrey TE,Ferris RL,Harris JM,Gooding W,Whiteside TL . Recent thymic emigrants and subsets of naïve and memory T cell in the circulation of patients with head and neck cancer. Clin Immunol.2005;116:27-36.

[47] Khong HT, Wang QJ, Rosenberg SA. Identification of multiple antigens recognized by tumor-infiltrating lymphocytes from a single patient: tumor escape by antigen loss and loss of MHC expression. J Immunother.2004;27:184-190.

[48] Campoli M,Chang CC, Ferrone S. HLA class I antigen loss, tumor immune escape and immune selection.Vaccine.2002;20 Suppl 4:A40-A45.

[49] Valmori D, Dutoit V, Schnuriger V, Quiquerez AL, Pittet MJ, Guillaume P, Rubio-Godoy V, Walker PR, Rimoldi D, Lienard D,Cerottini JC,Romero P,Dietrich PY.Vaccination with a Melan-A peptide selects an oligoclonal T cell population with increased functional avidity and tumor reactivity. J Immunol.2002 Apr;168(8): 4231-4240.

[50] Lanier LL.NK Cell Recognition. Annu Rev Immunol.2005 Apr; 23:225-274.

[51] Degli-Esposti MA,Smyth MJ. Close encounters of different kinds: dendritic cells and NK cells take centre stage. Nat Rev Immunol. 2005;5:112-124.

[52] Lee JC, Lee KM, Kim DW, Heo DS. Elevated TGF-beta1 secretion and down-modulation of NKG2D underlies impaired NK cytotoxicity in cancer patients. J Immunol. 2004;172:7335-7340.

[53] Poggi A, Massaro AM, Negrini S, Contini P, Zocchi MR. Tumor-induced apoptosis of human IL-2-activated NK cells: role of natural cytotoxicity receptors. J Immunol. 2005;174:2653-2660.

[54] Khong HT, Wang QJ, Rosenberg SA. Identification of multiple antigens recognized by tumor-infiltrating lymphocytes from a single patient: tumor escape by antigen loss and loss of MHC expression. J Immunother.2004;27:184-190.

[55] Andriance MC,Gendler SJ.Downregulation of Muc1 in MMTV-c-Neu tumors.Oncogene.2004 Jan; 23(3):697-705.

[56] Zamarron B,Wanjun C. Dual Roles of Immune Cells and Their Factors in Cancer Development and Progression. Int J Biol Sci. 2011;7(5):651-658.

[57] Sharma P,Wagner K,Wolchok DJ,Allison PJ. Novel cancer immunotherapy agents with survival benefit:recent successes and next steps. Nat Rev Cancer.2011 Oct; 11(11):805-812.

[58] Suzuki HI ,Yamagata K,Sugimoto K,Iwamoto T,Kato S,Miyazono K.Modulation of microRNA processing by p53.Nature.2009 Jul;460(7254):529-533.

[59] Youn JI,Kumar V,Collazo M,Nefedova Y,Condamine T,Cheng P,Villagra A,Antonia S,McCaffrey CJ,Fishman M,Sarnaik A,Horna P,Sotomayor E,Gabrilovich ID.Epigenetic silencing of retinoblastoma gene regulates pathologic differentiation of myeloid cells in cancer.Nature Immunol.2013;14:211-220.

[60] Pinzon-Charry A,Maxwell T,Lopez JA. Dendritic cell dysfunction in cancer: A mechanism for immunosuppression.Immunology and Cell Biology.2005;83:451-461.

[61] Demoulin S, Herfs M, Delvenne P,Hubert P. Tumor microenvironment converts plasmacytoid dendritic cells into immunosuppressive/tolerogenic cells: insight into the molecular mechanisms.J Leukoc.Biol.2013;93:343-352.

[62] Zhao X, Lapalombella R, Joshi T, Cheney C, Gowda A, Hayden-Ledbetter MS, Baum PR, Lin TS, Jarjoura D, Lehman A, Kussewitt D, Lee RJ, Caligiuri MA, Tridandapani S, Muthusamy N, Byrd JC.Targeting CD37-positive lymphoid malignancies with a novel engineered small modular immunopharmaceutical.Blood.2007 Apr;110(7): 2569-2577.

[63] Allard B, Turcotte M, Spring K, Pommey S, Royal I, Stagg J. Anti-CD73 therapy impairs tumor angiogenesis.Int J Cancer.2014; 134(6):1466–1473

[64] Beckwith K,Frissora F, Stefanovski M,Towns W,Cheney C, Mo X,Deckert J,Croce C,Flynn J,Andritsos L,Jones J, Maddocks K,Lozanski G,Byrd J,Muthusamy N. The

CD37-targeted antibody–drug conjugate IMGN529 is highly active against human CLL and in a novel CD37 transgenic murine leukemia model.Leukemia.2014 Jan; 28(7):1501-1510.

[65] Allard B,Turcotte M,Stagg J. CD73-Generated Adenosine: Orchestrating the Tumor-Stroma Interplay to Promote Cancer Growth Journal of Biomedicine & Biotechnology.2012 Oct;1-8.

[66] Zhang B.CD73 promotes tumor growth and metastasis. OncoImmunology.2012 Jan; 1(1):67-70.

[67] Antonia SJ, Larkin J, Ascierto PA. Immuno-oncology combinations: a review of clinical experience and future prospects. Clin Cancer Res. 2014 Dec;20(24):6258-6268

[68] Vannema M,Dranoff G. Combining immunotherapy and targeted therapies in cancer treatment.Nature Reviews Cancer.2012 Apr;12:237-251.

[69] Miller RE,Jones J,Le T,Whitmore J,Boiani N,Gliniak B,Lynch DH. 4-1BB-specific monoclonal antibody promotes the generation of tumor-specific immune responses by direct activation of CD8 T cells in a CD40-dependent manner. J.Immunol.(2002); 169:1792–1800.

[70] Curran MA, Montalvo W, Yagita H, Allison JP. PD-1 and CTLA-4 combination blockade expands infiltrating T cells and reduces regulatory T and myeloid cells within B16 melanoma tumors. Proc Natl Acad Sci USA. 2010;107:4275–4280.

[71] Kocak E, Lute K, Chang X,May Jr K,Exten K,Zhang H,Abdessalam S,Lehman A,Jarjoura D,Zheng P,Liu Y. Combination therapy with anti-CTL antigen-4 and anti-4-1BB antibodies enhances cancer immunity and reduces autoimmunity. Cancer Res. 2006;66:7276-7284.

[72] Hodi FS,Butler m,Oble D,Seiden M,Haluska F,Kruse A,MacRae S,Nelson M,Canning C,Lowy I,Korman A,Lautz D,Russel S,Jaklitsch M,Ramaiya N,Chen T,Neuberg D,Allison J,Mihm M,Dranoff G. Immunologic and clinical effects of antibody blockade of cytotoxic T lymphocyte-associated antigen 4 in previously vaccinated cancer patients.Proc Natl Acad Sci USA.2008;105:3005-3010.

[73] Rakhra K,Bachireddy P,Zabuawala T,Zeiser R,Xu L,Kopelman A,Fan AC,Yang Q,Braunstein L,Crosby E,Ryeom S,Felsher DW. CD4(+) T cells contribute to the remodeling of the microenvironment required for sustained tumor regression upon oncogene inactivation. Cancer Cell.2010;18:485-498.

[74] Nefedova Y,Cheng P,Gilkes D,Blaskovich M,Beg A,Sebti S,Gabrilovich D. Activation of dendritic cells via inhibition of Jak2/STAT3 signaling.J Immunol. 2005;175:4338-4346.

[75] Ko JS, AH, Rini BI, Ireland JL, Elson P,Cohen P,Golshavan A,Rayman PA,Wood L,Garcia J,Dreicer R,Bukowski r,Finke JH. Sunitinib mediates reversal of myeloid-de-

rived suppressor cell accumulation in renal cell carcinoma patients.Clin Cancer Res. 2009;15:2148-2157.

[76] Hahnel PS,Thaler S,Antunes E,Huber C,Theobald M,Schuler M. Targeting AKT Signaling sensitizes cancer to cellular immunotherapy. Cancer Res.2008;68:3899-3906.

[77] Osisami M,Keller E.Mechanisms of Metastatic Tumor Dormancy. J Clin Med. 2013;2(3):136-150.

[78] Seeger JM, Schmidt P, Brinkmann K, Hombach AA, Coutelle O, Zigrino P, Wagner-Stippich D, Mauch C, Abken H, Kronke M, Kashkar H. The proteasome inhibitor bortezomib sensitizes melanoma cells toward adoptive CTL attack. Cancer Res. 2010;70:1825–1834.

[79] Nefedova Y,Nagaraj S,Rosenbauer A,Muro-Cacho C,Sebti SM,Gabrilovich DI.Regulation of dendritic cell differentiation and antitumor immune response in cancer by pharmacologic-selective inhibition of the janus-activated kinase 2/signal transducers and activators of transcription 3 pathway. Cancer Res. 2005;65:9525–9535.

[80] Zou W. Regulatory T cells, tumour immunity and immunotherapy. Nature Reviews Immunology.2006;6:295-307.

[81] Mellman I ,Coukos G,Dranoff G.Cancer immunotherapy comes of age.Nature. 2011;480:480-489.

[82] Schreiber RD,Old LJ,Smyth MJ. Cancer immunoediting: integrating immunity's roles in cancer suppression and promotion. Science. 2011 Mar;331(6024):1565-1570.

[83] Kaukonen KM, Bailey M, Pilcher D, Cooper DJ, Bellomo R. Systemic inflammatory response syndrome criteria in defining severe sepsis. N Engl J Med. 2015;372:1629-1638.

[84] Barksdale AR, Bernard AC, Maley ME, Gellin GL, Kearney PA, Boulanger, BR, Tsuei BJ, Ochoa JB 2004. Regulation of arginase expression by T-helper II cytokines and isoproterenol. Surgery.135: 527-535.

[85] Angele MK, Faist E. Clinical review: Immunodepression in the surgical patient and increased susceptibility to infection. Crit Care. 2002;6:298–305.

[86] Mannick JA,Rodrick ML,Lederer JA.The immunologic response to injury.J Am Coll Surg. 2001;193:237–244.

[87] Giannoudis PV, Smith RM, Perry SL,Windsor AJ,Dickson RA,Bellamy MC. Immediate IL-10 expression following major orthopaedic trauma: relationship to anti-inflammatory response and subsequent development of sepsis. Intensive Care Med. 2000;26:1076–1081.

[88] heeran P,Hall G.Cytokines in anaesthesia.Br J Anaesth.1997;78:201-219.

[89] reund H, Atamian S, Holroyde J, Fischer JE. Plasma amino acids as predictors of the severity and outcome of sepsis. Ann Surg.1979 Nov; 190(5):571–576.

[90] Luiking YC,Poeze M,Ramsay G,Deutz N. Reduced citrulline production in sepsis is related to diminished de novo arginine and nitric oxide production. Am J Clin Nutr. 2009 Jan;89(1):142-152.

[91] Davis JS, Anstey NM. Is plasma arginine concentration decreased in patients with sepsis? A systematic review and meta-analysis. Crit Care Med. 2011;39(2):380–385.

[92] Kao CC, Bandi V, Guntupalli KK,Wu M,Castillo L,Jahoor F. Arginine, citrulline and nitric oxide metabolism in sepsis. Clin Sci (Lond) 2009;117:23–30.

[93] Bronte V, Zanovello P. Regulation of immune responses by L-arginine metabolism. Nat Rev Immunol.2005 Aug;5(8):641-654.

[94] Mocellin S, Bronte V, Nitti D. Nitric oxide, a double edged sword in cancer biology: searching for therapeutic opportunities. Med Res Rev. 2007;27(3):317–352.

[95] Ochoa JB, Bernard AC, O'Brien WE,Griffen M,Maley M,Rockich A,Tsuei B,Boulanger B,Kearney P,Morris S. Arginase 1 expression and activity in human mononuclear cells after injury. Ann Surg. 2001;233:393–399.

[96] Ochoa JB,Udekwu AO,Billiar TR,Curran RD,Cerra FB,Simmons RL,Peitzman AB. Nitrogen oxide levels in patients after trauma and during sepsis. Ann Surg.1991 Nov; 214(5):621-626.

[97] Ariel A,Serhan CN. Resolvins and protectins in the termination program of acute inflammation. Trends Immunol.2007 Apr;28(4):176-183.

[98] Popovic PJ,Zeh HJ,Ochoa JB. Arginine and immunity. J Nutr.2007 Jun;137(6 Suppl 2): 1681S-1686S.

[99] Menger M,Vollmar B. Surgical trauma: hyperinflammation versus immunosuppression? Langenbecks Arch Surg.2004 May;389(6):475-484.

[100] Ben-Eliyahu S,Page G,Yirmiya R,Shakhar G.Evidence that stress and surgical interventions promote tumor development by suppressing natural killer cell activity.Int J Cancer.1999;80:880-888.

[101] Colacchio TA, Yeager MP, Hildebrandt LW. Perioperative immunomodulation in cancer surgery. Am J Surg. 1994;167:174–179.

[102] Wada H, Seki S,Takahashi T,Kawarabayashi N,Higuchi H,Habu Y,Sugahara S,Kazama T. Combined Spinal and General Anesthesia Attenuates Liver Metastasis by Preserving Th1/Th2 Cytokine Balance. Anesthesiology.2007 Mar;106:499-506.

[103] Forget P, Collet V, Lavand'homme P, De Kock M.Does analgesia and condition influence immunity after surgery? Effects of fentanyl, ketamine and clonidine on natural killer activity at different ages. Eur J Anaesthesiol .2010;27: 233-240

[104] Kurosawa S,Kato M. Anesthetics, immune cells, and immune responses. J Anesth. 2008 Aug;22(3):263-277.

[105] Melamed R, Bar-Yosef S, Shakhar G, Shakhar K, Ben-Eliyahu S. Suppression of natural killer cell activity and promotion of tumor metastasis by ketamine, thiopental, and halothane, but not by propofol: mediating mechanisms and prophylactic measures. Anesth Analg.2003;97:1331-1339.

[106] Percival S,Nelson S,Milner J.Immunonutrition:Enhancing Tumoricidal Cell Activity.The Journal of Nutrition.2005; 135: 2898S-2907S.

[107] Wada H, Seki S,Takahashi T,Kawarabayashi N,Higuchi H,Habu Y,Sugahara S,Kazama T. Combined Spinal and General Anesthesia Attenuates Liver Metastasis by Preserving Th1/Th2 Cytokine Balance. Anesthesiology.2007 Mar;106:499-506.

[108] Kaur S,Chang T,Singh S,lim L,Mannan P,Garfield S,Pendrak M,Soto-Pantoja D,Rosenberg a,Jin S,Roberts D.CD47 Signaling Regulates the Immunosuppressive Activity of VEGF in T-cells.J Immunol.2014 Sept;193(8):3914-3924.

[109] Carson J, Grossman B, Kleinman S, Tinmouth A, Marques M, Fung M, Holcomb J, Illoh O, Kaplan L, Katz L, Rao S, Roback J, Shander A, Tobian A, Weinstein R, McLaughlin L, Djulbegovic B. Red Blood Cell Transfusion: A Clinical Practice Guideline From the AABB.Ann Intern Med.2012 Jul:157:49-58.

[110] Goodnough LT,Shander A. Patient blood management. Anesthesiology.2012 Jun; 116(6):1367-1376.

[111] O'Flaherty L,Bouchier-Hayes DJ. Immunonutrition and surgical practice. Proc Nutr Soc.1999;58:831-837.

[112] Li K,Dan Z,Nie YQ. Gastric cancer stem cells in gastric carcinogenesis, progression, prevention and treatment. World Journal of Gastroenterology.2014 May;20(18): 5420-5426.

[113] Villa-Morales M, Fernandez-Piquerar J. Targeting the Fas/FasL signaling pathway in cancer therapy. Expert Opin Ther Targets.2012 Jan;16(1):85-101.

[114] Bukur J,Jasinski S, Seliger B.The role of classical and non-classical HLA class I antigens in human tumors.Seminars in Cancer Biology. 2012;22(4);350-358.

[115] Kochan E,Escors D,Breckpot K,Guerrero-Setas D. Role of non-classical MHC class I molecules in cancer immunosuppression. Oncoimmunology.2013 Nov;2(11):e26491.

[116] Gajewski T,Schreiber H,Fu YX.Innate and adaptive immune cells in the tumor microenvironment. Nature Immunology.2013 Sept;14(10): 1014-1022.

[117] Zhou Y, Piao K, Zheng H,Hou W,Xiong L,Pei Y,Qi X. Influence on DC stimulating LPAK anti-tumor activity by feiliuping extract and its decomposed recipe.Cancer Research on Prevention and Treatment.2013; 40(1):3-6.

[118] Chen G, Li KK,Fung CH,Liu CL,Wong HL,Leung PC,Ko CH. Er-Miao-San, a traditional herbal formula containing Rhizoma Atractylodis and Cortex Phellodendri inhibits inflammatory mediators in LPS-stimulated RAW264.7 macrophages through inhibition of NF-κB pathway and MAPKs activation. J Ethnopharmacol.2014 Jul; 154(3):711-718.

[119] Wan C,Gao L,Hou L,Yang X,He P,Yang Y,Tang W,Yue J,Li J,Zuo J. Astragaloside II triggers T cell activation through regulation of CD45 protein tyrosine phosphatase activity. Acta Pharmacologica Sinica.2013;34(4):522-530.

[120] Wei H, Sun R, Xiao W,Feng J,Zhen C,Xu X,Tian Z. Traditional Chinese medicine Astragalus reverses predominance of Th2 cytokines and their up-stream transcript factors in lung cancer patients. Oncol Rep.2003 Sep-Oct;10(5):1507-1512.

[121] Wei H, Sun R, Xiao W,Feng J,Zhen C,Xu X,Tian Z .Type two cytokines predominance of human lung cancer and its reverse by traditional Chinese medicine TTMP. Cellular & Molecular Immunology.2004;1(1):63-70.

Chapter 3

Positron Emission Tomography in Autoimmune Disorders of the Central Nervous System

Ara Kaprelyan

Additional information is available at the end of the chapter

http://dx.doi.org/10.5772/61171

Abstract

This chapter covers the basic knowledge on interactions between the central nervous system and immunity. It presents information about the main factors and mechanisms that refer to the traditional and new concepts on immune privilege of the brain. In addition, the immune surveillance and tolerance are discussed in context of the central nervous system homeostasis, production of autoreactive lymphocytes, and neurons vulnerability.

Certain general aspects in principles of positron emission tomography (PET) technique, radiotracer characteristics, and specificities of the cerebral glucose uptake are provided. The chapter also offers an overview of the current clinical application of (18F)-FDG PET imaging in the detection and differential diagnosis of different autoimmune disorders of the central nervous system.

This chapter reviews the autoimmune underlying mechanisms and main abnormalities in cerebral glucose metabolism in patients with multiple sclerosis, late-onset ataxias, and limbic encephalitis. Own clinical observations and results are presented in accordance to previous publications. Neuroimaging findings are discussed in context of PET sensitivity and accuracy for assessment of disease localization and characterization.

Keywords: (18F)-FDG PET/CT, autoimmunity, CNS disorders

1. Introduction

1.1. Central nervous system and immunity

Advances in scientific research and accumulated working knowledge of anatomo-functional subsystems of the central nervous system (CNS) and their relationship with the downregulation of the immune system play a crucial role in the understanding of underlying mechanisms and treatment of immune-mediated neurological disorders [19, 37].

Traditionally, CNS is considered an immunologically-privileged site, meaning the brain and spinal cord can tolerate the introduction of foreign antigens without eliciting an afferent immune response [29, 34]. Immune privilege is believed to be an active process aiming to protect the brain structures from the harming effect of an inflammation. This immune privilege is thought to be due to a lack of lymphatic drainage and the integrity of blood-brain barrier (BBB) [21]. It varies throughout the different parts of the CNS, being most pointed in the white matter. Among the other factors that also contribute to the maintenance of brain immune privilege are local production of immunosuppressive cytokines, increased expression of surface molecules inhibiting complement activation, low expression of major histocompatibility complex (MHC) class Ia molecules, presence of neuropeptides, etc. [26].

Over the last two decades the concept of CNS as an immunologically-privileged site has been reevaluated. Today, experimental and clinical data show evidence suggesting the presence of resident CNS macrophages known as microglia [42]. Although the separation and isolation of CNS from the peripheral immune cells throughout the BBB, certain unique interactions exist due to the sequestration of neuronal antigens in "partially" immune-privilege sites, presence of antigen determinants shared by the nervous and immune systems, and secretion of immunoregulatory mediators by specific nerve cells [19, 29, 34]. Nowadays, it is known that activated lymphocytes are able to pass through the BBB regardless of their antigen specificity, directed by cytokines and adhesion molecules that are expressed on the brain endothelial cells (ICAM-1, VCAM-1) [2]. Normally, MHC class 1 and class 2 molecules are minimally expressed in the CNS, but in pathology the expression induced by proinflammatory cytokines IFN-γ is much higher. Immune surveillance in the CNS is under strong control and its major role is to provide constancy of the homeostasis in relation to the raised vulnerability of the neurons [26].

Immune tolerance is known to protect normal tissues from immune damage by prevention of immune response against a particular antigen to which the human organism is normally responsive. In the past, it was thought that the break of immune tolerance causes the production of autoantibodies and/or sensitized cytotoxic T-lymphocytes, attacking own tissues, the so-called autoreactive lymphocytes. Today, it is evident that these autoreactive cells normally exist in the immune system in a state of anergy and areactivity toward own antigens. Respectively, the immune tolerance is considered as a result from suppression and elimination of autoreactive T-lymphocytes [2].

It is known that autoimmunity represents an abnormal immune response directed against the cells and tissues of the organism. Autoimmune responses are considered an integral part of the immune system and present a survival self-defense mechanism. It is postulated that this aberrant immune response refers to the development of different diseases. The mechanisms of autoimmune disorders of the CNS are associated with molecular mimicry, upregulation of heat shock proteins, the release of so-called "sequestrated" antigens (brain tissue antigens hidden behind the BBB), bystander activation, and production of neoantigens [13, 42]. Most commonly T- and B-cell mediated autoimmune diseases result from the elimination and inhibition of regulatory T-cells or the dysregulation of humoral immunity.

2. Positron emission tomography in neurology

In recent years, a large number of scientific reports confirm the increasing influence of nuclear medicine in the diagnosis and treatment of patients with various neurological diseases [10, 23, 25, 33, 43]. Accordingly, positron emission tomography presents a modern non-invasive technique for investigation in vivo of basic biochemical processes and physiological functions of the CNS [36]. This method provides important information about the cerebral blood flow, permeability of BBB, activity of brain enzymes, and metabolism of glucose, amine and fatty acids, as well as synthesis and metabolism of neurotransmitters, gene expression and density of neuromediators receptors.

PET has a wide clinical application in the understanding of underlying mechanisms of neurological diseases, early and correct diagnosis, monitoring of clinical course and prognosis of outcome, studying of drugs pharmacokinetics and pharmacodynamics, and assessment of therapeutic response. In addition to structural neuroimaging, PET improves the diagnostic accuracy of localization, characterization, and distribution of anatomical and functional cerebral disturbances [17, 33, 36].

PET is realized through intravenous injection of radiotracer, which is a biological marker, labeled with positron emitting isotope [7]. Carbone (^{11}C), nitrogen (^{13}N), oxygen (^{15}O), and fluorine (^{18}F) are among the most frequently used in clinical practice due to their relatively short half-life (up to 110 min) and constant body spread, without prolonged radiation exposure [40].

It is well known that the human brain presents only 2% of body weight, but utilizes about 20% of absorbed oxygen and 60% of glucose, which is a major energy source for the nerve cells. Respectively, (18F)-FDG is the most appropriate radiotracer for functional study of cerebral tissue, because it reflects the level of glucose assimilation by brain neurons. ^{18}F-Fluorodeoxy-glucosae - (18)FDG represents deoxyglucosae that is labeled with ^{18}F. FDG is a glucose analogue that biodistribution fully reflects the glucose consumption of different organs and tissues [44]. Its cell's influx is realized through active transport, by means of glucose transporters in mechanisms that are similar and competing with glucose. After entering the cytosol, the molecule is phosphorylated into a stable form, which has a slower metabolism and prolonged cell's retention than glucose.

The brain tissue is characterized by high glucose activity, mainly in the cortical, thalamic, cerebellar, and basal ganglia gray matter, and relatively lower in the white matter [23]. The distribution in the cerebral cortex is not homogeneous, as the highest activities are realized in the occipital lobes.

New data support the notion that PET is a useful technique for diagnosis, planning treatment, and prognosis in various neurological diseases, including autoimmune disorders of the CNS [3, 8, 24]. By measuring brain and spinal cord metabolism, FDG-PET may demonstrate extensive regions of neurologic dysfunction in patients with multiple sclerosis (MS), immune-mediated cerebellar ataxias and autoimmune limbic encephalitis [4, 10, 15, 33, 41].

3. PET in diagnosis of autoimmune neurological disorders

3.1. Multiple sclerosis

MS is an immune-mediated inflammatory, demyelinating disease of the CNS [22]. The etiology is not known, but it is supposed to involve a combination of genetic predisposition and certain triggers (e.g., various viral infections, low vitamin D levels) that cause recurrent immune attacks [28]. MS is supposed to be associated with certain genetic loci, which are known to influence the regulation of the immune system and higher susceptibility to this autoimmune disease [12]. Strong relationship exists with class II alleles (HLA-DR2, HLA-DR15), T-cell receptor gene, genes synthesizing immunoglobulins, tumor necrosis factor-α (TNF-α), and myelin basic protein (MBP).

MS is an inflammatory disease of the CNS characterized by the dissemination lesions of demyelination, called plaques, in the brain and spinal cord [32]. The main pathological changes include the degeneration of axons, astrocytes-induced gliosis, and sclerosis [22]. The stepwise lesion formation enlists the activation of myelin-reactive T cells in the periphery, breakdown of the BBB, penetration of activated inflammatory cells (lymphocytes and macrophages), and B-cell activation (generation of antibodies to MBP). Evidence exist that MS plaques are associated with expression of high levels of Interleukin (IL)-12 and B7-1, stimulating the release of proinflammatory cytokines [28]. Functionally-decreased T-lymphocytes with regulatory role (Tregs), microglia, dendritic cells, natural killer (NK) cells, and nonimmune (endothelial) cells are also involved in the mechanisms of CNS inflammation.

MS is diagnosed on the basis of clinical findings, brain magnetic resonance imaging (MRI), and cerebrospinal fluid examination (CSF) [31, 32]. Additionally, (18F)-FDG PET scans reveal the localization and distribution of cerebral hypometabolism in relation to demyelinating lesions in the white matter and their remote influence over the glucose metabolism of cortex, basal ganglia, and cerebellum [5, 10]. This method is also useful in MS patients with cognitive dysfunction for investigation of global and regional cerebral glucose metabolism in comparison to MRI findings [35]. According to Bakshi R et al. [3] and Derache N et al. [9], (18F)-FDG PET scans have clinical application as a marker for assessment of disease activity and response to immunotherapy. Although, cerebral imaging studies show variable results [6, 15, 16, 27], our (18F)-FDG PET findings in MS patients with certain cognitive impairment reveal areas of hypometabolism, corresponding to the white matter lesions and brain atrophy (Clinical case 1).

Clinical case 1. A 44-year-old male with relapsing-remitting MS and cognitive impairment. Neuroimaging findings (Fig. 1, 2, and 3).

3.2. Autoimmune cerebellar ataxia

Late-onset progressive cerebellar disorders can result from various pathologic processes, including malformations, degenerative and vascular disorders, infections, neoplasms, paraneoplastic syndromes, toxic/metabolic disorders, and demyelinating disease [1]. It is known that the immune system plays an important role in the development of paraneoplastic

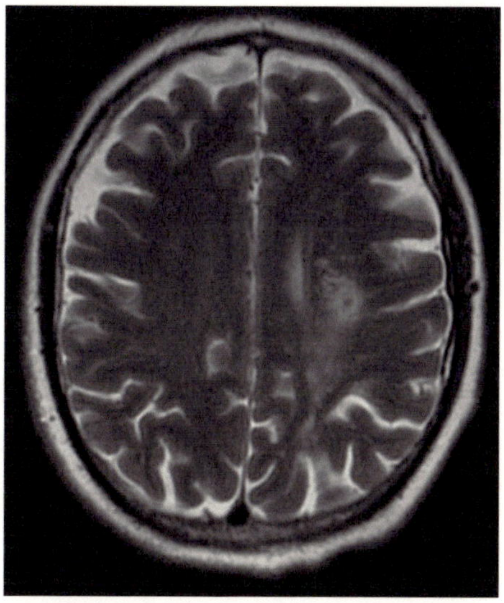

Figure 1. MRI shows MS lesions expressed in the left cerebral hemisphere.

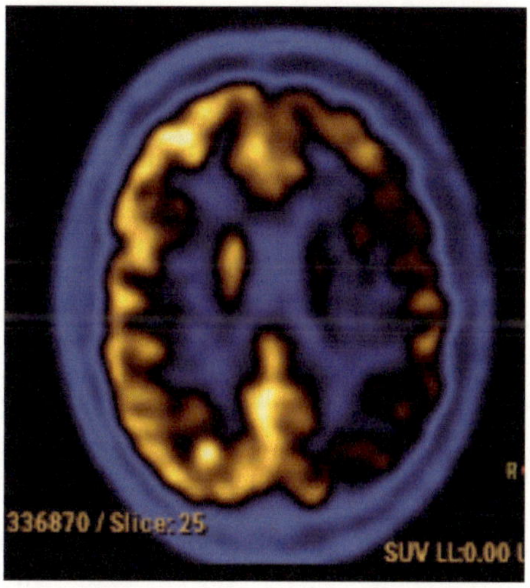

Figure 2. (18F)-FDG PET reveals areas of hypometabolism related to MS lesions and brain atrophy expressed mainly in the left cerebral hemisphere.

and nonparaneoplastic types of cerebellar ataxia [38]. Clinical data suggest that immune-mediated cerebellar ataxia may be caused by autoantibodies to various cerebellar targets [39]. Anti-voltage-gated calcium channel (VGCC), -Yo (Purkinje cell antigen), -ANNA-3, -Ri, -Hu, -Ma, -PCA-2, and -mGluR antibodies are found in patients with paraneoplastic cerebellar ataxia. In contrast, nonparaneoplastic ataxia is associated with anti-GAD, -gliadin, and -thyroid antibodies. Cross-reaction between tumor and cerebellar antigens is thought to be an underlying mechanism of autoimmune paraneoplastic ataxia [33]. The detection of circulating

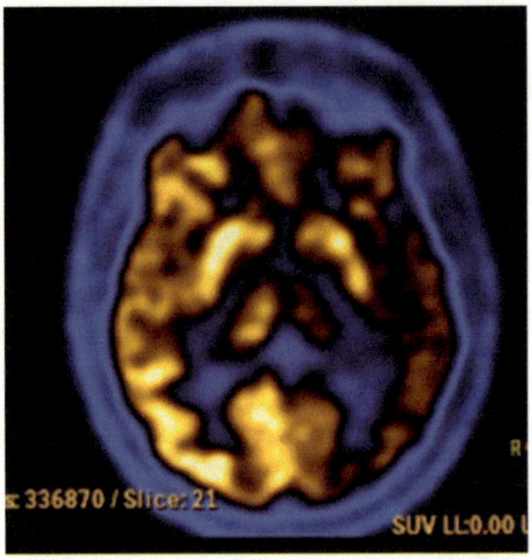

Figure 3. (18F)-FDG PET reveals areas of hypometabolism related to MS lesions and brain atrophy expressed mainly in the left cerebral hemisphere.

autoantibodies in patients with nonparaneoplastic cerebellar ataxia supports the notion that the immune system is also involved in the pathogenesis of these sporadic cases.

The diagnosis is usually suggested by the presence of atrophy of the cerebellum and brainstem on computed tomography scans (CT) and magnetic resonance imaging (MRI) [1, 38]. In addition, PET is useful in the investigation of patients with acute or chronic ataxias [33]. Functional neuroimaging with (18F)-FDG improves the detection of etiology and understanding of underlying pathophysiologic mechanisms in patients with late-onset cerebellar ataxia. Certain investigations reveal a reduction in absolute values of regional cerebral glucose metabolism in the cerebellar hemispheres and vermis, as well as in the brainstem or dentate nuclei [24, 25]. We report similar (18F)-FDG PET observations on our patient with anti-Yo antibody-positive late-onset cerebellar ataxia, associated with two different types of tumors (Clinical case 2). In contrast, Wang P et al. [41] show various patterns of cerebral glucose metabolism in patients with ataxia.

Clinical case 2. A 49-year-old female with skin melanoma and ovarian cyst in accordance with autoimmune (paraneoplastic) cerebellar ataxia. (18F)-FDG PET findings (Fig. 4 and 5).

3.3. Autoimmune limbic encephalitis

Limbic encephalitis is a severe, neuropsychiatric disorder that affects the limbic system, which is responsible for the basic autonomic functions [14]. Based on the etiology, it is divided into two clinical forms: viral and autoimmune. The inflammation in the latter is caused by the autoimmune process that involves medial temporal lobes. Autoimmune limbic encephalitis (ALE) may be either paraneoplastic, which is associated with a large number of cancers (lung, breast, testicular, thymoma, Hodgkin lymphoma) or idiopatic (non-paraneoplastic) [18, 20]. ALE can be associated with the presence of autoantibodies to two groups of antigens: intracellular neuronal and cell-surface [39]. The first group includes Hu, Mu2, Ri, glutamic acid

http://dx.doi.org/10.5772/61171

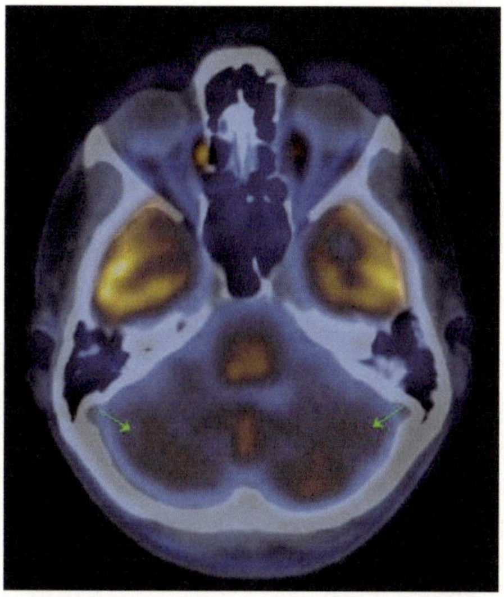

Figure 4. (18)F-FDG PET reveals strongly reduced metabolic activity in the cerebellum.

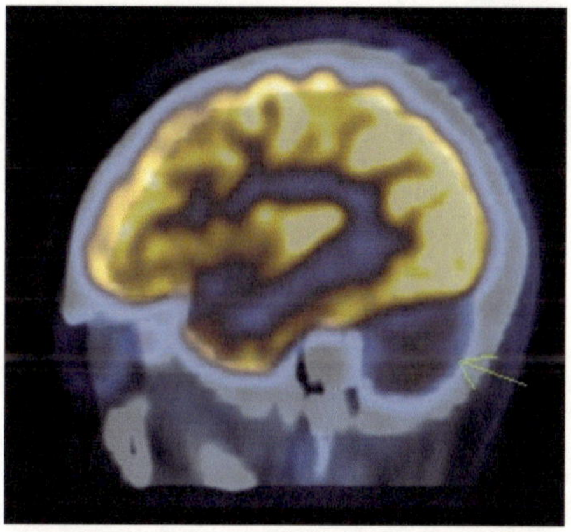

Figure 5. (18)F-FDG PET reveals strongly reduced metabolic activity in the cerebellum.

dexcarboxylase (GAD), amphiphysin, and collapsing responce-madiator protein 5. Voltage-gated potassium channels (VGKC), N-methyl-d-aspartate receptor (NMDAR), α-amino-3-hydroxy-5-methyl-4-isoxazoleproprionic acid (AMRAR) belong to the latter antigen group.

The diagnosis of ALE is based upon clinical features (memory loss, temporal lobe epilepsy, and psychiatric syndrome), MRI, electroencephalography (EEG), and cerebrospinal fluid analysis [14]. Cerebral (18F)-FDG PET studies describe different scan patterns in patients with ALE [4, 8]. According to Fisher R et al. [11], one is specific to the disease and presents a combination of pronounced occipital hypometabolism and hypermetabolism in the temporal and orbitofrontal cortex. We describe the similar findings in one patient with idiopathic ALE (Clinical case 3). The other pattern closely resembles a diffuse neurodegenerative disease. Rey

C et al. [30] report three cases with non-paraneoplastic limbic encephalitis characterized by (18F)-FDG PET bilateral striatal hypermetabolism, in contrast to diffused hypometabolism in the rest of the brain.

Clinical case 3. A 35-year-young male with idiopathic autoimmune limbic encephalitis. Neuroimaging findings (Fig. 6 and 7).

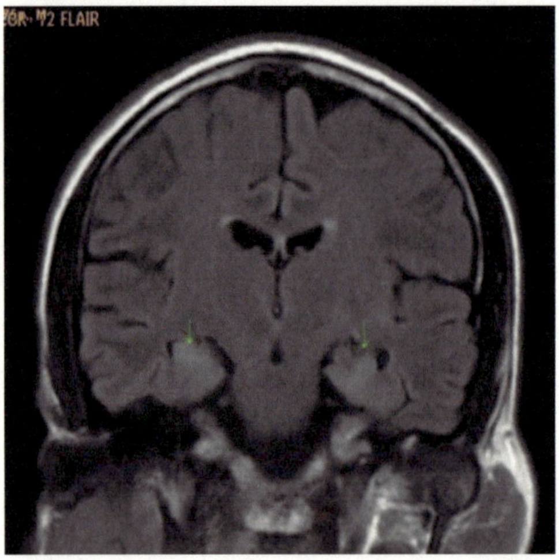

Figure 6. Coronal magnetic resonance-fluid attenuated inversion recovery (MRI-FLAIR) shows bilateral increased signal of hypothalamus and amygdala.

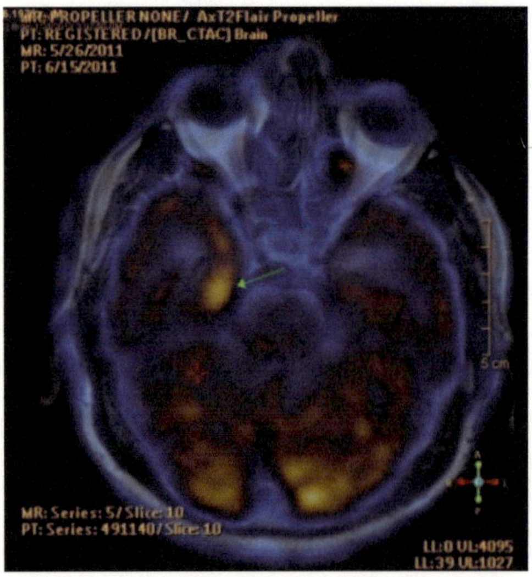

Figure 7. The (18F)-FDG PET scan reveals the nonhomogeneous distribution of cortical metabolic activity with discreet reduction in the left parietal region; hypermetabolism in both medial temporal lobes to hippocampi.

4. Summary

Although there are recent advances in molecular and cellular neurobiology, achievements of neurogenetics, and application of modern anatomical and functional neuroimaging techniques, the human brain is still an "enigma" and several immune-mediated inflammatory and neurodegenerative diseases of the CNS remain diagnosed late and unsuccessfully treated. Accordingly, a future research in basic neuroimmunology and innate mechanisms of autoimmunity is necessary to provide more precise immunodiagnostic assays and modern therapeutic approaches in patients with neurological autoimmune diseases. Furthermore, the development of new radiology methods and specific radiotracer biomarkers for the needs of neuroinflammation and degeneration imaging is another serious precondition to guarantee the early detection and adequate treatment of immune-mediated damages of the CNS. Respectively, existing clinical data support the notion that PET scanning improves the medical diagnosis, differentiation, monitoring, and prognosis of certain debilitating autoimmune diseases that affect the brain and spinal cord tissue.

Author details

Ara Kaprelyan*

Address all correspondence to: arakapri07@yahoo.co.uk

Department of neurology and neurosciences, "Prof. D-r P. Stoyanov" Medical University of Varna, Varna, Bulgaria

References

[1] Abele M, Burk K, Schols L et al. The aetiology of sporadic adult-onset ataxia. Brain, 2002; 125:961-8.

[2] Arima Y, et al. Regional neural activation defines a gateway for autoreactive T cells to cross the blood-brain barrier. Cell, 2012; 148:447-457.

[3] Bakshi R, Miletich R, Kinkel P, Emmet M, Kinkel W. High-resolution fluorodeoxyglucose positron emission tomography shows both global and regional cerebral hypometabolism in multiple sclerosis. J Neuroimaging, 1998; 8(4):228-34.

[4] Baumgartner A, Rauer S, Mader I, Meyer P. Cerebral FDG-PET and MRI findings in autoimmune limbic encephalitis: Correlation with autoantibody types. J Neurol, 2013; 260(11): 2744-2753.

[5] Blinkenberg M, Jensen C, Holm S, Paulson O, Sørensen P. A longitudinal study of cerebral glucose metabolism, MRI, and disability in patients with MS. Neurology, 1999; 53(1):149-53.

[6] Bolcaen J, Acou M, Mertens K, et al. Structural and metabolic features of two different variants of multiple sclerosis: A PET/MRI study. J Neuroimaging, 2013; 23:431-436.

[7] Bybel B, Wu G, Brunken R, et al. PET and PET/CT imaging. Cleve Clin J Med, 2006; 73:1075-1087.

[8] Chatzikonstantinou A, Szabo K, Ottomeyer C, et al. Successive affection bilateral temporomesial structures in a case of non-paraneoplastic limbic encephalitis demonstrated by serial MRI and FDG-PET. J Neurol, 2009; 256:1753-1755.

[9] Derache N, Marié R, Constans J, Defer G. Reduced thalamic and cerebellar rest metabolism in relapsing-remitting multiple sclerosis, a positron emission tomography study: Correlations to lesion load. J Neurol Sci, 2006; 245(1-2):103-9.

[10] Faria D, Copray S, Buchpiguel C, Dierckx R, de Vries E. PET imaging in multiple sclerosis. J Neuroimm Pharm, 2014; 9(4):468-482.

[11] Fisher R, Patel N, Lai E, Schulz P. Two different 18F-FDG brain PET metabolic patterns in autoimmune limbic encephalitis. Clin Nucl Med, 2012; 37:213-218.

[12] Gajofatto A, Bongianni M, Zanusso G, et al. Clinical and biomarker assessment of demyelinating events suggesting multiple sclerosis. Acta Neurol Scand, 2013; doi: 10.1111/ane.12123.

[13] Goverman J. Autoimmune T cell response in the central nervous system. Nature Reviews Immunol, 2009; 9(6):393. doi:10.1038/nri2550

[14] Haberlandt E, Bast T, Ebner A, et al. Limbic encephalitis in children and adolescents. Arch Dis Child, 2011; 96:186-191.

[15] Il'ves A, Prakhova L, Kataeva G, et al. Changes of cerebral glucose metabolism in patients with multiple sclerosis and their role in formation of the clinical picture and progression of the disease. Zh Nevrol Psikhiatr Im S S Korsakova, 2003; 2:53-60.

[16] Il'ves A, Prakhova L, Kataeva G, Petrov A, et al. Clinical and radiological (PET, MRI) correlations depending on disease progression in patients with multiple sclerosis. Zh Nevrol Psikhiatr Im S S Korsakova, 2006; 3:81-6.

[17] Javdar H, Colleti P. Competitive advantage of PET/MRI. Eur J Rad, 2014, 83(1):84-94.

[18] Kaira K, Okamura T, Takahashi H, et al. Small-cell lung cancer with voltage-gated calcium channel antibody-positive paraneoplastic limbic encephalitis: A case report. J Med Case Rep, 2014; 8:119.

[19] Kamimura D, Yamada M, Harada M, et al. The gateway theory: Bridging neural and immune interactions in the CNS. Front Neurosci, 2013; 7:204.

[20] Kondziella D. Case report on non-paraneoplastic autoantibody-negative limbic encephalitis. Neuropenews, 2012.

[21] Kubo T, Tokita S, Yamashita T. Crosstalk between the immune and central nervous system with special reference to drug development. In: Drug development - a case study based insight into modern strategies, C. Rundfeldt (Ed.), In Tech, 2011; 365-380.

[22] Lassman H. Pathology and disease mechanisms in different stages of multiple sclerosis. J Neurol Sci, 2013; doi:10.1016/j.jns.

[23] Mishina M. Positron emission tomography for brain research. J Nippon Med Sch, 2008; 75:68-76.

[24] Mishina M, Senda M, Ohyama M, et al. Regional cerebral glucose metabolism associated with ataxic gait - an FDG-PET activation study in patients with olivopontocerebellar atrophy. Rinsho Shinkeigaku, 1995; 35(11):1199-204.

[25] Otsuka M, Ichiya Y, Kuwabara Y, Hosokawa S, et al. Striatal 18F-dopa uptake and brain glucose metabolism by PET in patients with syndrome of progressive ataxia. J Neurol Sci, 1994; 124(2):198-203.

[26] Ousman S, Kubes P. Immune surveillance in the central nervous system. Nat Neurosci, 2012; 15:1096-1101.

[27] Padma M, Adineh M, Pugar K, et al. Functional imaging of a large demyelinating lesion. J Clin Neuroscie, 2005; 12(2):178-182.

[28] Pittock S, Lucchinetti C. The pathology of MS. New insights and potential clinical applications. Neurologist, 2007; 13:45-56.

[29] Ransohoff R, Brown M. Innate immunity in the central nervous system. J Clin Invest, 2012; 122(4):1164-1171.

[30] Rey C, Koric L, Guedj E, et al. Striatal hypermetabolism in limbic encephalitis. J Neurol, 2012; 259:1106-1110.

[31] Rubin S. Management of multiple sclerosis: An overview. Dis Mon, 2013; 59:253-260.

[32] Sand I, Lublin F. Diagnosis and differential diagnosis of multiple sclerosis. Continuum (Minneap Minn), 2013; 19:922-943.

[33] Sherry S, Tahari A, Mirpour S, Colucci A, Subramaniam R. FDG-PET/CT in the evaluation of paraneoplastic neurologic syndromes. Imaging in medicine, 2014; 6(1): 117-126.

[34] Shrestha R, Millington O, Brewer J, Bushell T. Is Central Nervous System an immune-privileged Site? Kathmandu Univ Med J, 2013; 41(1):102-107.

[35] Sørensen P, Jønsson A, Mathiesen H, Blinkenberg M, Andresen J, Hanson L, Ravnborg M. The relationship between MRI and PET changes and cognitive disturbances in MS. J Neurol Sci, 2006; 245(1-2):99-102.

[36] The Royal College of Physicians and The Royal College of Radiologists. Evidence-based indications for the use of PET-CT in the UK. London: RCP, RCR, 2013.

[37] Tian L, Ma L, Kaarela T, Li Z. Neuroimmune crosstalk in the central nervous system and its significance for neurological diseases. J Neuroinflamm, 2012; 9:155.

[38] van Gaalen J, van de Warenburg B. A practical approach to late-onset cerebellar ataxia. Pract Neurol, 2012; 12(1):14-24.

[39] Vincent A, Bien C, Irani S, Waters P. Autoantibodies associated with diseases of the CNS: New developments and future challenges. Lan Neurol, 2011; 10:759-772.

[40] Wadsak W, Mitterhauser M. Basics and principles of radiopharmaceuticals for PET/CT. Eur J Radiol, 2010; 73:461-469.

[41] Wang P, Liu R, Yang B, Soong B. Regional patterns of cerebral glucose metabolism in spinocerebellar ataxia type 2, 3 and 6: A voxel-based FDG-positron emission tomography analysis. J Neurol, 2007; 254(7):838-45.

[42] Wraith D, Nicholson L. The adaptive immune system in diseases of the central nervous system. J Clin Invest, 2012; 122(4):1172-1179.

[43] Wu C, Li F, Niu G, Chen X. PET imaging of inflammation biomarkers. Theranostics, 2013; 3:448-466.

[44] Zanzonico P. Principles of nuclear medicine imaging: Planar, SPECT, PET, multi-modality, and autoradiography systems. Radiation Reseach, 2012; 177:349-364.

Section 2

Reviews

Chapter 4

Tuberculosis and HIV — Doubling the Fatality

Tatina T. Todorova, Gabriela Tsankova, Neli Lodozova and Tcvetelina Kostadinova

Additional information is available at the end of the chapter

http://dx.doi.org/10.5772/61138

Abstract

Tuberculosis (TB) and HIV/AIDS infection are one of the most ubiquitous and deadliest communicable diseases in the world. They cause millions of deaths each year and are recognized as major threats for public health worldwide. The corresponding pathogens (*Mycobacterium tuberculosis* and HIV) share overlapping epidemiology—they affect low-income countries and place an immense burden on their feeble health care systems. Over the last decades, the natural history of both diseases has changed; in addition to devastating single HIV and TB infections, the coinfection with both pathogens has emerged and has spread in pandemic scale. When present as dual infection in an individual, *Mycobacterium tuberculosis* and HIV potentiate each other and kill in cooperation the host. TB is the leading cause of death in HIV-positive patients and in turn HIV infection is the strongest risk factor for the development of new or reactivation of dormant TB disease. Both pathogens (as single or dual infection) provoke a robust immune response in the infected host but the immune system does not achieve to eliminate the infectious agent(s). The failure of immune defense results in vulnerable immune balance between the micro- and the macroorganism and often ends up in a fatal outcome.

Keywords: Tuberculosis, HIV, immunity, co-infection

1. Introduction

Human immunodeficiency virus (HIV) and tuberculosis (TB) represent, respectively, the first and the second leading cause of death from infectious disease in the world. Both are responsible for approximately 3 million deaths annually [1].

Either HIV or TB, when present as a single infection, irreversibly affects and exhausts the immune system of the infected person. Moreover, if they simultaneously coexist in an individual (coinfection), they act in synergy to deteriorate the defense mechanisms of the host's immunity and to accelerate the fatal scenario.

In this chapter, we will review current knowledge of innate and adaptive immune responses against TB and HIV infections. We will discuss in detail the immunological basis behind the dual threat of TB/HIV coinfection.

2. Epidemiology

2.1. Epidemiology of HIV pandemic

HIV infection is a viral disease that affects host immune system and makes the host strongly susceptible to opportunistic infections. It spreads among human population via sexual contact, sharing needles during drug injection, transfusion of contaminated blood products, or during births from HIV-infected women.

Since the late 20th century, HIV infection has become a global pandemic and a major challenge for public health authorities at the national and international levels. At the end of 2013, 35 million people were living with HIV worldwide [2]. During the same year, approximately 2.1 million people were newly infected with HIV. Sub-Saharan Africa is the most affected region in the world—almost 70% of the prevalent and the new HIV-positive cases are diagnosed there. The socio-economic status of the countries in the core of HIV pandemic determines the low number of infected people currently on adequate antiretroviral therapy (only 36% of overall cases).

2.2. Epidemiology of tuberculosis

Tuberculosis (TB) is an infectious disease caused by bacterial species grouped in *Mycobacterium tuberculosis* complex—MBTC (*M. bovis, M. africanum, M. canetti, M. caprae, M. microti, M. pinnipedii*). Among these mycobacterial species, the most important and major cause of human tuberculosis is *Mycobacterium tuberculosis*. It is a widespread microorganism that readily colonizes and infects humans. Primary infection represents clinical manifestation in only 10% of infected individuals, while in the remaining 90%, *M. tuberculosis* stays in latent form without showing any obvious clinical signs—latent (dormant) tuberculosis [3].

The World Health Organization (WHO) recognizes TB as "a global public health emergency" and "one of the world's deadliest communicable diseases" [1]. At least one-third of the world population (approx. 2 billion people) is currently infected with latent mycobacteria and has a risk, although low (5–10%), to develop an active disease during the life course [1]. In 2013, 9 million new TB cases occurred worldwide (TB incidence: 126 cases per 100,000 population) and the prevalent cases were 11 million (TB prevalence: 159 cases per 100,000 population). Despite the efforts at the international, national, and regional level and the significant progress in the detection and management of TB infection, still the incidence, prevalence, and mortality rate of TB are unacceptably high.

2.3. Epidemiology of TB/HIV coinfection

People living with HIV have 26–31 times higher risk to develop active TB than the normal population [1]. Both diseases are epidemiologically and biologically connected—TB is the leading cause of death in HIV-positive patients and in turn HIV infection exacerbates the gravity of TB. Due to the global circulation of HIV, the incidence of TB —an infection previously thought to be almost eliminated at least in developed countries—is still high in both developing and high-income countries. HIV disrupts the host immune system through significant depletion of CD4+ lymphocytes, a mechanism that readily facilitates the reactivation of latent TB to an active disease. Therefore, HIV is the strongest risk factor for the development of new or the reactivation of dormant TB disease, including multidrug-resistant TB, an infection resistant to at least two of the first choice drugs for TB treatment, isoniazid and rifampicin. HIV infection predisposes TB-infected patients to antibiotic (rifampicin) resistance through gastrointestinal malabsorption of TB medications [4]. On the other hand, *M. tuberculosis* enhances HIV replication [5] and decreases the CD4+ T cell counts in HIV-positive patients [6].

As one-third of the total world population is currently infected with latent *M. tuberculosis* [1] and almost 1% of the adult population is living with HIV, it is not surprising that 1.1 million (13%) of the 9 million people who developed TB in 2013 were at the same time HIV-positive and 360,000 of the overall 1.5 million TB deaths for 2013 were HIV-positive. Most of them (78%) were living in low-income economies in Sub-Saharan Africa, a region where 50–80% of TB patients have HIV coinfection[1].

WHO recommends regular screening of TB for all people living with HIV at every visit to a health care specialist [7]. WHO also recommends that routine HIV testing should be offered to all patients with presumptive and diagnosed TB, as well as to partners of known HIV-positive TB patients.

In addition to the increase in TB incidence, the worldwide HIV pandemic changed the average age of TB-infected people. In contrast to normal populations where TB is most prevalent among elderly people, in regions with significant number of HIV-positive cases, the most affected age by TB is the reproductive age (20–45 years). This leads to the consecutive increase in the number of TB-infected children [8].

3. Immunology of tuberculosis

3.1. The first date

Primary infection with *M. tuberculosis* occurs after inhalation of aerosolized infectious nuclei containing mycobacterial cells [9]. Any person with active TB can transmit the pathogen through coughing or sneezing, infecting 2–10 healthy individuals. Tubercle bacilli survive in the air for a short time (few hours), but the infective dose is relatively low (only 1–10 living cells). Infectious nuclei bigger than 10 μm gravitate in the nasal conchae and the nasopharynx. Those measuring between 5 and 10 μm enter the lower respiratory tract and mucociliary escalator eliminates them. Only infectious droplets smaller than 5 μm persist in the distal lung alveoli and can cause infection.

In most cases, the non-immune mechanisms do not allow the development of the infectious process. If infection occurs, the immune system in the lungs activates the first-line innate defense and then, several weeks later, an adaptive anti-mycobacterial immune response is activated. The strong immune response against *M. tuberculosis* works in two warring interests —on one hand, it restricts *M. tuberculosis* dissemination outside the initial infection place, and on the other hand, it supports its survival and silent presence for years in healthy individuals. The human immune system succeeds to completely eliminate *M. tuberculosis* in only 10% of infected cases, while in the remaining 90%, it fulfills in different degrees and controls the infection by turning it into the latent state [3].

3.2. Innate immunity

The early stages of TB infection consist of inhalation of tubercle bacilli and initial encounter between the immune system and the pathogen. Alveolar macrophages and sometimes nonprofessional phagocytic cells (alveolar epithelial cells) are the first to recognize *M. tuberculosis* cells [10, 11, 12]. Still, unknown intrinsic virulent features of *M. tuberculosis* strains and individual host immune differences are crucial for the fate of tubercle bacilli in the early days of infection. The most favorable outcome is the definitive destruction of *M. tuberculosis* by non-specific defense mechanisms in the macrophages. In this case, adaptive immunity does not develop and participate in the protection.

If bacteria survive bactericidal macrophage action, they can multiply intracellularly to destroy the infected macrophage and to release attractants for monocyte and dendritic cells accumulation. The attracted monocytes will differentiate into macrophages that in turn can recognize new *M. tuberculosis* cells to increase the population size of infected cells in the lung and sometimes in extra pulmonary locations. All these immune cells readily engulf *M. tuberculosis* cells but are unable to completely destroy them. Thus, the number of *M. tuberculosis* in the place of infection progressively increases.

Macrophages and dendritic cells bind *M. tuberculosis* cells via different receptors: toll-like receptors (TLRs), nucleotide-binding oligomerization domain (NOD-) like receptors (NLRs), mannose receptors (CD207), dendritic cell-specific intercellular adhesion molecule grabbing nonintegrins (DC-SIGN), Dectin-1 receptors, complement receptors, and others [3]. Among TLRs, the most important for pulmonary TB cases are TLR2, TLR4, and TLR9 [10–12]. TLR2 recognizes tubercle polysaccharides and via binding with TLR1 can identify tubercle cell wall 19 and 27 kDa lipoproteins—important *M. tuberculosis* cell surface ligands. Furthermore, bacterial DNA released after bacterial destruction in lisosomes activates TLR9.

The interaction between *M. tuberculosis* and TLRs induces a signal proinflammatory cascade and provokes secretion of cellular signals—TNF-alpha, IL-1, IL-6, IL-12, IL-18, IL-15, IL-23, IFN-gamma, and chemokinases. The infected macrophages also release small molecules—chemokines CCL, CCL3, CCL4, CCL5 (8–10 κDa)—to attract other blood monocytes and neutrophils [13], which after differentiation can directly display bactericidal action towards

M. tuberculosis. Interleukins and chemokines serve both to attract other immune cells (lymphocytes) and to activate them.

3.3. Cell-mediated immunity

A fundamental characteristic of *M. tuberculosis* infection is the considerable delay in the onset of adaptive immunity, achieved by efficient control and management of the innate immunity; the host establishes an effective cell-mediated immune response several weeks (2–8) after the initial infection [3]. Nonetheless, the initiation of cell-mediated adaptive immunity, though delayed, is crucial for efficient control of further TB invasion.

The matured dendritic cells move to the regional lymph nodes where they initiate specific cell immune response by presenting the ingested mycobacterial antigens to the naïve T cells. Dendritic cells are a primary target for *M. tuberculosis* after aerosolic lung infection [14, 15]. They are professional antigen presenting cells (more effective than macrophages) and strong T cell activators. One of the mechanisms used by *M. tuberculosis* to delay the cell-mediated immunity is the efficient postponement of the movement of dendritic cells towards regional lymph nodes. In the lymph nodes, infected dendritic cells produce IL-12 [16] for the activation of NK cells and stimulation of INF-gamma release from T-lymphocytes [17]. Antigen presenting dendritic cells prompts T cells to differentiate and to migrate, under the navigation of secreted adhesion molecules and chemokines, to the initial site of infection.

The concentration of macrophages, T-lymphocytes, dendritic cells, and other immune and lung cells (epithelial, giant multinuclear Langerhans' cells, plasma cells, neutrophils, fibroblasts) in the place of infection is known as granuloma. The process of granuloma formation limits the spread of *M. tuberculosis* to other organs and restricts tissue's damage by separating the infected place [18]. But at the same time, granuloma microenvironment ensures the needed conditions for mycobacterial growth and multiplication.

Both human and animal granulomas contain giant multinuclear Langerhans' cells produced after the fusion of macrophages [18, 19]. In these cells, tubercle bacilli cannot multiply and survive successfully.

Neutrophils are important for early control of acute bacterial infection [20] as they immediately migrate to the place of mycobacterial infection and start bacterial phagocytosis [21]. Infected neutrophils produce IL-8 and TNF for activation of alveolar macrophages and limitation of the infection [22].

Both CD4+ and CD8+[23] contribute to the stimulation of macrophages and lysis of chronically infected macrophages (via INF-gamma action). The principal role in cell-mediated immunity against tuberculosis is played by CD4+ T-lymphocytes. CD4+ express *a/b* T cell receptors to recognize mycobacterial antigens on the surface of antigen-presenting cells such as monocytes, macrophages, or dendritic cells [24]. Then, CD4+ lymphocytes efficiently induce apoptosis of macrophages [25] and stimulate the cytotoxic function of CD8+ [26].

CD8+ cells play an important role in IFN-gamma release, cell lysis and bacterial killing [27]. Some CD8+ lymphocytes may also recognize surface antigens presented by Class I MHC molecules—MHC class I-restricted cytotoxic T-lymphocytes (CTL). They are able to eliminate infected macrophages and also to kill intracellular bacteria via production of granulysin (a cytolytic and proinflammatory substance) [28].

Other immune cells—CD1 restricted T cells, γ/δ-T cells, and cytotoxic T-cells—also protect lung tissue against tuberculosis. T cells of type γ/δ are the first line of defense against microbial antigens and the connection between innate and adaptive immune response [29]. They have cytotoxic activity and may present mycobacterial antigens to CD8+ and CD4+ lymphocytes. In response to IL-23 secreted from infected dendritic cells, the γ/δ-T cells start to release IL-17 for accumulation of additional immune cells in the place of infection.

Activated macrophages represent higher phagocytic activity against extracellular mycobacteria. On the base of T-lymphocyte stimulation, two types of macrophages are known: classically activated macrophages (CAM) and alternatively activated macrophages (AAM). During the immune response against tubercle bacilli, activation of macrophages by T-lymphocytes is achieved mainly through release of IFN-gamma and other Th-1 cytokines. The Th-1 cytokines (INF-gamma, TNF-alpha, IL-1beta) induce CAM to kill tubercle bacilli via production of nitric oxide synthetase (iNOS). This enzyme catalyzes synthesis of nitric oxide (NO), a powerful antimicrobial substance. The Th-2 cytokines (IL-4 and IL-13) activate AAM to produce anti-inflammatory cytokines and arginase. They both compete for arginine utilization with iNOS [30]. The increased arginase activity stimulates tissue repair but at the same time restricts bacterial killing [31].

M. tuberculosis (particularly the virulent strains and not the attenuated ones) can survive in phagosomes of macrophages by suppressing the fusion between formed mycobacterial phagosome and lysosomes [32]. Other mechanisms to overcome bactericidal activity of macrophages include the prevention of phagosomal acidification and guidance of infected cells towards necrosis. Necrosis is a form of cellular death characterized by plasma and mitochondrial membrane disruption. In this way, tubercle bacilli leave infected macrophages and spread to other cells. Moreover, *M. tuberculosis* may inhibit the programmed cell death or apoptosis, a cellular death that protects further bacterial spread by preserving the cellular integrity of infected macrophage. Apoptotic macrophages transmit mycobacterial antigens to dendritic cells and induce more efficient T cell response.

3.4. Humoral immunity

In addition to cell-mediated immunity, humoral immune response plays a major role in TB infection control. The formed antibodies cannot transfer immunity but have an opsoning role and facilitate the phagocytosis by the macrophages and the cytotoxic function of T-lymphocytes [33]. Besides their antibody synthetic function [34], B-lymphocytes can present mycobacterial antigens to T cells [35]. They stimulate proliferation and differentiation of T-lymphocytes by the production of different cytokines. Specific effector B1-cells secrete Th1-cytokines—IFN-gamma and IL-12—while B2-cells secrete IL-4, typical for Th2-cells. Furthermore, activated B cells can produce IL-6 for T cell stimulation and IL-10 for inhibition of dendritic cells and macrophages.

3.5. Latent tuberculosis

The late stage of TB infection represents a prolonged (in many cases lifelong) suppression of mycobacterial cells as a result of the dynamic balance between the pathogen and the host immunity. *M. tuberculosis* persists within the granulomas and escapes total disruption by the immune system. In latent TB, the host and tubercle bacilli coexist in "perfect" synergy; the granuloma represents a place for bacterial survival and place for host attack [36]. Usually, the host immune system succeeds to manage the infectious process, but in extreme conditions (starving, diabetes, alcohol abuse, corticosteroid treatment, and especially supplementary HIV infection) the disease can progress. This progression is linked to granuloma disruption and further dissemination of *M. tuberculosis*. The late tuberculosis occurs in the presence of sensitized T-lymphocytes and already existing specific defense mechanisms. This determines rapid limitation of the process with strong caseous necrosis, cavern formation, and fibrosis.

4. Immunology of HIV

4.1. Entry through the mucosal barrier

The principal route of HIV entry into the human body is through the mucosal epithelial surfaces (mainly genital or rectal). The virus prefers to infect immune cells expressing CD4+ receptors on their surface—CD4+ helper T cells, macrophages, and dendritic cells—all present in activated state in the mucosal lymphoid tissues.

HIV crosses the intact epithelial layers via interaction with dendritic cells and/or CD4+ helper T cells. The CD4+ receptor of these cells recognizes the viral envelope glycoprotein 120 (gp120) and causes its conformational change. This makes possible the binding with one of the auxiliary co-receptors: CCR5 or CXCR4. The second binding allows viral glycoprotein 41 (gp41) to integrate within the cell membrane and viral genome to access the host cytoplasm.

After entry into the cell, viral RNA—under the action of reverse transcriptase and integrase—turns into double-strand DNA and integrates into the host DNA. The integrated copy of HIV nucleic acid (named provirus) can stay in latent form for years and can become active at any time to complete the viral life cycle and produce new virions.

The principal target for HIV is the activated CD4+ T-lymphocyte expressing CCR5 or CXCR4 co-receptor. The high number of CD4+ T cells (especially memory CD4+CCR5+ T-lymphocytes) in the mucosa is ideal for HIV replication [37]. In contrast, mucosal dendritic cells do not express CD4+ or CCR5 receptors [38] but they do express other receptors that successfully recognize HIV envelope proteins—dendritic cell-specific intercellular adhesion molecule grabbing nonintegrins (DC-SIGN) and langerin [39].

4.2. HIV expansion

Early after the entry of HIV, the primary infected T-lymphocytes attract and activate other immune cells to expand the initial place of infection. The infected local site starts to grow until the detachment of the infected cells. Thus, the virus disseminates from the mucosal surfaces to the regional lymph nodes (usually in 10 days after the infection) and then throughout the body. The virus can be detected in all lymphoid organs but the highest number of viral particles concentrates in the mucosal lymphoid tissues (such as gastro-intestinal associated lymphoid tissue). Dendritic cells in lymph nodes and mucosal lymphoid tissues present the HIV antigens to naïve B cells and T cells, prompting them to differentiate and activate. In these first stages, the viral load is significant and CD4+ T cells count starts to decline rapidly.

In many cases, the early events of viral expansion (acute stage) are not clinically manifested. In some people, influenza-like or mononucleosis-like symptoms may occur several weeks after the exposure to infection but they are not specific and often misdiagnosed.

4.3. T cell-mediated immune response during HIV latency

Several months after the initial infection, a precise balance between the virus and the immune response (both cell-mediated and humoral) is established. Host immune system (especially CD8+ lymphocytes) succeeds to control viral replication at some degree but the elimination of target CD4+ population continues. This represents the chronic (latent) phase in HIV infection, clinically manifested with decreased viral load and appearance of specific anti-HIV antibodies in the blood of infected individuals.

Although the major characteristic of HIV infection is the depletion of CD4+ T cells, other lymphocyte types are also affected. HIV notably influences naïve T cells (both CD4 T naïve cells and CD8 T naïve cells) during the asymptomatic phase of the infection [40]. Any T cell-mediated immune response requires new naïve T cells and their depletion results in progressively compromised immunity. The reduction in naïve T cell counts is probably due to decreased thymic output and increased T cell turnover in HIV-positive patients [41]. Furthermore, during HIV asymptomatic phase, the overall CD8+ count remains the same as before infection but significant alteration in the ratio memory/naïve CD8+ cells occurs, the normal predominance of naïve CD8+ is replaced by the domination of memory cells (in many patients, the compartment of CD8+ memory cells represents more than 80% of all CD8+ circulating cells) [40].

The cellular immune response mediated by CD8+ cytotoxic T-lymphocytes (CTLs) plays a crucial role in HIV infection [42]. The precursor CTLs recognize viral antigens expressed on the surface of presenting cells. They become active with the help of IL-2, IFN-gamma, and TNF-alpha (produced from CD4+ T cells) and can directly eliminate infected CD4+ lymphocytes via secretion of perforin (a cytolytic protein) and granzymes (serine proteases). The increased ability to secrete perforin is specific for CD8+ T cells from small group HIV-positive individuals who maintain HIV replication in undetectable levels (elite controllers) [43] and who do not progress immunologically towards AIDS in the absence of antiretroviral treatment.

Simultaneously with the host response, the virus starts a mutation process to escape CD8+ recognition by changing epitopes and to correct the present viral variant. At this moment, a balance between host elimination and replication of new HIV variants is established. However,

CD8+ immune response, as well as humoral response, strongly needs CD4+ T helpers and gradually with CD4+ depletion, the CD8+ control fails to maintain the viremia.

The loss of effective antiviral response leads to a constant stimulation and repeated activation of HIV specific CD8+ T cells. This chronic activation soon exhausts the pool of CD8+ lymphocytes together with CD4+ T cell one.

The elevated activation is characteristic not only for CD8+ and CD4+ T cells, but also for B cells, NK cells, and monocytes. In HIV-seropositive patients, even in early stages of infection, high levels of proinflammatory cytokines (TNF-alpha, IL-6 and IL-1β) and chemokines (MIP-1alpha, MIP-1beta and RANTES) are detected [37].

The HIV life cycle is closely related to the extent of immune system activation. Activation of the immune cells enhances the entry of HIV into the cytoplasm because the auxiliary co-receptors are upregulated under immune stimulation [44]. It also increases the level of provirus transcription together with the normal cellular transcription [45]. The exhausted CD8+ T cells diminish secretion of immune-stimulatory cytokines, slow down proliferation and suspend killing of infected cells [46]. HIV infection stimulates upregulation of CD8+ inhibitory receptors (Programmed Death-1 (PD-1), T cell immunoglobulin, and mucin-domain-containing molecule-3 (Tim-3) [47,48]) that downregulate CD8+ immune response and maintain T cell tolerance.

4.4. Humoral immune response against HIV

The humoral immune response against HIV is mediated by specific anti-HIV antibodies produced from B-lymphocytes several weeks to several months after the initial infection. HIV cannot replicate into B-lymphocytes but influences their activation and apoptosis. Unmatured B-lymphocytes differentiate under the action of Th1 cytokines (IL-4, IL-5, IL-6, IL-10, TGF-beta) into plasma cells producing large amounts of binding and virus-neutralizing antibodies. Antibodies target free viral particles in the HIV-positive blood and a small quantity of them can also eliminate infected cells.

HIV specific antibodies recognize viral envelope (envelope proteins gp120 and gp41) and protect host cells from viral entry, but the virus successfully escapes the antibodies' binding via continual mutations. Memory B cells constantly produce new variants of antibodies and soon become exhausted.

4.5. AIDS

The latent phase can last several years (usually up to ten) and terminates finally with the development of AIDS and death. In the final stage, HIV infection completely exhausts the host immune system and especially the CD4+ T cell pool. AIDS is immunologically diagnosed by a CD4+ count less than 200 per μL or/and clinically by the occurrence of opportunistic HIV-related diseases.

5. Immunology of TB/HIV coinfection

5.1. HIV impact on TB infection

TB is the leading opportunistic infection and major cause of death in HIV-seropositive people. There is some evidence that both HIV-negative and HIV-positive persons have the same chance to be infected with TB [49]. In contrast, other studies have found that already existing HIV infection increased the risk of newly acquired TB [50, 51] and relapse of dormant *M. tuberculosis* [52]. However, there is unanimity that HIV exacerbates TB progress and accelerates the fatal end in coinfected individuals.

Existing data outlines two main hypotheses how HIV influences the course of TB infection: 1. HIV manipulates bactericidal activity of macrophages against *M. tuberculosis*; and 2. HIV kills CD4+ T cells within granulomas and facilitates *M. tuberculosis* survival and dissemination.

HIV impairs macrophages in HIV-positive patients turning them more susceptible to *M. tuberculosis* invasion [53]. First, HIV upregulates some of *M. tuberculosis* receptors on macrophages to favor tubercle bacilli entering into the cell [54]. Second, HIV modulates oxidative stress-dependent bactericidal activity in monocytes by diminishing their capacity to produce ROS [55]. As a result of increased levels of IL-10 (an anti-inflammatory interleukin) and decreased TNF-alpha production, infected macrophages escape apoptosis [53, 56]. Thus, more macrophages are directed towards necrosis, a mechanism that increases the *M. tuberculosis* survival and dissemination in the lungs and other extra pulmonary locations. Furthermore, HIV alters the acidification of phagosomes in *M. tuberculosis*-infected macrophages [57], changing the rate of tubercle bacilli elimination.

HIV manifests its presence by gradual depletion of CD4+ T cells, a main feature of HIV infection and clinical sign for progression towards AIDS. The low CD4+ cell count makes the host more susceptible to tubercle bacilli as the immune system cannot establish an efficient cell-mediated immune response. The risk of reactivation of latent TB, acquirement of new TB infection, and/or of dissemination of TB towards extra pulmonary locations increases with the decrease of CD4+ cell count; patients with CD4+ counts >350 cells/μL have unaltered clinical and radiographic presentation as HIV seronegative patients, while patients with CD4+ counts <350 cells/μL have atypical chest X-ray findings and frequent extra pulmonary TB. HIV-positive patients in South Africa with CD4+ counts <200 cells/μL are more susceptible to *M. tuberculosis* infection than HIV-positive individuals with CD4+ counts >500 cells/μL regardless of antiretroviral therapy applied [58].

The insufficient CD4+ T number fails to control granuloma formation and maintenance, therefore leading to higher incidence of extra pulmonary TB and enlarged risk of reactivation of latent infection in HIV-positive patients. Caseous necrotic granulomas—typical for single TB infection—are rare in TB/HIV coinfected patients. Despite the same number of granulomas and acid-fast stained bacilli in TB infected and TB/HIV coinfected persons [59], granulomas from dual-infected individuals are easy disrupted and infection can readily disseminate into multiple organs to form diffuse lesions [60].

However, HIV influence on TB course may only partially depend on CD4+ depletion, as HIV-positive miners in South Africa had an increased risk (2 to 3 times higher) of developing active TB in the first and second year after HIV seroconversion, when the number of CD4+ T-cell was still high [61]. HIV-positive individuals with preserved CD4+ T cell counts (during an antiretroviral treatment) also have an increased risk of developing TB infection. This suggests that additional immunological changes could happen during HIV infection, making the host more susceptible to TB. Such possible mechanism is the observed uniform distribution of CD8+ T cells within the granuloma, in contrast to the peripheral findings in the single TB infection [62]. HIV also specifically diminishes production of IFN-gamma, IL-2, and IL-12 [63], and suppresses proliferation of TB-specific T cells. Several months after HIV seroconversion, the number of *M. tuberculosis* specific CD4+ memory cells decreases significantly [64].

5.2. TB importance in HIV infection

HIV recognizes immune cells expressing CD4+ glycoprotein on their surface: CD4+ T-cells, macrophages, and dendritic cells. All of these cellular types are involved in TB pathogenesis and immune response. HIV also needs activated immune cells for replication and propagation; such cells are abundantly present during *M. tuberculosis* primary or latent infection. In this way, it can be speculated that TB infection areas (granulomas) create the optimal environment for HIV propagation.

HIV-positive patients who developed TB have an increased viral load during the acute phase of TB disease [65, 66]. Lung tissue samples from patients with TB have increased HIV viral load when compared to HIV-positive patients without lung disease or plasma samples from the same TB patients [67]. This suggests that a TB-infected lung has elevated local HIV replication in vivo. In addition, HIV replication is activated in TB-infected alveolar macrophages [68], lymphocytes, and CD14+ macrophages of the pleural space [69].

Infection with *M. tuberculosis* also enhances the level of inflammatory cytokines and chemokines. Their release stimulates HIV replication and increases viral load. Pleural fluids from patients with active TB provoke HIV replication in vitro via production of TNF-alpha, IL-6, and IFN-gamma [70].

Coinfected individuals have increased incidence and death rate of HIV-related opportunistic infections comparing to HIV-positive but TB-negative patients with the same level of immunosuppression (absolute CD4+ count) [71], indicating that *M. tuberculosis* accelerates the clinical course and outcome of HIV infection.

6. Concluding remarks

TB/HIV coinfection represents a leading threat to public health worldwide. Despite the extreme research effort, many aspects of the exceptionally complicated immunology of concurrent TB and HIV infections still need to be elucidated. Diagnosis of HIV/TB coinfection is challenging as both infections have overlapping clinical manifestations, which often lead to late or misdiagnosis. Furthermore, TB and HIV as well the coinfection mostly affect poor and developing regions where competent health care is hardly accessible.

Changes in both innate and adaptive immune response demand well-organized clinical and laboratory studies to understand possible mechanisms by which HIV and TB disrupt in perfect and fatal cooperation the immune system of the host.

Abbreviatons

AAM – Alternatively activated macrophages

AIDS – Acquired immune deficiency syndrome

CAM – Classically activated macrophages

CCL – CC chemokine ligand

CTL – Cytotoxic T-lymphocytes

DC-SIGN – Dendritic cell-specific intercellular adhesion molecule grabbing nonintegrins

HIV – Human immuno deficiency virus

IFN – Interferon

IL – Interleukin

iNOS – Nitric oxide synthetase

MBTC – *Mycobacterium tuberculosis* complex

MHC – Major histocompatibility complex

MIP – Macrophage inflammatory protein

NK – Natural killer cells

NLR – NOD-like receptors

NO – Nitric oxide

NOD – Nucleotide-binding oligomerization domain

PD-1 – Programmed death-1

RANTES – Regulated on activation, normal T cell expressed and secreted

ROS – Reactive oxygen species

TB – Tuberculosis

TGF – Transforming growth factor

Tim-3 – T cell immunoglobulin and mucin-domain-containing molecule

TLRs – Toll-like receptors

TNF – Tumor necrosis factor

WHO – World Health Organization

Author details

Tatina T. Todorova[1*], Gabriela Tsankova[1], Neli Lodozova[1,2] and Tcvetelina Kostadinova[2]

*Address all correspondence to: tatina.todorova@abv.bg

1 Department of Preclinical and Clinical Sciences, Faculty of Pharmacy, Medical University Varna, Bulgaria

2 TRS "Medical laboratory assistant", Medical College, Medical University Varna, Bulgaria

References

[1] WHO I Global tuberculosis report 2014. World Health Organization; [cited 2015 Jan 15]; Available from: http://www.who.int/tb/publications/global_report/en/.

[2] WHO I HIV/AIDS. World Health Organization; [cited 2015 Jan 15]; Available from: http://www.who.int/mediacentre/factsheets/fs360/en/.

[3] Ahmad S. Pathogenesis, immunology, and diagnosis of latent Mycobacterium tuberculosis infection. Clin Dev Immunol [Internet]. 2011 Jan [cited 2015 Jan 15]; 2011:814943. Available from: http://www.pubmedcentral.nih.gov/articlerender.fcgi?artid=3017943&tool=pmcentrez&rendertype=abstract.

[4] Frieden TR, Sterling T, Pablos-Mendez A, Kilburn JO, Cauthen GM, Dooley SW. The emergence of drug-resistant tuberculosis in New York City. N Engl J Med [Internet]. 1993 Feb 25 [cited 2015 Jan 15];328(8):521–6. Available from: http://www.ncbi.nlm.nih.gov/pubmed/8381207.

[5] Olczak A, Grąbczewska E. Tuberculosis in HIV-infected patients in the HAART era. HIV AIDS Rev [Internet]. 2010 Jan [cited 2015 Jan 15];9(2):41–4. Available from: http://www.sciencedirect.com/science/article/pii/S1730127010600689.

[6] Golub JE, Saraceni V, Cavalcante SC, Pacheco AG, Moulton LH, King BS, et al. The impact of antiretroviral therapy and isoniazid preventive therapy on tuberculosis incidence in HIV-infected patients in Rio de Janeiro, Brazil. AIDS [Internet]. 2007 Jul 11 [cited 2015 Jan 15];21(11):1441–8. Available from: http://www.pubmedcentral.nih.gov/articlerender.fcgi?artid=3063947&tool=pmcentrez&rendertype=abstract.

[7] World Health Organization. Guidelines for intensified tuberculosis case-finding and isoniazid preventive therapy for people living with HIV in resource-constrained settings. World Health [Internet]. 2011;01:142. Available from: http://whqlibdoc.who.int/publications/2011/9789241500708_eng.pdf.

[8] Marais BJ, Rabie H, Cotton MF. TB and HIV in children - advances in prevention and management. Paediatr Respir Rev [Internet]. 2011 Mar [cited 2015 Jan 15];12(1):39–45. Available from: http://www.sciencedirect.com/science/article/pii/S1526054210000709.

[9] Schwander S, Dheda K. Human lung immunity against Mycobacterium tuberculosis: Insights into pathogenesis and protection. Am J Respir Crit Care Med [Internet]. 2011 Mar 15 [cited 2015 Jan 2];183(6):696–707. Available from: http://www.pubmedcentral.nih.gov/articlerender.fcgi?artid=3081283&tool=pmcentrez&rendertype=abstract.

[10] Andersson M, Lutay N, Hallgren O, Westergren-Thorsson G, Svensson M, Godaly G. Mycobacterium bovis bacilli Calmette-Guerin regulates leukocyte recruitment by modulating alveolar inflammatory responses. Innate Immun [Internet]. 2012 Jun 12 [cited 2015 Jan 15];18(3):531–40. Available from: http://ini.sagepub.com/content/early/2012/01/11/1753425911426591.

[11] Jo E-K, Yang C-S, Choi CH, Harding C V. Intracellular signalling cascades regulating innate immune responses to Mycobacteria: Branching out from Toll-like receptors. Cell Microbiol [Internet]. 2007 May [cited 2015 Jan 15];9(5):1087–98. Available from: http://www.ncbi.nlm.nih.gov/pubmed/17359235.

[12] Akira S, Uematsu S, Takeuchi O. Pathogen recognition and innate immunity. Cell [Internet]. 2006 Feb 24 [cited 2014 Jul 9];124(4):783–801. Available from: http://www.ncbi.nlm.nih.gov/pubmed/16497588.

[13] Algood HMS, Chan J, Flynn JL. Chemokines and tuberculosis. Cytokine Growth Factor Rev [Internet]. Elsevier; 2003 Dec 12 [cited 2015 Jan 15];14(6):467–77. Available from: http://www.cgfr.co.uk/article/S1359610103000546/fulltext.

[14] Saunders BM, Cooper AM. Restraining mycobacteria: Role of granulomas in mycobacterial infections. Immunol Cell Biol [Internet]. 2000 Aug [cited 2015 Jan 15];78(4): 334–41. Available from: http://www.ncbi.nlm.nih.gov/pubmed/10947857.

[15] Wolf AJ, Linas B, Trevejo-Nunez GJ, Kincaid E, Tamura T, Takatsu K, et al. Mycobacterium tuberculosis Infects Dendritic Cells with High Frequency and Impairs Their Function In Vivo. J Immunol [Internet]. American Association of Immunologists; 2007 Aug 3 [cited 2014 Nov 28];179(4):2509–19. Available from: http://www.jimmunol.org/content/179/4/2509.full.

[16] Giacomini E, Iona E, Ferroni L, Miettinen M, Fattorini L, Orefici G, et al. Infection of Human Macrophages and Dendritic Cells with Mycobacterium tuberculosis Induces a Differential Cytokine Gene Expression That Modulates T Cell Response. J Immunol [Internet]. American Association of Immunologists; 2001 Jun 15 [cited 2015 Jan 15]; 166(12):7033–41. Available from: http://www.jimmunol.org/content/166/12/7033.full.

[17] Tailleux L, Neyrolles O, Honore-Bouakline S, Perret E, Sanchez F, Abastado J-P, et al. Constrained Intracellular Survival of Mycobacterium tuberculosis in Human Dendritic Cells. J Immunol [Internet]. American Association of Immunologists; 2003 Feb 15 [cited 2015 Jan 15];170(4):1939–48. Available from: http://www.jimmunol.org/content/170/4/1939.full.

[18] Co DO, Hogan LH, Kim S-I, Sandor M. Mycobacterial granulomas: keys to a long-lasting host-pathogen relationship. Clin Immunol [Internet]. 2004 Nov [cited 2015 Jan 15];113(2):130–6. Available from: http://www.ncbi.nlm.nih.gov/pubmed/15451467.

[19] Peyron P, Vaubourgeix J, Poquet Y, Levillain F, Botanch C, Bardou F, et al. Foamy macrophages from tuberculous patients' granulomas constitute a nutrient-rich reservoir for M. tuberculosis persistence. PLoS Pathog [Internet]. 2008 Nov 11 [cited 2014 Dec 27];4(11):e1000204. Available from: http://journals.plos.org/plospathogens/article?id=10.1371/journal.ppat.1000204.

[20] Fulton SA, Reba SM, Martin TD, Boom WH. Neutrophil-Mediated Mycobacteriocidal Immunity in the Lung during Mycobacterium bovis BCG Infection in C57BL/6 Mice. Infect Immun [Internet]. 2002 Sep 1 [cited 2015 Jan 15];70(9):5322–7. Available from: http://iai.asm.org/content/70/9/5322.full.

[21] Lowe DM, Redford PS, Wilkinson RJ, O'Garra A, Martineau AR. Neutrophils in tuberculosis: friend or foe? Trends Immunol [Internet]. 2012 Jan [cited 2015 Jan 9];33(1):14–25. Available from: http://www.ncbi.nlm.nih.gov/pubmed/22094048.

[22] Sawant K V, McMurray DN. Guinea pig neutrophils infected with Mycobacterium tuberculosis produce cytokines which activate alveolar macrophages in noncontact cultures. Infect Immun [Internet]. 2007 Apr [cited 2015 Jan 15];75(4):1870–7. Available from: http://www.pubmedcentral.nih.gov/articlerender.fcgi?artid=1865707&tool=pmcentrez&rendertype=abstract.

[23] Segovia-Juarez JL, Ganguli S, Kirschner D. Identifying control mechanisms of granuloma formation during M. tuberculosis infection using an agent-based model. J Theor Biol [Internet]. 2004 Dec 7 [cited 2014 Dec 29];231(3):357–76. Available from: http://www.ncbi.nlm.nih.gov/pubmed/15501468.

[24] Schluger NW, Rom WN. The host immune response to tuberculosis. Am J Respir Crit Care Med [Internet]. 1998 Mar [cited 2015 Jan 7];157(3 Pt 1):679–91. Available from: http://www.ncbi.nlm.nih.gov/pubmed/9517576.

[25] Oddo M, Renno T, Attinger A, Bakker T, MacDonald HR, Meylan PR. Fas ligand-induced apoptosis of infected human macrophages reduces the viability of intracellular Mycobacterium tuberculosis. J Immunol [Internet]. 1998 Jun 1 [cited 2015 Jan 15];160(11):5448–54. Available from: http://www.ncbi.nlm.nih.gov/pubmed/9605147.

[26] Serbina N V., Lazarevic V, Flynn JL. CD4+ T Cells Are Required for the Development of Cytotoxic CD8+ T Cells During Mycobacterium tuberculosis Infection. J Immunol [Internet]. American Association of Immunologists; 2001 Dec 15 [cited 2015 Jan 7];

167(12):6991–7000. Available from: http://www.jimmunol.org/content/167/12/6991.full.

[27] Cho S, Mehra V, Thoma-Uszynski S, Stenger S, Serbina N, Mazzaccaro RJ, et al. Antimicrobial activity of MHC class I-restricted CD8+ T cells in human tuberculosis. Proc Natl Acad Sci U S A [Internet]. 2000 Oct 24 [cited 2015 Jan 15];97(22):12210–5. Available from: http://www.pubmedcentral.nih.gov/articlerender.fcgi?artid=17320&tool=pmcentrez&rendertype=abstract.

[28] Stenger S, Hanson DA, Teitelbaum R, Dewan P, Niazi KR, Froelich CJ, et al. An antimicrobial activity of cytolytic T cells mediated by granulysin. Science [Internet]. 1998 Oct 2 [cited 2015 Jan 15];282(5386):121–5. Available from: http://www.ncbi.nlm.nih.gov/pubmed/9756476.

[29] Brandes M, Willimann K, Bioley G, Lévy N, Eberl M, Luo M, et al. Cross-presenting human gammadelta T cells induce robust CD8+ alphabeta T cell responses. Proc Natl Acad Sci U S A [Internet]. 2009 Feb 17 [cited 2015 Jan 15];106(7):2307–12. Available from: http://www.pnas.org/content/106/7/2307.full.

[30] Silva Miranda M, Breiman A, Allain S, Deknuydt F, Altare F. The tuberculous granuloma: An unsuccessful host defence mechanism providing a safety shelter for the bacteria? Clin Dev Immunol [Internet]. 2012 Jan [cited 2015 Jan 10];2012:139127. Available from: http://www.pubmedcentral.nih.gov/articlerender.fcgi?artid=3395138&tool=pmcentrez&rendertype=abstract.

[31] Benoit M, Desnues B, Mege J-L. Macrophage polarization in bacterial infections. J Immunol [Internet]. 2008 Sep 15 [cited 2015 Jan 15];181(6):3733–9. Available from: http://www.ncbi.nlm.nih.gov/pubmed/18768823.

[32] Behar SM, Martin CJ, Booty MG, Nishimura T, Zhao X, Gan H-X, et al. Apoptosis is an innate defense function of macrophages against Mycobacterium tuberculosis. Mucosal Immunol [Internet]. 2011 May [cited 2014 Dec 15];4(3):279–87. Available from: http://www.pubmedcentral.nih.gov/articlerender.fcgi?artid=3155700&tool=pmcentrez&rendertype=abstract.

[33] De Vallière S, Abate G, Blazevic A, Heuertz RM, Hoft DF. Enhancement of innate and cell-mediated immunity by antimycobacterial antibodies. Infect Immun [Internet]. 2005 Oct [cited 2015 Jan 15];73(10):6711–20. Available from: http://www.pubmedcentral.nih.gov/articlerender.fcgi?artid=1230956&tool=pmcentrez&rendertype=abstract.

[34] Abebe F, Bjune G. The protective role of antibody responses during Mycobacterium tuberculosis infection. Clin Exp Immunol [Internet]. 2009 Aug [cited 2015 Jan 15];157(2):235–43. Available from: http://www.pubmedcentral.nih.gov/articlerender.fcgi?artid=2730849&tool=pmcentrez&rendertype=abstract.

[35] Maglione PJ, Chan J. How B cells shape the immune response against Mycobacterium tuberculosis. Eur J Immunol [Internet]. 2009 Mar [cited 2014 Dec 30];39(3):676–86.

Available from: http://www.pubmedcentral.nih.gov/articlerender.fcgi?artid=2760469&tool=pmcentrez&rendertype=abstract.

[36] Diedrich CR, Flynn JL. HIV-1/mycobacterium tuberculosis coinfection immunology: How does HIV-1 exacerbate tuberculosis? Infect Immun [Internet]. 2011 Apr [cited 2014 Sep 5];79(4):1407–17. Available from: http://www.pubmedcentral.nih.gov/articlerender.fcgi?artid=3067569&tool=pmcentrez&rendertype=abstract.

[37] Appay V, Sauce D. Immune activation and inflammation in HIV-1 infection: Causes and consequences. J Pathol [Internet]. 2008 Jan [cited 2015 Jan 15];214(2):231–41. Available from: http://www.ncbi.nlm.nih.gov/pubmed/18161758.

[38] Poonia B, Wang X, Veazey RS. Distribution of simian immunodeficiency virus target cells in vaginal tissues of normal rhesus macaques: implications for virus transmission. J Reprod Immunol [Internet]. 2006 Dec [cited 2015 Jan 15];72(1-2):74–84. Available from: http://www.ncbi.nlm.nih.gov/pubmed/16956666.

[39] Hussain LA, Lehner T. Comparative investigation of Langerhans' cells and potential receptors for HIV in oral, genitourinary and rectal epithelia. Immunology [Internet]. 1995 Jul [cited 2015 Jan 15];85(3):475–84. Available from: http://www.pubmedcentral.nih.gov/articlerender.fcgi?artid=1383923&tool=pmcentrez&rendertype=abstract.

[40] Roederer M, Dubs JG, Anderson MT, Raju PA, Herzenberg LA. CD8 naive T cell counts decrease progressively in HIV-infected adults. J Clin Invest [Internet]. 1995 May [cited 2015 Jan 15];95(5):2061–6. Available from: http://www.pubmedcentral.nih.gov/articlerender.fcgi?artid=295794&tool=pmcentrez&rendertype=abstract.

[41] Douek DC, Betts MR, Hill BJ, Little SJ, Lempicki R, Metcalf JA, et al. Evidence for Increased T Cell Turnover and Decreased Thymic Output in HIV Infection. J Immunol [Internet]. American Association of Immunologists; 2001 Dec 1 [cited 2015 Jan 15]; 167(11):6663–8. Available from: http://www.jimmunol.org/content/167/11/6663.full.

[42] Schmitz JE, Kuroda MJ, Santra S, Sasseville VG, Simon MA, Lifton MA, et al. Control of viremia in simian immunodeficiency virus infection by CD8+ lymphocytes. Science [Internet]. 1999 Feb 5 [cited 2015 Jan 15];283(5403):857–60. Available from: http://www.ncbi.nlm.nih.gov/pubmed/9933172.

[43] Hersperger AR, Pereyra F, Nason M, Demers K, Sheth P, Shin LY, et al. Perforin expression directly ex vivo by HIV-specific CD8 T-cells is a correlate of HIV elite control. PLoS Pathog [Internet]. 2010 May 27 [cited 2015 Jan 15];6(5):e1000917. Available from: http://journals.plos.org/plospathogens/article?id=10.1371/journal.ppat.1000917.

[44] Levy JA. Wiley: HIV and the Pathogenesis of AIDS, 3rd Edition - J. A. Levy [Internet]. [cited 2015 Jan 15]. Available from: http://eu.wiley.com/WileyCDA/WileyTitle/productCd-1555813933.html.

[45] Cron RQ, Bartz SR, Clausell A, Bort SJ, Klebanoff SJ, Lewis DB. NFAT1 enhances HIV-1 gene expression in primary human CD4 T cells. Clin Immunol [Internet]. 2000

Mar [cited 2015 Jan 15];94(3):179–91. Available from: http://www.ncbi.nlm.nih.gov/pubmed/10692237.

[46] Wherry EJ, Ahmed R. Memory CD8 T-cell differentiation during viral infection. J Virol [Internet]. 2004 Jun [cited 2015 Jan 15];78(11):5535–45. Available from: http://www.pubmedcentral.nih.gov/articlerender.fcgi?artid=415833&tool=pmcentrez&rendertype=abstract.

[47] Jin H-T, Anderson AC, Tan WG, West EE, Ha S-J, Araki K, et al. Cooperation of Tim-3 and PD-1 in CD8 T-cell exhaustion during chronic viral infection. Proc Natl Acad Sci U S A [Internet]. 2010 Aug 17 [cited 2015 Jan 9];107(33):14733–8. Available from: http://www.pubmedcentral.nih.gov/articlerender.fcgi?artid=2930455&tool=pmcentrez&rendertype=abstract.

[48] Tandon R, Giret MTM, Sengupta D, York VA, Wiznia AA, Rosenberg MG, et al. Age-related expansion of Tim-3 expressing T cells in vertically HIV-1 infected children. PLoS One [Internet]. 2012 Jan [cited 2015 Jan 15];7(9):e45733. Available from: http://www.pubmedcentral.nih.gov/articlerender.fcgi?artid=3454343&tool=pmcentrez&rendertype=abstract.

[49] Whalen CC, Zalwango S, Chiunda A, Malone L, Eisenach K, Joloba M, et al. Secondary attack rate of tuberculosis in urban households in Kampala, Uganda. PLoS One [Internet]. 2011 Jan 14 [cited 2015 Jan 15];6(2):e16137. Available from: http://journals.plos.org/plosone/article?id=10.1371/journal.pone.0016137.

[50] Crampin AC, Mwaungulu JN, Mwaungulu FD, Mwafulirwa DT, Munthali K, Floyd S, et al. Recurrent TB: relapse or reinfection? The effect of HIV in a general population cohort in Malawi. AIDS [Internet]. 2010 Jan 28 [cited 2015 Jan 7];24(3):417–26. Available from: http://www.pubmedcentral.nih.gov/articlerender.fcgi?artid=2917772&tool=pmcentrez&rendertype=abstract.

[51] Sonnenberg P, Murray J, Glynn JR, Shearer S, Kambashi B, Godfrey-Faussett P. HIV-1 and recurrence, relapse, and reinfection of tuberculosis after cure: a cohort study in South African mineworkers. Lancet [Internet]. Elsevier; 2001 Nov 17 [cited 2014 Dec 28];358(9294):1687–93. Available from: http://www.thelancet.com/article/S0140673601067125/fulltext.

[52] Selwyn PA, Hartel D, Lewis VA, Schoenbaum EE, Vermund SH, Klein RS, et al. A prospective study of the risk of tuberculosis among intravenous drug users with human immunodeficiency virus infection. N Engl J Med [Internet]. 1989 Mar 2 [cited 2015 Jan 15];320(9):545–50. Available from: http://www.ncbi.nlm.nih.gov/pubmed/2915665.

[53] Patel NR, Swan K, Li X, Tachado SD, Koziel H. Impaired M. tuberculosis-mediated apoptosis in alveolar macrophages from HIV+ persons: Potential role of IL-10 and BCL-3. J Leukoc Biol [Internet]. 2009 Jul [cited 2015 Jan 15];86(1):53–60. Available

from: http://www.pubmedcentral.nih.gov/articlerender.fcgi?artid=2704623&tool=pmcentrez&rendertype=abstract.

[54] Rosas-Taraco AG, Arce-Mendoza AY, Caballero-Olín G, Salinas-Carmona MC. Mycobacterium tuberculosis upregulates coreceptors CCR5 and CXCR4 while HIV modulates CD14 favoring concurrent infection. AIDS Res Hum Retroviruses [Internet]. 2006 Jan [cited 2015 Jan 15];22(1):45–51. Available from: http://www.ncbi.nlm.nih.gov/pubmed/16438645.

[55] Spear GT, Kessler HA, Rothberg L, Phair J, Landay AL. Decreased oxidative burst activity of monocytes from asymptomatic HIV-infected individuals. Clin Immunol Immunopathol [Internet]. 1990 Feb [cited 2015 Jan 15];54(2):184–91. Available from: http://www.ncbi.nlm.nih.gov/pubmed/1688521.

[56] Patel NR, Zhu J, Tachado SD, Zhang J, Wan Z, Saukkonen J, et al. HIV impairs TNF-alpha mediated macrophage apoptotic response to Mycobacterium tuberculosis. J Immunol [Internet]. 2007 Nov 15 [cited 2014 Dec 23];179(10):6973–80. Available from: http://www.ncbi.nlm.nih.gov/pubmed/17982088.

[57] Mwandumba HC, Russell DG, Nyirenda MH, Anderson J, White SA, Molyneux ME, et al. Mycobacterium tuberculosis resides in nonacidified vacuoles in endocytically competent alveolar macrophages from patients with tuberculosis and HIV infection. J Immunol [Internet]. 2004 Apr 1 [cited 2015 Jan 15];172(7):4592–8. Available from: http://www.ncbi.nlm.nih.gov/pubmed/15034077.

[58] Lawn SD, Myer L, Edwards D, Bekker L-G, Wood R. Short-term and long-term risk of tuberculosis associated with CD4 cell recovery during antiretroviral therapy in South Africa. AIDS [Internet]. 2009 Aug 24 [cited 2015 Jan 15];23(13):1717–25. Available from: http://www.pubmedcentral.nih.gov/articlerender.fcgi?artid=3801095&tool=pmcentrez&rendertype=abstract.

[59] Heyderman RS, Makunike R, Muza T, Odwee M, Kadzirange G, Manyemba J, et al. Pleural tuberculosis in Harare, Zimbabwe: The relationship between human immunodeficiency virus, CD4 lymphocyte count, granuloma formation and disseminated disease. Trop Med Int Health [Internet]. 1998 Jan [cited 2015 Jan 15];3(1):14–20. Available from: http://www.ncbi.nlm.nih.gov/pubmed/9484963.

[60] De Noronha ALL, Báfica A, Nogueira L, Barral A, Barral-Netto M. Lung granulomas from Mycobacterium tuberculosis/HIV-1 co-infected patients display decreased in situ TNF production. Pathol Res Pract [Internet]. 2008 Jan [cited 2015 Jan 15];204(3): 155–61. Available from: http://www.ncbi.nlm.nih.gov/pubmed/18096327.

[61] Sonnenberg P, Glynn JR, Fielding K, Murray J, Godfrey-Faussett P, Shearer S. How soon after infection with HIV does the risk of tuberculosis start to increase? A retrospective cohort study in South African gold miners. J Infect Dis [Internet]. 2005 Jan 15 [cited 2015 Jan 15];191(2):150–8. Available from: http://www.ncbi.nlm.nih.gov/pubmed/15609223.

[62] Shen JY, Barnes PF, Rea TH, Meyer PR. Immunohistology of tuberculous adenitis in symptomatic HIV infection. Clin Exp Immunol [Internet]. 1988 May [cited 2015 Jan 15];72(2):186–9. Available from: http://www.pubmedcentral.nih.gov/articlerender.fcgi?artid=1541541&tool=pmcentrez&rendertype=abstract.

[63] Zhang M, Gong J, Iyer D V, Jones BE, Modlin RL, Barnes PF. T cell cytokine responses in persons with tuberculosis and human immunodeficiency virus infection. J Clin Invest [Internet]. 1994 Dec [cited 2015 Jan 15];94(6):2435–42. Available from: http://www.pubmedcentral.nih.gov/articlerender.fcgi?artid=330075&tool=pmcentrez&rendertype=abstract.

[64] Geldmacher C, Schuetz A, Ngwenyama N, Casazza JP, Sanga E, Saathoff E, et al. Early depletion of Mycobacterium tuberculosis-specific T helper 1 cell responses after HIV-1 infection. J Infect Dis [Internet]. 2008 Dec 1 [cited 2015 Jan 15];198(11):1590–8. Available from: http://www.pubmedcentral.nih.gov/articlerender.fcgi?artid=2650495&tool=pmcentrez&rendertype=abstract.

[65] Toossi Z, Mayanja-Kizza H, Hirsch CS, Edmonds KL, Spahlinger T, Hom DL, et al. Impact of tuberculosis (TB) on HIV-1 activity in dually infected patients. Clin Exp Immunol [Internet]. 2001 Feb [cited 2015 Jan 15];123(2):233–8. Available from: http://doi.wiley.com/10.1046/j.1365-2249.2001.01401.x.

[66] Goletti D, Weissman D, Jackson RW, Graham NM, Vlahov D, Klein RS, et al. Effect of Mycobacterium tuberculosis on HIV replication. Role of immune activation. J Immunol [Internet]. 1996 Aug 1 [cited 2015 Jan 15];157(3):1271–8. Available from: http://www.ncbi.nlm.nih.gov/pubmed/8757635.

[67] Nakata K, Rom WN, Honda Y, Condos R, Kanegasaki S, Cao Y, et al. Mycobacterium tuberculosis enhances human immunodeficiency virus-1 replication in the lung. Am J Respir Crit Care Med [Internet]. 1997 Mar [cited 2015 Jan 15];155(3):996–1003. Available from: http://www.ncbi.nlm.nih.gov/pubmed/9117038.

[68] Hoshino Y, Hoshino S, Gold JA, Raju B, Prabhakar S, Pine R, et al. Mechanisms of polymorphonuclear neutrophil-mediated induction of HIV-1 replication in macrophages during pulmonary tuberculosis. J Infect Dis [Internet]. 2007 May 1 [cited 2015 Jan 15];195(9):1303–10. Available from: http://www.ncbi.nlm.nih.gov/pubmed/17396999.

[69] Lawn SD, Pisell TL, Hirsch CS, Wu M, Butera ST, Toossi Z. Anatomically compartmentalized human immunodeficiency virus replication in HLA-DR+ cells and CD14+ macrophages at the site of pleural tuberculosis coinfection. J Infect Dis [Internet]. 2001 Nov 1 [cited 2015 Jan 15];184(9):1127–33. Available from: http://jid.oxfordjournals.org/content/184/9/1127.long.

[70] Garrait V, Cadranel J, Esvant H, Herry I, Morinet P, Mayaud C, et al. Tuberculosis generates a microenvironment enhancing the productive infection of local lympho-

cytes by HIV. J Immunol [Internet]. 1997 Sep 15 [cited 2015 Jan 15];159(6):2824–30. Available from: http://www.ncbi.nlm.nih.gov/pubmed/9300705.

[71] Whalen C, Horsburgh CR, Hom D, Lahart C, Simberkoff M, Ellner J. Accelerated course of human immunodeficiency virus infection after tuberculosis. Am J Respir Crit Care Med [Internet]. 1995 Jan [cited 2015 Jan 15];151(1):129–35. Available from: http://www.ncbi.nlm.nih.gov/pubmed/7812542.

Chapter 5

Principles of Cancer Immunobiology and Immunotherapy of Solid Tumors

Assia Konsoulova

Additional information is available at the end of the chapter

http://dx.doi.org/10.5772/61211

Abstract

The immune system and cancer coexist in close relationship which is an indispensable part of the processes of tumorigenesis, tumor growth, and metastatic spread. The elucidation and understanding of this continuous process could provide opportunities to develop strategies to impact the prognosis, and eventually to improve the cancer treatment process. Such strategies have been already implicated and proven efficient in the treatment of several tumor localizations such as malignant melanoma, lung and renal cancer. The present publication reviews the principles of cancer-related immune response, types and mechanisms of immune response and suppression, immunotherapy of solid tumors. We also discuss the pathways and the signaling molecules, participating in those immune response/suppression processes, turning them into potential targets and their actual and potential future role in the management of solid tumors. We focus on potential role and rationale for combination of immunotherapeutic and chemotherapeutic/targeted agents and radiotherapy in one treatment strategy.

Keywords: immune response, immune suppression, checkpoint inhibitors, immunotherapy, solid tumors

1. Introduction

The relationship between the immune system and cancer has recently become a "modern topic" of interest in cancer research even though it was back in the early 1800s, when Virchow first described the presence of inflammatory cells in pathohistological tumor samples. Subsequently, Coley demonstrated that the use of bacterial products induced certain regression in inoperable tumors [1]. It has been known for decades that the immune system plays an important role in the processes of inflammation, chronic inflammation, and cancer. Thus, scientific researchers continued the struggle to understand the role of Virchow's findings, aiming to link those processes. The elucidation of such relation could give an insight into the processes of tumorigenesis, tumor growth, and metastatic spread; it could potentially provide subsequent opportunities to develop strategies to impact the diagnosis, prognosis, and eventually to improve the cancer treatment process. The synallagmatic reciprocal talk between the host immune system and the tumor has been intensively studied. The processes of the host immune control over the tumor, immunoediting by the tumor, the immune escape, and the development of immune tolerance and suppression are described in this chapter. Our aim is also 1) to highlight the principles of cancer-related immune mechanisms, immunotherapy, and their role in the process of treatment of solid tumors; - and 2) to discuss the options to combine immunotherapeutic and chemotherapeutic agents trying to overcome the mechanisms of immune or inflammatory suppression and potentially improve cancer treatment strategies.

The initial immune-related therapies were aiming to activate the immune system and were represented by non-specific immunotherapies that didn't aim towards a specific target in the cancer cell (cytokines, interleukins, interferons, etc.). Subsequent efforts tried to identify antigens of the cancer cell and to design monoclonal antibodies (MAB), targeting those antigens. However, it has become clear that these therapies are failing because of the ability of cancers to induce immune tolerance, evasion, and suppression of the immune system, which created a new direction of research - to discover the pathways and the signaling molecules, participating in those immune suppression processes, thus turning them into potential targets as anticancer treatments.

2. Basic principles of immune response

There has been major growth in the understanding of the immune role and its relationship to cancer progression and therapy. The immune system comprises of a multitude of interconnected cells and tissues, distributed in the body. It basically consists of three general categories of blood cells: 1) lymphocytes (T, B cells and natural killer (NK) cells); 2) myeloid cells (macrophages, dendritic cells, and antigen presenting cells); and 3) granulocytes (neutrophils, basophils, and eosinophils). Simplified, the immune system protects the organism from harmful foreign agents (antigens) by producing specific proteins (antibodies). Those antibodies circulate until they find and attach to the targeted antigen, thus triggering immune response and destruction of the antigen-containing cells.

2.1. Principles of immune response in solid tumors

The anti-cancer immune response could be largely divided into two types: innate and adaptive immune response. The innate immunity includes the granulocytes, macrophages, dendritic cells, mast cells, and NK cells serving as a first-line protective mechanism, recognizing stressed mutating cells of the organism, and triggering effector mechanism, aiming their eradication. Subsequently, the adaptive immune response is triggered - it consists of specific immune activation of B cells, CD 4- and CD 8-expressing T-lymphocytes.

2.1.1. Innate antitumor response

Normal cells of the organism could become subject of malignant genetic and epigenetic transformation and thus acquire additional characteristics, permitting their uncontrolled proliferation, survival, and dissemination. Such genetic injuries stimulate the innate immune system, which normally serves as a front-line surveillance mechanism, reacting immediately. The NK cells distinguish normal from tumor cells by a complex process of expression of different inhibitory and stimulatory molecules. Specific MHC inhibitory receptors have been described, shedding light over the molecular basis of the activation of the NK cell during the process of natural cytotoxicity of the innate antitumor response. Different receptors frequently referred to as natural cytotoxicity receptors (NCR) are expressed at the surface of the NK cell; they comprise of molecules such as NKp46, NKp30, NKp44, and NKG2D, which bind to their ligands of the MHC class I [2]. NKG2D appears to play either a complementary or a synergistic role with NCRs. The expression of those ligands is induced on the surface of the stressed transformed tumor cells [3,4]. The binding of the MHC-I related ligands to the NKG2D triggers activation of NK cells, NKT and $\gamma\delta$ T cells, and CD 8 T cells, which inhibit tumor cytotoxicity and IFN-γ production. Extracellular release of cytoplasmic stress molecules, such as HSP-70, HMGB1, and uric acid, activates macrophages and dendritic cells, resulting in IL-12 production and transition to the adaptive immunity [5].

2.1.2. Adaptive antitumor responses

The adaptive immune response could be described as the "second-line" response. As a highly specific response to a specific pathogen, it starts relatively later after the initial rapid innate reaction. It is triggered by the dendritic cells, which capture, process, and present tumor antigens to the class I and II MHC, thus stimulating the antigen-specific T- and B-lymphocytes (cellular response) and the specific production of antibodies (humoral component).

Macrophages, dendritic cells, and antigen-presenting cells (APCs) recognize foreign cells and participate in the immune response as they are one of the first responders, approaching a potential harmful antigen. They internalize those extracellular antigens via phagocytosis or receptor-mediated endocytosis; they process and fragment the proteins into peptide sequences that are subsequently presented back at the extracellular membrane surface of the APCs within the context of the Major Histocompatibility Complex (MHC) class II (Figure 1). They also produce large amounts of different cytokines, thus promoting immune response. In cases of inadequately directed immune reaction towards self-antigens, the dendritic cells particularly prevent further autoimmune reaction [6]. In order to prevent self-destruction, the immune system uses endogenous crosstalks—"immune checkpoints"—that normally terminate immune responses after antigens activation of T-cells.

Once the immune response is triggered, the foreign antigen is presented to other cells of the immune complex. More specialized cells, the lymphocytes, encounter the foreign antigen and respond by proliferation and differentiation into different subpopulations. B-lymphocytes arise and differentiate in the bone marrow and enter into the blood stream as functional mature cells. They express a receptor for the antigen on their surface and following encounter with that specific antigen, they start to divide, differentiate into plasma cells, and produce soluble

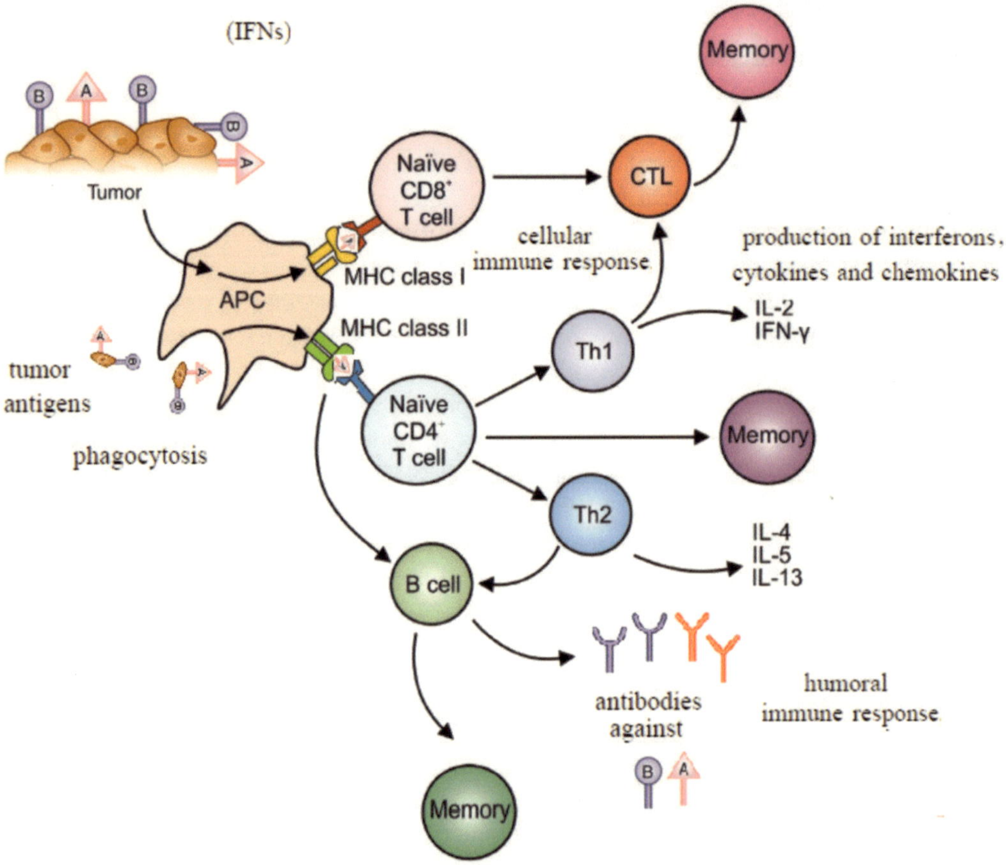

Figure 1. Induction of rapid innate and retarded adaptive immune response (humoral and cellular T- and B-cell response). Tumor cell proteins are degraded into smaller peptides in endosomes/lysosomes in the APCs and are subsequently expressed on the cell surface in MHC class II peptide complexes, which can be recognized by CD4+ T helper lymphocyte cells. T helpers assist B cells to proliferate and mature into antibody-producing plasma cells. Via this route of antigen acquisition, DCs can also present epitopes to CD8+ T cells. This is also known as cross-presentation.

immunoglobulin molecules—antibodies in the circulation. T cells arise in the bone marrow and migrate to the thymus (named thereafter) where they undergo a process of maturation. Immunocompetent T cells leave the thymus and enter into the circulation. There are different T cells classified by their function and phenotype. The largest part of T cells expresses CD 4 glycoprotein and are called T helpers. They enhance the immune process by secreting cytokines and direct cell-to-cell contact [7]. Other numerous specific functional T-lymphocytes are called cytotoxic (CTLs). They express CD8 glycoprotein and are capable of direct killing of the antigen-containing cells (virally infected or cancerous). Upon encounter of their target, they kill it by induction of apoptosis in the infected or cancerous cell. A part of the lymphocytes remain as sensitized long-living memory cells, recognizing only a single antigen, posed to respond if it is encountered again. The regulatory T cells (T regs) are a small population of T cells and express CD 25 glycoprotein, which participate in the process of self-antigen recognition, preventing autoimmune reactions [8, 9]. If the immune system functions correctly, its work remains unnoticed, efficiently protecting the individual from a variety of foreign pathogens. In cases of dysfunction, however, severe consequences appear, presented either as immunodeficiency or autoimmunity.

3. Principles of cancer immunobiology: Immunoediting, surveillance, and immune escape

The importance of intact immune surveillance in controlling the outgrowth of neoplastic transformation has been known for decades [10]. With the discovery of the cellular oncogenes, it became evident that human cancers arise from normal cells and harbor various genetic and epigenetic alterations, generating potentially recognizable by the immune system cancer neoantigens [11]. Being of host origin, cancer cells share features of the host. The plastic nature of tumors makes them adaptive in rebounding from clinical regimens of radiotherapy/ chemotherapy that are traditionally used. The tumor progression can be described as a continuum of multiple clonal expansions, each of which triggered by the fortunate acquisition of an enabling mutant genotype. Even when the vast majority of cancer cells are killed by a cytotoxic chemotherapy drug, a small number of residual cells are primarily or become secondarily resistant to that agent. They can be sufficient enough to seed the subsequent tumor regrowth that is resistant to the previously used chemotherapy agent. This leads to the concept of selection of tumor cells and evolving resistance that becomes a key disease progression feature; development and progression of cancer is driven by the selection of cells that survive conditions that are normally lethal. Resistance to any normally lethal condition (radiotherapy, chemotherapy, etc.) can be selected by the cancer cell population evolution because of the genetic plasticity, which is an important feature of the cancer cell [12].

The tumor development is a multi-step process, requiring the acquisition of several biological features: 1) sustained proliferation signaling; 2) evasion of growth suppression; 3) apoptosis escape; 4) uncontrolled growth and reproduction; 5) angiogenesis induction; and 6) invasion and metastasizing potential. These hallmarks of the tumor cells ensure their survival, proliferation, and dissemination [13]. There are other characteristics that facilitate the acquisition of these hallmarks by the cancer cells, such as the tumor-associated stromal microenvironment and inflammation, genomic instability, and mutations, mediating the process of tumorigenesis [14]. There are two more features that are functionally important for the development of cancer hallmarks. The first feature involves major reprogramming and deregulation of cellular energy metabolism in order to continuously ensure cell growth and proliferation. The second feature involves active tumor escape of the immune system destruction and elimination. This capability highlights the dichotomous role of the immune system that both suppresses and enhances cancer initiation, promotion, and progression [15-17]. Both of these features may well prove to facilitate the initiation and progression of many forms of malignant human solid tumors [14].

There is a theory suggesting that cells and tissues are constantly monitored by an ever-alert immune system, and that such immune surveillance is responsible for recognizing and eliminating the vast majority of incipient cancer cells and thus nascent tumors. According to this logic, solid tumors that do appear have somehow managed to avoid detection by the immune system or have been able to limit the extent of immunological killing, thereby escaping eradication. This is a process called immunoediting—a tumor mechanism, exerting an extrinsic suppression; it occurs only after a malignant cancerous transformation has already occurred and the intrinsic tumor suppressor mechanisms have already failed. The cancer immunoediting roughly consists of three sequential phases: elimination, equilibrium, and escape. In the first phase, the body immune system successfully detects cancer cells and eliminates them efficiently [18,19]. In the equilibrium phase the immune system obstructs tumor growth, but is unable to completely eradicate the tumor. This step is thought to be continuous in time and it could either progress to the last escape phase or reverse backwards, leading to complete tumor eradication by the immune system. If this second phase continues for a longer period of time, the immune system is incapable of tumor eradication and continuously interacts with the tumor, thus sculpturing or editing the tumor genetics [20-22]. In the last phase, the tumor growth is no longer controlled and blocked by the immune system and the tumor spreads and produces clinically apparent diseases [23].

4. Targets and types of immunotherapy in solid tumors

Immunotherapy is defined as an interaction with the immune system aiming to treat/cure cancer. Immunotherapy could be largely divided into passive and active.

4.1. Active immunotherapy

Active immunotherapy has recently undergone active clinical research. As tumors express multiple tumor-associated antigens or neonatigens, the immune system should respond by adaptive activation of T-lymphocytes against those potential targets as previously described in section 3.1.2. Any mechanism leading to activation of the immune system is considered as active immunotherapy. Active immunotherapy has been developed in order to induce and stimulate the individual's own immune response. An example of this still-developing branch of immunotherapy represents Sipuleucel-T, which is the first active cellular immunotherapy approved for clinical use by the American Food and Drug Agency (FDA) in the treatment of prostate cancer based on the data that a benefit in survival was observed in the group of asymptomatic or minimally symptomatic patients with Castrate-resistant prostate cancer (CRPC) [24]. It consists of autologous peripheral-blood mononuclear cells obtained by leucopheresis, cultured and activated ex vivo with a recombinant human fusion protein PA2024 consisting of prostatic acid phosphatase linked to granulocyte-macrophage colony-stimulating factor (PAP-GM-CSF). GM-CSF stimulates the maturation process of APCs to mature DCs, while PAP peptides functions with MHC I and II. Upon reinfusion in the patient, an immune response against PAP-containing cells is triggered [24,25].

Another example of active immunotherapy is the cellular adoptive immunotherapy using transfusion of the patient's own T-lymphocytes previously stimulated ex vivo and currently tested in phase I/II trials. There is also a wealth of trials with autologous or donor dendritic cells, autologous tumor cell lysate, activated lymphocytes, or vaccines (DNA, peptide, recombinant viral vector vaccines, etc.) used as monotherapy or in combination with chemotherapy or other passive immunotherapy options such as anti-CTLA 4 MAB, anti-PD-1 MAB, and anti-PD-L1 MAB [26-30].

4.2. Passive immunotherapy

At present, passive immunotherapy is still more commonly used as it refers to the delivery of previously synthesized agents that could be used by the immune system; typical examples are the use of non-specific immunomodulatory cytokines IFN-α, IL-2, or the specific MAB. Early clinical studies demonstrated that the use of immunomodulatory cytokines such as interferon alpha (IFN α) or interleukin 2 (IL-2) may induce antitumor immune-mediated effects as tumor regression in some solid malignancies [31,32]. Cytokines have been used as cancer immunotherapy for long decades and they work either by exerting a direct antitumor effect or by indirectly enhancing the antitumor immune response [33]. Multiple in vitro studies have shown that TNF-α and IL-6 exert direct antitumor effect suppressing cancer cell growth and survival. However, clinical use of these cytokines in cancer patients has led to less successful results because of significant toxicity and the controversial influence of a single molecule such as TNF-α and IL-6. Although they are able to suppress tumor growth, they actually promote growth of other tumors; further on, IL-6 may also exert immunosuppression. Therefore, the use of the direct antitumor effect of cytokines remains exclusively an academic pursuit.

In contrast, other cytokines may enhance the antitumor immune response through a variety of different pathways and thus they are more widely used in the clinical practice. For example, IL-2 and IFN-α promote T-lymphocytes and NK cells growth and activation, while granulocyte-macrophage colony-stimulating factor (GM-CSF) acts on APCs, increasing the processes of antigen processing and presentation as well as the production of co-stimulatory cytokines. These cytokines are nowadays well-established cancer immunotherapies, e.g., IL-2 is used in the treatment of metastatic melanoma and metastatic renal cell carcinoma, and IFN-α is approved for the treatment of malignant melanoma [34,35]. There are reports in the literature where recombinant IL-2 has also been used in the treatment of other solid tumor malignancies, including neuroendocrine tumors [36]. This led to the introduction of immunotherapy as an anticancer treatment for metastatic renal cell carcinoma in 1992 and metastatic melanoma in 1998. Subsequently, immunotherapy with interferon was also approved in the adjuvant setting in patients with high-risk malignant melanoma as it was considered a beneficial approach [37,38]. Some other cytokines, such as IL-7, IL-11, IL-12, IL-15, IL-21, IFN-β, and IFN-γ, are also currently evaluated as cancer immunotherapies.

Another typical example of passive immunotherapy is the use of MAB. There are multiple MAB used in the treatment of solid malignancies such as the MAB against the Epidermal Growth Factor (EGFR antibody) *cetuximab* or the antibody targeting the Human Epidermal Receptor type 2 (HER 2) *trastuzumab*. These MAB specifically target their receptor at the cancer cell surface and by binding to it, they prevent the signal cascade, transmitted intracellularly, thus preventing further tumor growth or reproduction. MAB may also target soluble circulatory factors that are important for the tumor such as the MAB *bevacizumab*, which targets the vascular endothelial growth factor (VEGF).

MAB may target not only tumor pathways. More recent research focused on the "communication" between the host and the tumor, targeting the immune system as a mechanism and controlling this process. The PD-1/PD-L1 interaction is a major pathway hijacked by tumors to suppress immune control. The normal function of PD-1 under healthy conditions is to downmodulate unwanted or excessive immune responses, including autoimmune reactions. PD-1 is expressed by activated T cells, mediating immunosuppression (Figure 2).

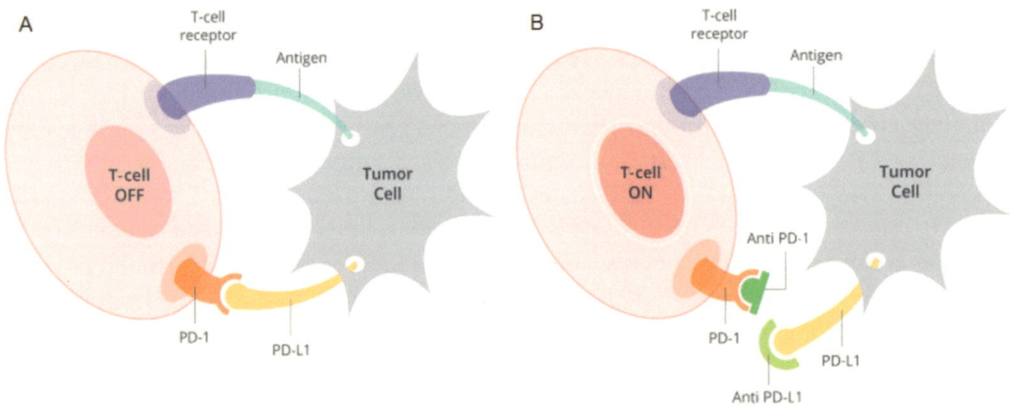

Figure 2. Immunosuppression, mediated via PD-1/PD-L1 pathway. A) PD-1 is expressed by activated T cells; by binding to PD-L1, it mediates T-lymphocyte suppression. B) The use of immune checkpoint inhibitors (anti-PD-1 or anti-PD-L1 MAB) leads to the interruption of this immunosuppression and potential cytotoxicity exerted by the T cells.

PD-1 functions in peripheral tissues where T cells encounter immunosuppressive PD-1 ligands PD-L1 and PD-L2 that are expressed by tumor cells, stromal cells, or both [39-42]. Inhibition of the interaction between PD-1 and PD-L1 enhances T cell responses in vitro and mediates preclinical antitumor activity [39,43]. PD-L1 leads to inhibition of the T-lymphocyte proliferation, survival and effector functions (cytotoxicity, cytokine release), inducing apoptosis of tumor-specific T cells, and promoting the differentiation of $CD4^+$ T cells into regulatory T cells. The blockade of PD-1/PD-L1 results in a potent and durable tumor regression and prolonged stabilization in patients with advanced malignancies [44]. Therefore, inhibition of PD-L1 binding to PD-1 represents an attractive strategy to restore tumor-specific T cell immunity.

The mechanism by which PD-1 down modulates T cell responses is similar to, but distinct from, that of CTLA-4 as both molecules regulate an overlapping set of signaling protein. PD-1 was shown to be expressed on T cells, B cells, monocytes, and natural killer T cells, following their activation [45,46]. PD-L1 and PD-L2 are expressed in a variety of cell types, including non-hematopoietic tissues, as well as in various malignancies. PD-L1 is expressed at low levels on non-hematopoietic tissues, whereas PD-L2 protein is only detectably expressed on antigen-presenting cells in lymphoid tissue or chronic inflammatory environments. PD-L2 controls immune T cell activation in lymphoid organs, whereas PD-L1 serves to protect healthy tissues from unwarranted T-cell immune-mediated damage.

Although healthy organs express little (if any) PD-L1, many cancers express abundant levels of this T cell inhibitor. High expression of PD-L1 on tumor cells (and to a lesser extent, PD-L2) has been found to correlate with poor prognosis and survival in various cancers, including RCC [47], pancreatic carcinoma [48], hepatocellular carcinoma [49], and ovarian carcinoma [50]. Furthermore, PD-1 has been suggested to regulate tumor-specific T cell expansion in melanoma patients [51].

The observed correlation of clinical prognosis with PD-L expression in multiple cancers suggests that the PD-1/PD-L1 pathway plays a critical role in tumor immune evasion and should be considered as an attractive target for therapeutic intervention.

Over the past several decades, these observations have resulted in intensive efforts to develop immunotherapeutic approaches as cancer treatment options. Such agents include immune-checkpoint-pathway inhibitors such as anti-cytotoxic T-lymphocyte antigen-4 (anti-CTLA-4) antibody (ipilimumab), anti-programmed death 1 (anti-PD-1) inhibitor (pembrolizumab, nivolumab, pidilizumab), anti-PD-L1 inhibitors (MPDL3280A, BMS-936559, MEDI4736), etc. (Table 1).

So far, passive immunotherapy has had limited success in the treatment of solid tumors, except in the treatment of malignant melanoma and renal cell cancer (RCC) [52-55]. The therapeutic options for advanced disease in RCC comprise of tyrosine-kinase inhibitors, m-TOR inhibitors, IL-2, antiangiogenic VEGF inhibitors, and IFNα. Spontaneous remissions and durable responses have been largely described as a result of this non-specific immune response. The prognosis of those patients unfortunately remains poor with a 5-year overall survival below 5% [56]. Thus, new options appear on the horizon involving the new specific targeted immunotherapies, focusing on the blockade of T cell regulation and functions, as well as activation of the dendritic cells (a form of active immunotherapy, described below). There are also phase I/II trials, studying the potential benefit of cellular adoptive immunotherapy using transfusion of stimulated patient's own T-lymphocytes. This adoptive T-lymphocyte therapy consists of infusion of ex vivo isolated, activated, or expanded tumor-specific T-lymphocytes [57]. There are different types of adoptive therapy, including TILs, engineered T-cells, expressing a specific cancer-related receptor (TCRs) or chimeric antigen receptor (CAR). Each of these approaches has its own advantages and disadvantages.

4.3. Immunotherapy as cancer prevention

Tumor cells express neoantigens that are expressed as a consequence of the malignant transformation of the host cell. The expression of neoantigens could also be the result of a

Target	Drug name	Biological description	Phase of the trial by tumor site		
			Phase I	Phase II	Phase III
CTLA-4	*Ipilimumab (BMS-734016)*	MAB	Pancreatic tumors	Ovarian Gastric	NSCLC CRPC
	Tremelimumab	MAB	MEL	MEL	-
PD-1	*Nivolumab (BMS-936558)*	Fully human IgG4 MAB	CRPC	Esophageal carcinoma	MEL, NSCLC
	Pembrolizumab Lambrolizumab (MK-3475)	Humanized IgG4 MAB	CRC, HCC, prostate cancer	RCC, CRC	MEL NSCLC RCC
	Pidilizumab (CT-011)	Humanized IgG1 MAB	-	MEL	-
	AMP-224	IgG1 fusion protein	Solid malignancies	-	-
PD-L1	*BMS-936559*	Fully human IgG4 MAB	NSCLC, MEL, CRC, RCC, ovarian, pancreatic, breast cancer	-	-
	MPDL3280A	MAB	NSCLC, MEL, CRC, ovarian, pancreatic, breast cancer	RCC, bladder carcinoma	NSCLC
	MEDI4736 Medimmune-AZ	IgG4 MAB	SCCHN	MEL	NSCLC

This is not an entirely comprehensive list of all trials that have been listed in www.clinicaltrials.com. (Source www.clinicaltrials.com)

Abbreviations:

CTLA-4: Cytotoxic T-lymphocyte-associated protein 4

PD-1: Programmed death 1

PD-L1: Programmed death 1 ligand

MAB: Monoclonal antibody

MEL: Melanoma

CRPC: Castrate-resistant prostate cancer

RCC: Renal cell carcinoma

NSCLC: Non-small cell lung cancer

CRC: Colorectal cancer

SCCHN: Squamous cell carcinoma of the head and neck

Table 1. Immune-checkpoint-pathway inhibitors and their targets in currently running clinical trials.

viral or (more rarely) bacterial infection that induced and provoked this malignant transformation and thus the idea to vaccinate against those pathogens and prevent the associated cancer. More than 15% of all cancers are considered to be related to infectious agents [58]. Infection with human papilloma viruses (HPVs) is associated in about 30% of those cases (5% of all cancers) and hepatitis B and C viruses together with *Helicobacter pylori* (*H. Pylori*) account for 60% more of all infectious-agent-related cancers. It is logical that the success of conventional antimicrobial vaccines could encourage potential cancer vaccine prevention research. This approach has proven its efficacy in hepatitis B-induced hepatocellular carcinoma [59]. In carcinoma of the uterine cervix, it is a well-known fact that about 70% of them are caused by HPV types 16 and 18, and it is expected that HPV-vaccination could decrease the incidence not only of cervical cancer [60,61], but also of head-and-neck squamous cell carcinoma [62]. The mechanism, by which HPV induces malignant transformation, is by provoking the synthesis of two oncogene products, encoded by the virus, which degradate the tumor suppressor protein p53 and block other tumor suppressor proteins cells in the premalignant dysplasia cells, as well as the cell in the in situ and the invasive carcinomas. The recombinant vaccination against HPV leads to secretion of specific antibodies, protecting the non-infected organisms from HPV-infections, and the subsequent development of HPV-infection-related cancer sites [63]. No significant effect was demonstrated in already HPV-infected individuals [64].

4.4. Immunotherapy as anticancer treatment

There are 271 trials that are recruiting patients as assessed on 23 Apr 2015 at www.clinicaltrials.com. They include different DNA-vaccines, dendritic cell vaccines, peptide vaccines, allogeneic GM-CSF-secreting vaccines, recombinant vaccines, vaccines, targeting different auto-antigens as targets, etc. They are carried in patients with various solid malignancies, predominantly in melanoma, renal cell carcinoma, non-small cell carcinoma and other solid tumors. The immunotherapy approach was also implemented in the treatment of neuroendocrine tumors, e.g., vaccination with tumor lysate-pulsed DCs that induced a significant antitumor immune response in a neuroendocrine carcinoma of the pancreas [65].

A common example of the vaccine's use as treatment is the Bacillus Calmette-Guerin (BCG), which represents an attenuated mycobacterium, originally developed as anti-tuberculosis vaccine. It was only subsequently proven in 1976 that its immunostimulation characteristics led to antitumor effects in preventing recurrence in patients who underwent transurethral resection of superficial non-muscle invasive bladder carcinoma and carcinoma in situ when used as local repeated intravesical instillations [66]. Besides the non-specific immune activation, there is a theory suggesting that its anticancer effect might be attributed to specific BCG internalization in the tumor cells by the integrins and fibronectins of the tumor cells [67,68], provoking antigen-specific adaptive immune response as well [69-71].

A list of some of the more important clinical trials using cancer vaccines as therapeutic options are listed in Table 2.

Vaccine class	Name and target of the vaccine	Biological description	Phase of the trial by tumor site		
			Phase I	Phase II	Phase III
Tumor cell	Pancreatic tumor cell vaccine	GM-CSF gene-transfected tumor cell vaccine	MEL	Pancreas	
	Algenpantucel-L	Allogeneic human pancreatic cancer vaccine	RCC, prostate	MEL, NSCLC	Pancreas adenocarcinom a
	SL-701	Multivalent glioma-associated antigen vaccine	-	GBM	-
DC / APCs	Ovapuldencel-T	Autologous PBMCs in GM-CSF	-	Ovarian, peritoneal carcinoma	-
	AGS-003	Autologous DCs transfected with tumor and CD40L RNAs	-	-	RCC
	DCVAC/Pca	Autologous DCs pulsed with killed prostate cancer line LNCap	-	Prostate	Prostate
	DCVax-L	Autologous DCs pulsed with tumor lysate antigen	-	-	GBM
	CVac	Autologous DCs pulsed with MUC1-mannan fusion protein	-	Ovarian	-
	ICT-107	Autologous DCs pulsed with antigens	-	GBM	-
	MelCancerVac	Autologous DCs pulsed with allogeneic melanoma cell lysate	-	CRC, NSCLC	-
Peptides/ proteins	GV1001	hTERT peptide	MEL, pancreatic	HCC	NSCLC, pancreatic
	Nelipepimut-S	HER2/*neu* peptide combined with GM-CSF	-	-	Breast
	L-BLP25 (Tecemotide)	Liposome-encapsulated synthetic peptide derived from MUC-1	-	Rectal, NSCLC, prostate, CRC	NSCLC
	Rindopepimut	hEGFR variant III specific peptide conjugated to KLH	-	GBM	GBM
	POL-103A	Protein antigens from 3 melanoma cell lines with alum adjuvant	-	-	MEL
	IMA901	Synthetic vaccine consisting of 10 different TUMAPs	-	-	RCC
	MAGE-A3	MAGE-A3 combined with GM-CSF	-	Bladder	MEL
	MAGE-A3 ASCI	MAGE-A3 antigen-specific cancer immunotherapeutic	-	NSCLC	NSCLC

Vaccine class	Name and target of the vaccine	Biological description	Phase of the trial by tumor site		
			Phase I	Phase II	Phase III
	Belange-pumatocel-L	Non-viral gene-based allogeneic tumor cell vaccine	-	NSCLC	NSCLC
	PVX-410	Multi-peptide vaccine	-	-	-
	IMA950	Multi-peptide glioma vaccine containing TUMAPs	GBM	GBM	-
	Racotumumab	Anti-idiotypic vaccine able to mimic the tumor-associated antigen NeuGcGM3	-	-	NSCLC
Genetic	Rilimogene galvacirepvec	Recombinant fowlpox/vaccinia virus encoding hPSA and TRICOM	Prostate	Prostate	Prostate
	CG0070	Oncolytic adenovirus encoding GM-CSF	-	Bladder	-
	TG4010	Recombinant modified vaccine virus strain Ankara, carrying coding sequences for human MUC1 antigen and human interleukin-2 and IL-2	Solid tumors	NSCLC	NSCLC

Abbreviations:

APC: Antigen-presenting cell

CRC: Colorectal cancer

DC: Dendritic cell

EGFR: Epidermal growth factor receptor

GBM: Glioblastoma

GM-CSF: Granulocyte-macrophage colony-stimulating factor

HCC: Hepatocellular carcinoma

hPSA: Human prostate specific antigen

hTERT: Human telomerase reverse transcriptase

IL-2: Interleukin-2

KLH: Keyhole limpet hemocyanin

MEL: Malignant melanoma

MUC1: Mucin 1

NSCLC: Non-small cell lung cancer

PBMC: Peripheral blood mononuclear cells

RCC: Renal cell carcinoma

TRICOM: Recombinant vaccinia virus vaccine encoding 3 co-stimulatory molecule transgenes B7.1, ICAM-1, and LFA-3

TUMAPs: Tumor-associated peptides

Table 2. Therapeutic use of cancer vaccines in clinical development in solid malignancies. This is not an entirely comprehensive list of all trials that have been listed in www.clinicaltrials.com. (Source www.clinicaltrials.com).

4.5. Predictive and prognostic biomarkers for immunotherapy

Research is ongoing in order to identify potential biomarkers for cancer immunotherapy. In order to optimize this process, we shall recently be in great demand of predictive/prognostic factors, justifying the selection of patients, who would be the best candidates for such novel, expensive, and potentially toxic treatments. PD-L1-positive cancers are associated with poorer prognoses than PD-1 negative. A correlation of PD-L1 expression and response rate was demonstrated in patients with the highest levels of PD-L1 expression and PD-L1-positive TILs [72]. The potential role of PD-L1 as well as TILs as a biomarkers remain to be elucidated.

The presence or absence of TILs also remains to be clarified. There are data that the immune system plays an important role in the process of recurrence of solid tumors. There is a multicenter study over 603 patients with colorectal cancer that showed the importance of the adaptive immune response and the presence/absence of T-lymphocytes in the resected tumor was a factor that correlated more accurately with clinical outcomes than the current parameters considered as gold standards for prognosis, histopathologically determined tumor stage (T) and nodal status (N), yielding a place for TILs as a potential prognostic marker in colorectal cancer [73] and potentially in other localizations of malignant tumors. It has also been proven for patients with large early-stage cervical cancer [74], muscle-invasive urothelial bladder carcinoma [75], and breast cancer [76]. All these findings suggest that assessment and consideration of the local intratumoral immune response in the primary tumor may have prognostic value and should be evaluated in the process of treatment decision taking.

5. Adverse effects of immunotherapy

Adverse events (AE) are graded using NCI Common Terminology Criteria for Adverse Events Version 4.0. Their management is important as the population of treated patients frequently consists of patients with disseminated disease or patients who have been previously treated with multiple treatment lines. Most frequent drug-related AEs with potential immune-related mechanism are hepatitis, pneumonitis, infusion reactions, colitis, arthralgia, and rash, necessitating sometimes the use of corticosteroids [77]. Fatigue, decreased appetite, nausea, dyspnea, diarrhea or constipation, vomiting, pyrexia, vitiligo, and headache are also described as immune-related AEs.

6. Classic chemotherapy and rationale for combination with immunotherapy

Introduction of immunotherapy into the classic chemotherapy regimens is undoubtedly a challenge. The use of chemotherapy aims complete direct cancer cell eradication, which frequently is not achieved. Post chemotherapy exposure to a tumor cell death may be induced, leading to cancer antigen release. These antigens could be subsequently processed by the APCs

http://dx.doi.org/10.5772/61211

and the cytotoxic CTLs. Besides a direct cytotoxic effect, such immune modulating effects have been proven for gemcitabine [78,79]; induction of immunogenic cancer cell death or immune sensitization for T-lymphocytes killing of the cancer cell has also been described for platinum compounds [29,80,81]. The effector cells of the immune system seem to remain unaffected [82], thus suggesting a possible rationale for searching of increased synergistic antitumor activity by combination of chemotherapy agents and immunotherapy. A large number of clinical trials are already running in multitude of solid tumor localizations. An example of a combination with chemotherapeutic agent is the emtansine/trastuzumab complex that is used in the treatment of HER-2 positive metastatic breast cancer.

Synergistic combinations with immunotherapy are also possible with radiotherapy [83], targeted agents [84], antiangiogenic drugs, or combining two immunotherapeutic agents with complementary mechanism of action [85]. There are multiple phase I–III trials, recruiting patients with solid tumors (MEL, NSCLC, RCC, CRC, etc.) where combinations of two immune checkpoint inhibitors are used in combination, e.g., anti-CTLA-4 MAB (ipilimumab) with PD-1 or PD-L1 inhibitors. CTLA-4 inhibitors stimulate the T cell activation in lymphatic tissues and increase the frequency of tumor-specific T cells, while the inhibition of the PD-1/PD-L1 axis modulates the T cell effector phase in order to overcome T cell anergy present in the tumor microenvironment [86].

A theory hypothesizes that combining immunotherapy with targeted agents could be synergistic as targeted agents promote apoptosis in tumor cells, thus enhancing tumor antigen presentation without adversely effecting immune effector cells; they can also directly modulate the immune response and improve immune-cell function, essentially acting as immune-sensitizing agents through different mechanisms [84]. The combination of immunotherapy with anti-angiogenic agents (e.g., *bevacizumab, sunitinib,* or *pazopanib*) is also supported by a strong biologic rationale as it has been shown that *bevacizumab* increases the maturation of DCs and antigen presentation process while *sunitinib* decreases the number of MDSCs and Tregs in the tumor microenvironment [87].

The rationale behind combination with radiotherapy is multidimensional, including radiation-induced tumor cell damage, leading to the spill of tumor-associated antigens, attracting the immune effector cells [80,88]. Radiotherapy also sensitizes the tumor cells, thus making them more susceptible to immune-mediated killing; it is partially due to the expression of MHC class I and death receptors [88]. There is a phase II trial in metastatic malignant melanoma (NCT01689974), which compares the use of ipilimumab as monotherapy or in combination with radiotherapy. Another important issue to be addressed in order to optimize the effect of this strategy is related to the timing of radiotherapy related to the administration of the immunotherapy [89].

The combination of agents always upfronts the question of antitumor effects and potential additive toxicity that is largely considered today. Currently, the most frequent combination remains the administration of immune adjuvants, e.g., IL-2 or GM-CSF with MAB or cancer vaccines, in order to stimulate the recruitment/activation of immune effector cells.

7. Tumor response evaluation of immunotherapy

An issue that has been recently recognized is the measurement of antitumor effect of immunotherapy. The cytotoxicity of chemotherapeutic agents often produces a measurable change in the size of the target lesions within weeks of the initial administration. Response for solid tumors is most frequently assessed using WHO or RECIST criteria [90,91]. For cytotoxic agents, these guidelines assume that an early increase in tumor growth and/or appearance of new lesions signal progressive disease (PD) and the term "progression" became synonymous with drug failure. Cessation of the currently used chemotherapy is thus recommended once PD has been detected.

On the other hand, immunotherapeutic agents enhance antitumor immune responses [92] and achievement of stable disease (SD) may also be viewed as an indicator of meaningful therapeutic effect. Beyond that, additional novel response patterns, observed with these agents, raise concerns about the interpretation and characterization of WHO or RECIST criteria. In studies with cytokines, cancer vaccines, and monoclonal antibodies, response classified as CR, PR, or SD has been shown to occur after an initial increase in tumor burden characterized as PD by WHO or RECIST criteria [93-96]. Therefore, conventional response criteria may not adequately assess the activity of immunotherapeutic agents because PD (by initial radiographic evaluation) does not necessarily reflect therapeutic failure. Thus, in order to systematically characterize additional patterns of response in patients treated with immunotherapy, underlying WHO criteria were evolved into immune-related response criteria (irRC) [97]. The core novelty of the irRC is the incorporation of measurable new lesions into "total tumor burden" and comparison of this variable to baseline measurements (before and after WHO PD, but not after confirmed irPD). Clinical activity often appears to be delayed following immunotherapeutic treatment and a period of apparent progression (as defined by the existing response criteria) may occur, followed by response. Four types of distinct response patterns have been described (two conventional and two new, unique to immunotherapy): 1) immediate response; 2) durable stable disease; 3) response after tumor burden increase; and 4) response in the presence of new lesions. The apparent increase in tumor burden that sometimes precedes response in patients receiving immune therapy may reflect either continued tumor growth until a sufficient immune response develops or transient immune-cell infiltration into the tumor with or without edema [97].

The use of irRC for response evaluation with immunotherapeutic treatment is considered clinically meaningful as they appear to be related to favorable survival. However, they are still in early development and prospective trials need to evaluate their role and potential association with survival.

8. Conclusion

A lot of scientific evidence has been recently accumulated over the role of the immune system in the prevention, development and progression of solid tumors. All this knowledge is continuously enriched in order to implicate it into meaningful clinically relevant therapeutic strategies and use immunotherapy either alone or in combination with other systemic anticancer treatments. These new strategies will hopefully lead to improvement of the outcomes of patients with solid malignancies.

Author details

Assia Konsoulova[1,2]

Address all correspondence to: dr.konsoulova@gmail.com

1 Medical Oncology Clinic, University Hospital Sveta Marina, Varna, Bulgaria

2 University of Medicine, Prof. Dr. Paraskev Stoyanov, Varna, Bulgaria

References

[1] Nauts HC, Fowler GA, Bogatko FH: A review of the influence of bacterial infection and of bacterial products (Coley's toxins) on malignant tumors in man; a critical analysis of 30 inoperable cases treated by Coley's mixed toxins, in which diagnosis was confirmed by microscopic examination selected for special study. Acta Med Scand Suppl 276:1-103, 1953

[2] Moretta A, Bottino C, Vitale M, et al: Activating receptors and coreceptors involved in human natural killer cell-mediated cytolysis. Annu Rev Immunol 19:197-223, 2001

[3] Bauer S, Groh V, Wu J, et al: Activation of NK cells and T cells by NKG2D, a receptor for stress-inducible MICA. Science 285:727-9, 1999

[4] Diefenbach A, Jamieson AM, Liu SD, et al: Ligands for the murine NKG2D receptor: expression by tumor cells and activation of NK cells and macrophages. Nat Immunol 1:119-26, 2000

[5] Medzhitov R: Toll-like receptors and innate immunity. Nat Rev Immunol 1:135-45, 2001

[6] Steinman RM: Decisions about dendritic cells: past, present, and future. Annu Rev Immunol 30:1-22, 2012

[7] Pepper M, Jenkins MK: Origins of CD4(+) effector and central memory T cells. Nat Immunol 12:467-71, 2011

[8] Josefowicz SZ, Rudensky A: Control of regulatory T cell lineage commitment and maintenance. Immunity 30:616-25, 2009

[9] Shevach EM: CD4+ CD25+ suppressor T cells: more questions than answers. Nat Rev Immunol 2:389-400, 2002

[10] Disis ML: Immune regulation of cancer. J Clin Oncol 28:4531-8, 2010

[11] Sjoblom T, Jones S, Wood LD, et al: The consensus coding sequences of human breast and colorectal cancers. Science 314:268-74, 2006

[12] Prendergast GCe, Jaffee EMe: Cancer immunotherapy : immune suppression and tumor growth (ed Second edition.)

[13] Hanahan D, Weinberg RA: The hallmarks of cancer. Cell 100:57-70, 2000

[14] Hanahan D, Weinberg RA: Hallmarks of cancer: the next generation. Cell 144:646-74, 2011

[15] Negrini S, Gorgoulis VG, Halazonetis TD: Genomic instability--an evolving hallmark of cancer. Nat Rev Mol Cell Biol 11:220-8, 2010

[16] Luo J, Solimini NL, Elledge SJ: Principles of cancer therapy: oncogene and non-oncogene addiction. Cell 136:823-37, 2009

[17] Colotta F, Allavena P, Sica A, et al: Cancer-related inflammation, the seventh hallmark of cancer: links to genetic instability. Carcinogenesis 30:1073-81, 2009

[18] Dunn GP, Old LJ, Schreiber RD: The immunobiology of cancer immunosurveillance and immunoediting. Immunity 21:137-48, 2004

[19] Dunn GP, Old LJ, Schreiber RD: The three Es of cancer immunoediting. Annu Rev Immunol 22:329-60, 2004

[20] Koebel CM, Vermi W, Swann JB, et al: Adaptive immunity maintains occult cancer in an equilibrium state. Nature 450:903-7, 2007

[21] Eyles J, Puaux AL, Wang X, et al: Tumor cells disseminate early, but immunosurveillance limits metastatic outgrowth, in a mouse model of melanoma. J Clin Invest 120:2030-9, 2010

[22] Teng MW, Swann JB, Koebel CM, et al: Immune-mediated dormancy: an equilibrium with cancer. J Leukoc Biol 84:988-93, 2008

[23] Schreiber RD, Old LJ, Smyth MJ: Cancer immunoediting: integrating immunity's roles in cancer suppression and promotion. Science 331:1565-70, 2011

[24] Higano CS, Schellhammer PF, Small EJ, et al: Integrated data from 2 randomized, double-blind, placebo-controlled, phase 3 trials of active cellular immunotherapy with sipuleucel-T in advanced prostate cancer. Cancer 115:3670-9, 2009

[25] Small EJ, Schellhammer PF, Higano CS, et al: Placebo-controlled phase III trial of immunologic therapy with sipuleucel-T (APC8015) in patients with metastatic, asymptomatic hormone refractory prostate cancer. J Clin Oncol 24:3089-94, 2006

[26] Mellman I, Coukos G, Dranoff G: Cancer immunotherapy comes of age. Nature 480:480-9, 2011

[27] Mocellin S, Mandruzzato S, Bronte V, et al: Part I: Vaccines for solid tumours. Lancet Oncol 5:681-9, 2004

[28] Tartour E, Sandoval F, Bonnefoy JY, et al: [Cancer immunotherapy: recent breakthroughs and perspectives]. Med Sci (Paris) 27:833-41, 2011

[29] Lesterhuis WJ, Haanen JB, Punt CJ: Cancer immunotherapy--revisited. Nat Rev Drug Discov 10:591-600, 2011

[30] Turcotte S, Rosenberg SA: Immunotherapy for metastatic solid cancers. Adv Surg 45:341-60, 2011

[31] Kirkwood JM, Ernstoff MS: Interferons in the treatment of human cancer. J Clin Oncol 2:336-52, 1984

[32] Rosenberg SA, Lotze MT, Muul LM, et al: Observations on the systemic administration of autologous lymphokine-activated killer cells and recombinant interleukin-2 to patients with metastatic cancer. N Engl J Med 313:1485-92, 1985

[33] Dzivenu, O.K. and O'Donnell-Tormey, J. Cancer and the immune system: the vital connection. Cancer Research Institute. 2003

[34] Proleukin (aldesleukin) [prescribing information]. San Diego, CA: Prometheus Laboratories Inc.; July, 2012.

[35] Roferon-A (interferon alfa-2a, recombinant) [prescribing information]. Nutley, NJ: Hoffmann-La Roche Inc; June, 2011.

[36] Lissoni P, Barni S, Tancini G, et al: Immunoendocrine therapy with low-dose subcutaneous interleukin-2 plus melatonin of locally advanced or metastatic endocrine tumors. Oncology 52:163-6, 1995

[37] Creagan ET, Dalton RJ, Ahmann DL, et al: Randomized, surgical adjuvant clinical trial of recombinant interferon alfa-2a in selected patients with malignant melanoma. J Clin Oncol 13:2776-83, 1995

[38] Grob JJ, Dreno B, de la Salmoniere P, et al: Randomised trial of interferon alpha-2a as adjuvant therapy in resected primary melanoma thicker than 1.5 mm without clinically detectable node metastases. French Cooperative Group on Melanoma. Lancet 351:1905-10, 1998

[39] Dong H, Strome SE, Salomao DR, et al: Tumor-associated B7-H1 promotes T-cell apoptosis: a potential mechanism of immune evasion. Nat Med 8:793-800, 2002

[40] Dong H, Zhu G, Tamada K, et al: B7-H1, a third member of the B7 family, co-stimulates T-cell proliferation and interleukin-10 secretion. Nat Med 5:1365-9, 1999

[41] Freeman GJ, Long AJ, Iwai Y, et al: Engagement of the PD-1 immunoinhibitory receptor by a novel B7 family member leads to negative regulation of lymphocyte activation. J Exp Med 192:1027-34, 2000

[42] Topalian SL, Drake CG, Pardoll DM: Targeting the PD-1/B7-H1(PD-L1) pathway to activate anti-tumor immunity. Curr Opin Immunol 24:207-12, 2012

[43] Iwai Y, Ishida M, Tanaka Y, et al: Involvement of PD-L1 on tumor cells in the escape from host immune system and tumor immunotherapy by PD-L1 blockade. Proc Natl Acad Sci U S A 99:12293-7, 2002

[44] Brahmer JR, Drake CG, Wollner I, et al: Phase I study of single-agent anti-programmed death-1 (MDX-1106) in refractory solid tumors: safety, clinical activity, pharmacodynamics, and immunologic correlates. J Clin Oncol 28:3167-75, 2010

[45] Hodi FS, Dranoff G: The biologic importance of tumor-infiltrating lymphocytes. J Cutan Pathol 37 Suppl 1:48-53, 2010

[46] Kloor M: Lymphocyte infiltration and prognosis in colorectal cancer. Lancet Oncol 10:840-1, 2009

[47] Oble DA, Loewe R, Yu P, et al: Focus on TILs: prognostic significance of tumor infiltrating lymphocytes in human melanoma. Cancer Immun 9:3, 2009

[48] Polcher M, Braun M, Friedrichs N, et al: Foxp3(+) cell infiltration and granzyme B(+)/Foxp3(+) cell ratio are associated with outcome in neoadjuvant chemotherapy-treated ovarian carcinoma. Cancer Immunol Immunother 59:909-19, 2010

[49] Suzuki H, Chikazawa N, Tasaka T, et al: Intratumoral CD8(+) T/FOXP3 (+) cell ratio is a predictive marker for survival in patients with colorectal cancer. Cancer Immunol Immunother 59:653-61, 2010

[50] Chew V, Tow C, Teo M, et al: Inflammatory tumour microenvironment is associated with superior survival in hepatocellular carcinoma patients. J Hepatol 52:370-9, 2010

[51] Liotta F, Gacci M, Frosali F, et al: Frequency of regulatory T cells in peripheral blood and in tumour-infiltrating lymphocytes correlates with poor prognosis in renal cell carcinoma. BJU Int 107:1500-6, 2011

[52] Coppin C, Porzsolt F, Awa A, et al: Immunotherapy for advanced renal cell cancer. Cochrane Database Syst Rev:CD001425, 2005

[53] Escudier B, Pluzanska A, Koralewski P, et al: Bevacizumab plus interferon alfa-2a for treatment of metastatic renal cell carcinoma: a randomised, double-blind phase III trial. Lancet 370:2103-11, 2007

[54] Fyfe G, Fisher RI, Rosenberg SA, et al: Results of treatment of 255 patients with metastatic renal cell carcinoma who received high-dose recombinant interleukin-2 therapy. J Clin Oncol 13:688-96, 1995

[55] Hodi FS, O'Day SJ, McDermott DF, et al: Improved survival with ipilimumab in patients with metastatic melanoma. N Engl J Med 363:711-23, 2010

[56] Logan JE, Rampersaud EN, Sonn GA, et al: Systemic therapy for metastatic renal cell carcinoma: a review and update. Rev Urol 14:65-78, 2012

[57] Harris TJ, Drake CG: Primer on tumor immunology and cancer immunotherapy. J Immunother Cancer 1:12, 2013

[58] Pisani P, Parkin DM, Munoz N, et al: Cancer and infection: estimates of the attributable fraction in 1990. Cancer Epidemiol Biomarkers Prev 6:387-400, 1997

[59] Chang MH, Chen CJ, Lai MS, et al: Universal hepatitis B vaccination in Taiwan and the incidence of hepatocellular carcinoma in children. Taiwan Childhood Hepatoma Study Group. N Engl J Med 336:1855-9, 1997

[60] Harper DM, Franco EL, Wheeler C, et al: Efficacy of a bivalent L1 virus-like particle vaccine in prevention of infection with human papillomavirus types 16 and 18 in young women: a randomised controlled trial. Lancet 364:1757-65, 2004

[61] Schiffman M, Castle PE, Jeronimo J, et al: Human papillomavirus and cervical cancer. Lancet 370:890-907, 2007

[62] D'Souza G, Dempsey A: The role of HPV in head and neck cancer and review of the HPV vaccine. Prev Med 53 Suppl 1:S5-S11, 2011

[63] Lowy DR, Schiller JT: Prophylactic human papillomavirus vaccines. J Clin Invest 116:1167-73, 2006

[64] Schiller JT, Castellsague X, Villa LL, et al: An update of prophylactic human papillomavirus L1 virus-like particle vaccine clinical trial results. Vaccine 26 Suppl 10:K53-61, 2008

[65] Schott M, Feldkamp J, Lettmann M, et al: Dendritic cell immunotherapy in a neuroendocrine pancreas carcinoma. Clin Endocrinol (Oxf) 55:271-7, 2001

[66] Morales A, Eidinger D, Bruce AW: Intracavitary Bacillus Calmette-Guerin in the treatment of superficial bladder tumors. J Urol 116:180-3, 1976

[67] Ratliff TL, Kavoussi LR, Catalona WJ: Role of fibronectin in intravesical BCG therapy for superficial bladder cancer. J Urol 139:410-4, 1988

[68] Kuroda K, Brown EJ, Telle WB, et al: Characterization of the internalization of bacillus Calmette-Guerin by human bladder tumor cells. J Clin Invest 91:69-76, 1993

[69] Ratliff TL, Gillen D, Catalona WJ: Requirement of a thymus dependent immune response for BCG-mediated antitumor activity. J Urol 137:155-8, 1987

[70] Peuchmaur M, Benoit G, Vieillefond A, et al: Analysis of mucosal bladder leucocyte subpopulations in patients treated with intravesical Bacillus Calmette-Guerin. Urol Res 17:299-303, 1989

[71] Ratliff TL: Role of the immune response in BCG for bladder cancer. Eur Urol 21 Suppl 2:17-21, 1992

[72] Soria JC, Cruz C, Bahleda R, et al. Clinical activity, safety and biomarkers of PD-L1 blockade in non-small cell lung cancer: additional analyses from a clinical study of the engineered antibody MPDL3280A (anti-PDL1). European Cancer Congress. 2013; Amsterdam (abstr 3408).

[73] Galon J, Costes A, Sanchez-Cabo F, et al: Type, density, and location of immune cells within human colorectal tumors predict clinical outcome. Science 313:1960-4, 2006

[74] Piersma SJ, Jordanova ES, van Poelgeest MI, et al: High number of intraepithelial CD8+ tumor-infiltrating lymphocytes is associated with the absence of lymph node metastases in patients with large early-stage cervical cancer. Cancer Res 67:354-61, 2007

[75] Sharma P, Shen Y, Wen S, et al: CD8 tumor-infiltrating lymphocytes are predictive of survival in muscle-invasive urothelial carcinoma. Proc Natl Acad Sci U S A 104:3967-72, 2007

[76] Kohrt HE, Nouri N, Nowels K, et al: Profile of immune cells in axillary lymph nodes predicts disease-free survival in breast cancer. PLoS Med 2:e284, 2005

[77] Brahmer JR, Tykodi SS, Chow LQ, et al: Safety and activity of anti-PD-L1 antibody in patients with advanced cancer. N Engl J Med 366:2455-65, 2012

[78] Nowak AK, Lake RA, Marzo AL, et al: Induction of tumor cell apoptosis in vivo increases tumor antigen cross-presentation, cross-priming rather than cross-tolerizing host tumor-specific CD8 T cells. J Immunol 170:4905-13, 2003

[79] Nowak AK, Robinson BW, Lake RA: Gemcitabine exerts a selective effect on the humoral immune response: implications for combination chemo-immunotherapy. Cancer Res 62:2353-8, 2002

[80] Apetoh L, Ghiringhelli F, Tesniere A, et al: Toll-like receptor 4-dependent contribution of the immune system to anticancer chemotherapy and radiotherapy. Nat Med 13:1050-9, 2007

[81] Ramakrishnan R, Assudani D, Nagaraj S, et al: Chemotherapy enhances tumor cell susceptibility to CTL-mediated killing during cancer immunotherapy in mice. J Clin Invest 120:1111-24, 2010

[82] Lesterhuis WJ, de Vries IJ, Aarntzen EA, et al: A pilot study on the immunogenicity of dendritic cell vaccination during adjuvant oxaliplatin/capecitabine chemotherapy in colon cancer patients. Br J Cancer 103:1415-21, 2010

[83] Gough MJ, Crittenden MR: Combination approaches to immunotherapy: the radiotherapy example. Immunotherapy 1:1025-37, 2009

[84] Ribas A, Wolchok JD: Combining cancer immunotherapy and targeted therapy. Curr Opin Immunol 25:291-6, 2013

[85] Drake CG: Combination immunotherapy approaches. Ann Oncol 23 Suppl 8:viii41-6, 2012

[86] Ott PA, Hodi FS, Robert C: CTLA-4 and PD-1/PD-L1 blockade: new immunotherapeutic modalities with durable clinical benefit in melanoma patients. Clin Cancer Res 19:5300-9, 2013

[87] Vanneman M, Dranoff G: Combining immunotherapy and targeted therapies in cancer treatment. Nat Rev Cancer 12:237-51, 2012

[88] Higgins JP, Bernstein MB, Hodge JW: Enhancing immune responses to tumor-associated antigens. Cancer Biol Ther 8:1440-9, 2009

[89] Kalbasi A, June CH, Haas N, et al: Radiation and immunotherapy: a synergistic combination. J Clin Invest 123:2756-63, 2013

[90] Miller AB, Hoogstraten B, Staquet M, et al: Reporting results of cancer treatment. Cancer 47:207-14, 1981

[91] Eisenhauer EA, Therasse P, Bogaerts J, et al: New response evaluation criteria in solid tumours: revised RECIST guideline (version 1.1). Eur J Cancer 45:228-47, 2009

[92] Dougan M, Dranoff G: Immune therapy for cancer. Annu Rev Immunol 27:83-117, 2009

[93] Little RF, Pluda JM, Wyvill KM, et al: Activity of subcutaneous interleukin-12 in AIDS-related Kaposi sarcoma. Blood 107:4650-7, 2006

[94] van Baren N, Bonnet MC, Dreno B, et al: Tumoral and immunologic response after vaccination of melanoma patients with an ALVAC virus encoding MAGE antigens recognized by T cells. J Clin Oncol 23:9008-21, 2005

[95] Kruit WH, van Ojik HH, Brichard VG, et al: Phase 1/2 study of subcutaneous and intradermal immunization with a recombinant MAGE-3 protein in patients with detectable metastatic melanoma. Int J Cancer 117:596-604, 2005

[96] Di Giacomo AM, Danielli R, Guidoboni M, et al: Therapeutic efficacy of ipilimumab, an anti-CTLA-4 monoclonal antibody, in patients with metastatic melanoma unresponsive to prior systemic treatments: clinical and immunological evidence from three patient cases. Cancer Immunol Immunother 58:1297-306, 2009

[97] Wolchok JD, Hoos A, O'Day S, et al: Guidelines for the evaluation of immune therapy activity in solid tumors: immune-related response criteria. Clin Cancer Res 15:7412-20, 2009

Chapter 6

Viral Diseases in Transplant and Immunocompromised Patients

Liliya Ivanova, Denitza Tsaneva, Zhivka Stoykova and Tcvetelina Kostadinova

Additional information is available at the end of the chapter

http://dx.doi.org/10.5772/61232

Abstract

For the last few years, the number of immunocompromised individuals is growing fast, due to more intensive antitumor therapy, transplantations and the concomitant immunosuppressive therapy, and the HIV epidemic, as well. Immunosuppressed patients very often are affected with nosocomial infections in hospitals, and with infections in the society. The defense from viral diseases depends mainly on the immune system. When there is immune deficiency, the illness is taking severely longer and has complicated outcome. Usually immunocompromised individuals have one or more defects in the defensive mechanisms and leading cause of death is infection.The viruses taking part in this process are Epstein Barr virus (EBV), Cytomegalovius (CMV), Herpes simplex viruses (HSV1, HSV2), Varicella zoster virus (VZV), Hepatitis B virus (HBV), Hepatitis C virus (HCV), and Human Polyomaviruses (BKV, JC). Many viruses (HIV, CMV, EBV) are depressing the immune resistance and are leading to co-infections with other microbial agents. Some viruses (HSV1/2, HPV, CMV, EBV, BKV, JC) are at latent condition in the infected persons for life. They become activated when decline in the immunity occurs, leading to serious illnesses. For this reason, accurate screening and prompt and precise diagnosis can be performed to prevent exacerbation of diseases and provide appropriate treatment.

Keywords: immunosupression, immunocompromised individuals, transplantation, viral infections

1. Introduction

According to several studies during the last few years, a tendency toward decreasing immune protection in human population has been under review. In the second half of the 20th century, the number of immunocompromised individuals is growing fast, due to more intensive antitumor therapy, transplantations, and the concomitant application of immunosuppressors and the HIV epidemic, as well. New syndromes and diseases appear, such as post-transplant lymphoproliferative disease (PTLD), caused in most cases by Epstein-Barr virus (EBV), and pneumonia by Cytomegalovirus (CMV). Other viruses taking part in this process are Herpes simplex viruses (HSV1, HSV2), Varicella zoster virus (VZV), Hepatitis B virus (HBV), Hepatitis C virus (HCV), and Human Polyomaviruses (BKV, JC). Usually immunocompromised individuals have one or more defects in the defensive mechanisms and leading cause of death is infection. The problem with viral causers of infections and diseases has become complicated for a few reasons:

1. The defense from viral diseases depends mainly on the immune system. When there is immune deficiency, the illness is taking severely longer from its normal course and has complicated outcome. In such patients, the disease often becomes chronic or lead to neoplasms.

2. Many viruses (HIV, CMV, EBV) are depressing the immune resistance and are leading to co-infections with other microbial agents.

3. Some viruses (HSV1/2, HPV, CMV, EBV, BKV, JC) are at latent condition in the infected persons for life. They become activated when decline in the immunity occurs, leading to serious illnesses.

4. In seronegative pregnant women and those with immune deficiency, the risk for congenital infections rises substantially.

The immune deficiency can be primary (congenital) and secondary (acquired).

Primary immunodeficiency is developed because of genetic block in differentiation of immunocompetent cells and impairment of immune mechanisms in antibody and/or T-lymphocytes production. There are three groups of primary immune deficiency:

1. Combined immune deficiency affecting T and B cell population with insufficient cellular and humoral immunity (hypogammaglobulinaemia of Glanzmann-Riniker).

2. Immunodeficiency due to a defect in the function of B cells with hypo- and agammaglobulinaemia and especially IgA deficiency (agammaglobulinaemia of Bruton, common variable hypogammaglobulinaemia).

3. Immunodeficiency based on T cell insufficiency with thymus aplasia (DiGeorge Syndrome), defect in α- and γ-interferon synthesis.

Other than the primary immune deficits mentioned above, there are others, such as defect in the enzyme assuring purine nucleotides' phosphorylation and structural defects in the 14th chromosome.

The congenital B cell insufficiency leads to serious diseases after live vaccine application (poliomyelitis, measles, mumps, rubella). There is affecting of central nervous system and development of paresis and frequent recurrent viral infections of respiratory track. After infections caused by enteroviruses, encephalitis and myositis can occur. Chronic diarrhea is typical in rotavirus infection.

The congenital T-cell insufficiency brings about systematic infections caused by different viruses such as CMV, EBV, VZV, and by viruses of families ortho- and paramyxoviridae also.

Patients with interferon failure suffer from frequent respiratory diseases.

Secondary immune deficiency can be seen in:

1. Viral diseases as measles, mumps, and mononucleosis syndrome (EBV, CMV).
2. Autoimmune and malignant diseases, especially to the blood and reticuloendothelial system (myeloid leukemia, lymphoid leukemia, multiple myelomas, Morbus of Hodgkin), affecting T cell precursors and macrophages and causing deficiency in cell-mediated immunity.
3. Renal failure and uremia in patients on hemodialysis.
4. Viral infections of the immune system (HIV) affecting the function of CD4+ T-helper cells, humoral and cell-mediated immune response afterwords are suppressed.
5. Medical treatment with immunosuppressive therapy, treatment with glycocorticoids, radiotherapy are affected barrier function of the epithelium of upper respiratory track and intestinal mucosa. This results in severe respiratory and intestinal infections. Cell proliferation is suppressed, leading to neutropenia, lymphopenia, monocytopenia. The advance of PMN cells into the space of inflammation is also suppressed. There is also difference in the sensitivity of macrophages to macrophage-activating cytokine (α-interferons). Precursors of T cell and macrophages are affected, which leads to the deficiency of cell-mediated immunity.
6. Organ transplantation and immunosuppressive therapy during post-transplant period.

Etiology and pathogenesis of viral infections in immunocompromised patients depends on the type of the immune deficiency. Clinical disease usually includes nonspecific symptoms. In most cases, it cannot be differentiated from organ rejection in patients with transplantation. The specific laboratory virological and serological tests are important for diagnosis.

More significant viral infections and diseases in immunocompromised patients are described below.

2. Epstein-Barr Virus (EBV)

EBV is a herpesvirus that is thought to infect up to 95% of the adult population. Primary infection in childhood usually results in mild, self-limiting illness [1, 2]. Asymptomatic carriers in childhood are often seen. Immunocompetent older children and adult patients get sick from infectious mononucleosis with benign lymphoproliferation of B cells under the control of the cytotoxic T cells and cellular immune response consisting of CD4+ and CD8+ T cells, which control both primary infection ant periodic reactivation that occur in all EBV-seropositive persons [1, 3, 4]. The EBV causes nasopharyngeal carcinoma, Burkitt lymphoma, and other lymphoepithelic tumors (non-Hodgkin's lymphoma, B- and T-cellular lymphomas) [5]. Development of these diseases is based on some cellular factors, as well as 14th chromosome translocation. Once infected with EBV, the virus persists latently in a person for life, in B cell lymphocytes, and chronically replicating in the cells of the oropharynx [5, 6]. In patients with HIV and transplanted ones, EBV becomes a main problem because of the inability of the immune system to control B cell proliferation and immortalization. EBV infection is registered in nearly 75% of transplanted recipients as the source usually is the donor. Contagion can also occur after blood transfusion. In the course of the immunosuppression, the latent EBV infection can be reactivated. Clinical disease represent mononuclear syndrome with temperature, lymphadenopathy, hepatosplenomegaly and monocytosis. The central nervous system is rarely involved with symptoms of serous meningitis, encephalitis, Guillen Barre syndrome.

The immunosuppression required to prevent graft rejection post-transplantation impairs T cell immunity, potentially allowing for uncontrolled proliferation of EBV-infected B cells, which may result in a spectrum of B cell proliferations that range from hyperplasia to true lymphoma [7, 8]. In the initial stages of PTLD, prolypheration is polyclonal. With mutation and selective growth, the lesion becomes oligoclonal and later, monoclonal. Lymphocytes from patients treated with cyclosporine do not exhibit an appropriate T cell response to EBV-infected B cells in vitro. The activity of natural killer cells is reduced for several months following transplantation [9, 10].

PTLD is a well-recognized complication of both solid organ transplantation and allogeneic hematopoietic stem cell transplantation (HSCT). It is one of the most common post-transplant malignancies. In most cases, it is associated with EBV infection of B cells, either as a consequence of post-transplant reactivation of the virus or from primary EBV infection. The median onset of disease in solid organ transplant population is 6 months and in hematopoietic stem cell recipients 70–90 days [11, 12] after transplantation. The frequency of PTLD depends largely on the type of transplant received and the immunosuppression that the particular transplant requires [6, 11, 12]. Primary EBV infection may develop, such as in an EBV seronegative recipient who received an allograft from an EBV-seropositive donor. This is recognized as probably the most significant risk factor for developing PTLD and be higher in pediatric transplant recipients [12]. The incidence ranged from 0.6%–2.1% in adult kidney recipients to 4.4%–6.9% in pediatric kidney recipients [12, 13] at different time after transplantation. Lung and heart transplantation in adult population is associated with a relatively high rate of PTLD with an incidence of approximately 5% or more [14]. After liver transplantation, reported rate of incidence is approximately 1% in adult recipients and pediatric recipients [15]. In the setting of allogeneic hematopoietic stem cell transplantation, PTLD rates vary greatly depending on the conditioning regimen and the amount of T cell depletion. In pediatric recipients, PTLD occurs in less than 1% of non-T-cell-depleted grafts from matched siblings, compared with as high as 30% of patients with unrelated or HLA-mismatched donors when extensive T cell depletion of the donor bone marrow is performed. Treatment of graft versus host disease with antitimocyte globulin or anti-T-cell monoclonal antibodies is another risk factor for PTLD [16].

According to the laboratory data, PTLD is characterized by leukopenia, thrombocytopenia, atypical lymphocytosis, generalized lymphadenopathy. Also B-cell lymphoma, non-Hodgkin's lymphoma (90%), lung lymphoid hyperplasia and lymphoid interstitial pneumonia (after lung transplantation), oral "hairy" leukoplakia (in association with HPV), and malignant transformation are developed. Of note, PTLD may be very difficult to distinguish from episodes of organ rejection and infection. Cell factors take part in the progress of PTLD, as well as co-infection with CMV. Different clinical symptoms can go along with the functional disorder. Mortality rate after solid-organ transplantation is more than 50% and after hematopoietic stem cell transplantation early mortality rate approached 90% [17, 18].

PTLD is an often-fatal complication of transplanted patients. Early diagnosis is important. Good medical practice requires elucidating the serological status of the patients for EBV before transplantation or immunosuppression. ELISA and immunofluorescence are used. Those who have latent infection have positive results for IgG against capsid antigen of the virus (VCA), and in most cases, against nuclear Ag (EBNA). Patients with primary or activated latent infection may have IgM and IgG anti EBV VCA, and high titer against early Ag (EA), usually EBNA are not formed. Other special studies to confirm the diagnosis of PTLD include immunophenotyping by flow cytometry or immunohistochemistry and molecular studies such as fluorescent in situ hybridization for EBV early RNA (EBER). EBV PCR of peripheral blood may be useful at the time of diagnosis and during follow-up as a method of monitoring the patient's response to treatment [18]. Surveillance by monthly PCR for circulating EBV DNA may be appropriate in such high-risk settings as EBV-seromismatched (donor-positive, recipient-negative) solid organ transplants and T cell depleted, HLA-mismatched stem cell transplants [18, 19].

Reduction in immunosuppression remains the primary therapy and often results in permanent disease eradication (19). Antiviral drugs are used (acyclovir, valacyclovir, famcyclovir, gancyclovir) combined with immunotherapy with anti-B-cell antibodies or conventional chemotherapy. Adoptive immunotherapy with EBV-specific donor T cells is highly effective. There is some data for the prophylactic administration of gancyclovir before transplantation and immunosuppression (20).

3. Cytomegalovirus (CMV)

CMV is a ubiquitous herpesvirus that infects majority of humans and is transmitted via saliva, body fluids, cell, and tissue. Primary infection in immunocompetent individuals manifests as an asymptomatic or self-limited febrile illness or as mononucleosa-like syndrome in childhood and older age. The seroprevalence depends on the socioeconomic status and ranges from 30%–97% in Europe and North America [2, 21]. Following primary viral replication in seronegative individuals, CMV establishes non-replicative infection for life, named latency, in CD34+ myeloid progenitor cells as a major site [22] and in lymphoid organs and tissues as well (23). Various latently infected cells serve as reservoirs for reactivation and as carriers of infection to susceptible individuals [24]. After reactivation, CMV multiplies inside. In immunocompromised patients and especially after transplantation, CMV is one of the main clinical problems in almost all types of allograft recipients. Basic risk factor in the development CMV replication and disease is transmission via transplanted organs or tissues including the heart, kidney, lung, liver, and hematopoietic stem cells [25, 26]. CMV disease risk is highest when primary infection occurs in seronegative transplant recipients by the transplanted organ from the seropositive donor (27). On the other hand, secondary infection presumably occurs following the reactivation of the recipient's endogenous latent infection and is more common than primary infection. The frequency depends on the specific immunosuppression utilized. The third type of infection can be correlated with a presumed superinfection that is reinfection of the previously seropositive recipients by donor virus present in allograft [28].

The initial infection is dangerous for all immunosuppressed patients, because of numerous CMV indirect effects, due to the ability to modulate the immune system, and is an important contributor to active and chronic allograft injury [26, 29]. CMV can cause dysfunction of the transplanted organ or can participate in its rejection from the organism, which is often seen in recipients of liver, heart, and lungs. Infections and diseases with CMV are also typical for recipients of kidneys and bone marrow, as mortality is in the rate of 32–70%. Other risk factors are the overall state of immunosuppression as determined by the immunosuppressive protocol (e.g. type of drug, dose, timing, and duration), host factors (e.g. age, comorbidity, leucopenia and lymphopenia, genetic factors), and others [30]. The degree of immunosuppression correlates with the severity of the clinical symptoms of CMV infection. According to the data, conventional immunosuppressive therapy is increasing the gravity of the disease.

Source of primary infection and reinfection are also blood and blood products, which have not been checked for the presence of latent CMV virus in lymphocytes. A CMV seronegative recipient who received donor organ of a seronegative individual has the lowest risk of CMV disease when receiving CMV-negative blood or leuco-depleted blood products. The use of mTOR inhibitors (everolimus, sirolimus) is associated with a lower risk of CMV disease [31]. Transplant recipients who receive treatment with lymphocyte-depleted drugs, especially if given for the treatment of rejection, should be considered at high risk for CMV disease [32].

It is considered that in almost 100% of immunocompromised patients, the latent CMV infection will become reactivated. This reactivation refers, especially, to recipients from seropositive donors, although clinical manifestation is developed in 20–25 % of them [28, 33].

To assess the risk for CMV-related disease, serology testing of all donors and transplant candidates prior to transplantation can be performed. The clinical symptoms of active CMV infection are often nonspecific, also known as CMV syndrome (prolonged fever, weakness, hematological abnormalities such as thrombocytopenia, atypical lymphocytosis and leukopenia, and abnormalities of hepatic function). The symptoms occur 1–4 months after transplantation, in some cases, even later and sometimes it is difficult to differentiate them from those of organ rejection. The greatest risk for this condition is at the first 30 days after the immunosuppression. Tissue-invasive CMV disease is when it implicates the gastrointestinal tract, pneumonitis, hepatitis, nephritis, myocarditis, pancreatitis, retinitis, etc. [34]. In patients with transplanted liver, CMV hepatitis occurs in 17% of the cases. The "vanishing bile duct syndrome" (VBS) is related with CMV infection and organ rejection. Heart and lung recipients usually develop interstitial pneumonia, as those with bone marrow transplantation. Mortality is from 33–100% in a half of the patients. Atherosclerosis of coronary vessels develops three times faster in patients with active CMV infection in heart recipients [35–42].

Laboratory diagnosis of CMV infection and CMV disease can be accomplished with various methods. Preliminarily, before starting with the immunosuppression or transplantation, the serological status of the donor and recipient is defined. Generally, the method used for this purpose is ELISA, which detects specific IgG Ab in the serum of the patient. CMV infection after transplantation represents the presence of the virus and viral replication in body fluids or tissue samples regardless of clinical symptoms. CMV disease after transplantation represents the presence of any clinical symptoms in patients with CMV infection [43]. The laboratory methods to confirm CMV infections are histology, culture, serology, antigenemia (pp65 antigenemia), and molecular assay that detect and quantify CMV nucleic acid (NAT) [35]. Serology to detect CMV-IgM and IgG has limited use for diagnosis of CMV disease after transplantation (44). Molecular tests that detect CMV DNA or RNA are the preferred methods. Detection of CMV RNA is indicative of CMV replication. Detection of CMV DNA may or may not reflect CMV replication since a highly sensitive NAT may amplify latent viral DNA. Quantitative NAT (QNAT) assay have been developed to potentially differentiate active viral replication typically associated with high viral load from latent virus with low level CMV DNAemia [35, 45]. QNAT is useful for guiding preemptive therapy, for rapid and sensitive diagnosis of CMV infection, and to guide treatment responses [45]. Patients suspected to have tissue-invasive CMV disease but with negative QNAT or pp65 antgenemia should undergo tissue biopsy and histopathology to confirm the clinical suspicion of CMV disease [35].

The approaches to CMV prevention in recipients vary among different transplant population and risk profile. The two major strategies for CMV prevention are: antiviral prophylaxis and preemptive therapy. Antiviral prophylaxis is the administration of antiviral drug to "at-risk" patients for a defined period after transplantation. Preemptive therapy is the administration of antiviral drug only to asymptomatic patients with evidence of early CMV replication in order to prevent disease. Recipients are monitored at regular intervals (usually once weekly) using a laboratory assay such as CMV QNAT or pp65 antgenemia.

Antiviral prophylaxis has the advantage of preventing reactivation of other herpesviruses, and has been associated with lower incidence of indirect CMV effects [46]. Antiviral prophylaxis can be administered to any at-risk recipients. The duration varies depending on the CMV donor and recipient serostatus and the transplant types, extended between 100 days and 12 months in different group [35]. Valgancyclovir is the preferred drug. Alternative options are intravenous gancyclovir, oral gancyclovir, and for kidney recipients only valacyclovir. Unselected intravenous immunoglobulin (IVIG) may also be used but only as an adjunct to antiviral therapy in lung, heart, and intestinal transplant recipients. In general, antiviral prophylaxis should be started as early as possible and within the first 10 days after transplantation [35]. However, antiviral prophylaxis is associated with late-onset CMV disease particularly among CMV D+/R- patients, probably due to development of drug resistance [47]. The potential options for prevention and management of late-onset CMV disease are careful clinical follow up with early treatment of CMV disease when symptoms occur, CMV QNAT or pp65 antgenemia monitoring after completion of antiviral prophylaxis, and prolonged antiviral prophylaxis.

Preemptive therapy requires weekly patient monitoring for evidence of early CMV replication, which is then treated with valgancyclovir or intravenous gancyclovir. The recommended doses are valgancyclovir (900 mg twice daily) or intravenous ganciclovir (5 mg/kg every 12 h). Many authors prefer antiviral prophylaxis for D+/R- and lung transplant recipients while recognizing the clinical utility of preemptive therapy in CMV R+ kidney, liver, pancreas, and heart recipients [21, 35]. The same laboratory test for monitoring is recommended, with frequency of once weekly for 12 weeks after transplantation.

Indications of use of ganciclovir also include severe local (often eye damages) and life threatening conditions in patients with HIV, organ transplantations, and neoplasms. The use of lymphocyte-depleting therapy is a major risk factor for CMV disease when used for rejection treatment. The optimal duration of antiviral prophylaxis is given for 1–3 months with valgancyclovir (900 mg once daily, oral gancyclovir 1 g p.o. thrice daily) or intravenous gancyclovir (5 mg/kg every 24 h) [35].

Patients who develop CMV disease after prolonged courses of gancyclovir or vagancyclovir administration, and those failing to respond to standard gancyclovir treatment, should be suspected of having gancyclovir resistant virus. In these conditions, genotype testing should be performed. Immunosupression should be cautiously reduced. Therapeutic options for gancyclovir resistant CMV are limited. Foscarnet is often the first line for the treatment of UL97-mutant gancyclovir-resistent CMV (48). Switching to sirolimus-containing regimen may be an option for patients receiving mTOR inhibitors. Other therapeutic options are administration of cidofovir or its new oral formulation that may be available for compassionate release brinsidofovir (CMX001), compassionate release letermovir (AIC246), compassionate release maribavir, off-label leflunomid and off-label artesunate [49, 50]. Due to the virus, ability to evade host defenses of primary infection with CMV has not been shown to confer immunity from subsequent infections. Notwithstanding this, there are efforts to develop a CMV vaccine for prevention and therapy [51]. Due to some toxic effects of ganciclovir, patients need preliminary tests for renal function and blood count. Renal function is defined with the means of creatinine clearance, which has to be more than 70 ml/min. In blood, the number of neutrophiles has to be more than 1000 cells/mm^3, platelets –above 25000 cells/mm^3. During the treatment process these indicators are monitored every week and if they begin to decrease drastically, therapy is ceased. CMV therapy is not recommended in pregnant women, children under 12 years old and people more than 65 years old.

4. Varicella Zoster Virus (VZV)

VZV is a human herpesvirus that spreads through direct contact with skin lesions or through air from respiratory droplets. Primary exposure, usually in childhood, leads to varicella, typically presents with fever, constitutional symptoms, and widely disseminated vesicular rush that primary involves the trunk and face [52]. Symptoms usually resolve within 7–10 days in immunocompetent children and young adults. More than 90% of adults acquire the infection in childhood and will be seropositive for VZV [2]. After initial infection, VZV establishes lifelong latency in the cranial nerve and dorsal root ganglia, and can reactivate years to decades later as herpes zoster in some individuals [53]. In children with primary and secondary immunodeficiency because of immunosuppressive therapy (leukemia, lymphoma, solid tumors), after transplantation VZV causes progressive varicella characterized by the continuous development of vesicular rash because of high viral replication and inadequate immune response [54, 55]. The high mortality among these children and adult organ recipients is because of systematic infection with multiple organ involvement, especially in the lungs, liver, pancreas, and central nervous system and, in some cases, disseminated intravascular coagulopathy. Relapses are often seen. More recent reports have shown that pediatric renal and liver transplant recipients are at lower risk (4%–6.2%) for complication when given immediate antiviral therapy [56–60].

Herpes zoster is characterized by vesicular rash units all over the corresponding nerve and estimated to occur in up to 20% of the immunocompetent individuals during their lifetime. In immunosuppressed and transplanted patients, herpes zoster is a frequent infectious complication during the first four years after the transplantation [61, 62]. About half of the cases in the first year after the transplantation, a disseminated infection with mortality about 9% is observed, especially in the cases of organ rejection. Allogeneic stem cell transplantation is another procedure that greatly heightens the risk of herpes zoster. The incidence of VZV reactivation is 20.7%. VZV-related complications occur in 29% of patients with reactivation, most common of which is disseminated disease and postherpetic neuralgia. Radiotherapy can also become a reason for herpes zoster in about 15%–34 %. There is dissemination of the rash units outside the affected dermatome. In about 1% of all cases, encephalitis develops. This is typical, a second relapse that manifests, involving other body parts. In children with leukemia, herpes zoster or varicella develops more than one episode of clinical manifestation. Older transplant recipients are at greater risk for the development of herpes zoster and postherpetic neuralgia as secondary complication [62–65].

To determine the risks of VZV primary infection or reactivation after immunosupression and transplantation, all patients being considered for these procedures should undergo serologic testing (ELISA anti VZV IgG) to document prior exposure to VZV. Patients who are seronegative are at high risk for the development of primary VZV, and seropositive patients are at high risk for developing herpes zoster. In general, both primary varicella and herpes zoster have typical clinical presentations. Definitive laboratory testing can be used for atypical cases and should be used for suspected disseminated, visceral disease, or central nervous system disease. Rapid diagnostic methods, including polymerase chain reaction (PCR) and direct immunofluorescent assay, are the methods of choice. PCR can be used for detecting VZV in vesicle fluid, serum, spinal fluid, and other tissues. Viral culture is specific and can help distinguish VZV from other herpesvirus pathogens (herpes simplex virus - HSV) [66].

Post-transplant and immunosuppressive patients who develop primary varicella should be treated with intravenous (IV) acyclovir early in the course of the illness, especially within 24 hours of rash onset. Reduction of immunosuppressive therapy should be considered. However, IVIG or VZV immunoglobulin (VZIG) have been used in those with severe infection. Patients with disseminated or organ invasive herpes zoster should be treated with IV acyclovir. Localized nonsevere dermatomal herpes zoster can be treated with oral acyclovir, valacyclovir or famcyclovir [65].

Oral acyclovir and its pro-drugs have been shown to prevent VZV reactivation in immunosuppressed population. During the early post-transplant period, many current regimens used for CMV prevention will likely prevent VZV reactivation. In patients who do not receive CMV prophylaxis, short-term antivirals given for HSV prophylaxis may also be effective against VZV during the period immediately post-transplant [65]. Other authors recommended one year prophylactic with acyclovir, which has been shown to effectively prevent VZV-reactivation after allogeneic hematopoietic stem cell transplantation [61].

In the U.S., potential transplant recipients who are susceptible to VZV should be given varicella vaccination (one or two doses) with live attenuated Oka vaccine (Varivax, Merck & Co., Inc., Whitehouse Station, NJ, USA). There is currently a herpes zoster vaccine (Zostavax, Merck & Co., Inc.) that has not been studied in patients with end-organ disease awaiting transplantation. The Oka varicella vaccines have been shown to be safe in select children undergoing chemotherapy, and studies have shown that they can be given safely to posttransplant recipients receiving immunosupression. Inactivated VZV vaccines, which are in development, may eventually provide another option for this high-risk population [65–68].

5. Herpes simplex virus

Herpes simplex virus type 1 (HSV1) and herpes simplex virus type 2 (HSV2) are members of the Herpesvirus family and is transmitted via close personal contact. Seroprevalence studies indicated that infections are common worldwide and increases with age [2, 69]. More than 90% of adult have acquired HSV infection by their fifth decade of live, though only a minority develop clinically apparent disease at the time of acquisition [70]. After the first contagion, HSV stays in latent condition for a lifetime. HSV1 is acquired predominantly during childhood age, while HSV2 is acquired by sexual contact. A recent study indicated that HSV1 can also cause genital herpes (71). In immunocompetent individuals, symptomatic disease is presented as orolabial or genital herpes [72, 73]. Symptomatic disease may occur as a first episode that heals in 10–21 days, followed by the establishment of latency and the risk of subsequent episodes of reactivation. Cell-mediated immunity plays an important role in host defense and the containment of infection [74]. Individuals with impaired cell-mediated immunity, such as immunosupressed and transplanted patients, are subject to more frequent episodes of reactivation, prolonged duration of symptoms and shedding, increased severity of infection, and a greater potential for dissemination [75]. Solid organ transplant patients have had pre-transplant HSV seropositivity rates and age distributions similar to the general population. In the absence of antiviral prophylaxis, seropositive recipients often experience reactivation of latent infection within one or two months after transplantation [76]. Mucocutaneous lesions are the majority of HSV disease in transplant population, mainly with orolabial and anogenital localizations. HSV esophagitis, pneumonia, meningitis, and viremia dissemination either from reactivation or primary infection, may involve the spread to multiple organs such as the liver, adrenal glands, gastrointestinal tract, lungs, skin, and bone marrow [77].

To determine the risk of HSV primary infection or reactivation after immunosupression and transplantation, all patients being considered for these procedures should undergo serologic testing (ELISA anti HSV1 IgG and anti HSV2 IgG) to document prior exposure to the viruses. Patients who are seronegative are at high risk for the development of primary HSV, and seropositive patients are at high risk for developing reactivation. In the presence of characteristic mucocutaneous lesions, clinical diagnosis may be considered reliable. Laboratory testing can be used for atypical cases and should be used for suspected disseminated, visceral disease, or central nervous system disease. Viral culture is the definitive method of diagnosis for isolation of the virus from vesicles, urine, stool, nasopharynx, throat, conjunctive, and cerebrospinal fluid. Nucleic acid amplification method of DNA detection (PCR) is increasing utility, and has been shown to be 3 to 4 times more sensitive than viral culture [79]. Direct fluorescent antibody test is another mode of diagnosis of HSV; it offers rapid diagnosis and can also give type-specific diagnoses [75–79].

Acyclovir is the drug of choice for treatment of HSV infections in both immunocompetent and immunocompromized patients. Transplant patients with mucocutaneous lesions may be treated with IV acyclovir (5 mg/kg/dose given every 8 hours) for 7–14 days, oral acyclovir, or one of the alternative oral antiviral agents with better bioavailability (valacyclovir or famcyclovir). Disseminated infections and herpes simplex encephalitis, due to the potentially life-threatening nature of these infections, should be treated with a high dose IV acyclovir (10 mg/kg/dose given every 8 hours) for 7–14 days. Recently, in the last few years, some mutated acyclovir resistant strains of HSV have been isolated. These mutants are founded in patients with HIV and those with bone marrow transplantation and preventive treatment with acyclovir. These patients are treated according to a scheme with pencyclovir [76]. Gancyclovi, valgancyclovir, foscarnet or cidofovir are other antiviral agents with activity against herpesviruses, including HSV and CMV co-infections. Acyclovir can also be used for prophylaxis of the infection before immunosuppression and transplantation to prevent reactivation of the latent infection and considerably reduced incidence of disease in the early posttransplant period.

Numerous efforts have been made to develop an HSV vaccine using several different methods including inactivated virus, live attenuated virus, viral subunits and more recently, recombinant viruses. Many of these attempts shower promising results in their early phase of development [79–80].

6. Polyomaviruses (BKV, JCV)

Polyomaviruses are ubiquitous, infecting many different mammalian species including humans. Most human polyoma-diseases are caused by JCV and BKV. The prevalence of infections differs in geographical and age distribution, suggesting they circulate independently. BKV infection is acquired in early childhood, whereas JC presents later. Transmission of BKV occurs typically via oral and respiratory routes, but data suggests transmission via cells and tissues, in particular by kidney transplantation [81]. Approximately 50%–80% of humans have seropositivity to JCV and BKV viruses due to multiple routes of transmission [82, 83]. Clinically apparent diseases in immunocompetent hosts are extremely rare and are not associated with any well-defined clinical syndrome. After primary infection, viruses remain latent possibly in the lymphoid organs, neuronal tissue, kidney, and tubular epithelial cells. About 5% of healthy individuals intermittently reactivate BKV replication with detectible viruria [84]. Under the circumstances of severe immunosuppression both viruses reactivate. BKV can cause pneumonitis, hepatitis, retinitis, and meningoencephalitis [85]. Hemorrhagic cystitis is seen in 25–60% of bone marrow transplant patients, usually 2 weeks after transplantation [86]. Up to 80% of renal transplant patients have BK viruria, and 5%–10% progress to BKV nephropathy (BKVN) [87]. Given that polyomavirus is widely latent in the kidney, renal transplantation is believed to be an important mode of infection in patients with end stage kidney disease. Graft loss rate have been reported to be as high as 30%–50% following a diagnosis of BKVN [88]. More recent data indicate that with early diagnosis of BK viremia or viruria using regular screening, the majority of patients respond favorably [89, 90].

Serologic testing may be used in risk-assessment of virus transmission via organ transplantation. The greatest risk of post-transplant viral reactivation is associated with positive serostatus of both the donor and recipient. The presence of IgG antibody to BKV-VP-1 in serum is associated with increased risk of virus transmission and disease in renal allograft recipient [91]. To detect viral replication in urine and blood, real time PCR is the method of choice for diagnosis of BKVN [92] and screening every 3 months for the first two years after transplant or when allograft dysfunction occurs is recommended [93].

The first line of treatment of BKV nephropathy is reduction of immunosupression [92, 93]. A variety of drugs with possible anti-BKV activity that are being utilized as adjuvant therapy but fraught with side-effects are cidofovir, leflunomide, and intravenous immunoglobulin [94]. Fluoroguinolons have been reported to display anti-BK activity because of its large T-antigen helicase activity [95]. Further studies are needed to firmly establish the role of polyoma viruses in human cancer [96].

Other polyomavirus with importance of human pathology is JCV. Progressive multifocal leukoencephalopathy (PML) is a progressive demyelinating central nervous system disorder involving cerebral white matter caused by the JCV. It most often presents as an opportunistic infection in HIV patients with lymphopenia but has recently been seen with new immunosuppressives. After reactivation in severely immunosuppressed states, the virus travels to the central nervous system through infected B-lymphocytes, where it produces lytic destruction of myelin producing glial cells (i.e., oligodendrocytes) and non-lytic infection of astrocytes, causing progressive disease in central nervous system. Typical PML patients have very low CD4+T cell counts even less than 200/mm^2 [97, 98]. The estimated incidence of PML in HIV patients is 5%, but is decreasing with the introduction of highly active anti-retroviral therapy (HAART) [99]. The differential diagnosis of PML is HIV-associated encephalopathy and primary CNS lymphoma. Brain biopsy is the gold standard for diagnosis. Staining with immunohistochemistry using antibodies directed to SV40-T antigen is confirmatory. Analysis of cerebrospinal fluid for JCV by PCR has a sensitivity of to 92% and specificity up to 100% (100). For patients with PML and HIV, introduction or optimization of HAART needs to be implemented to decrease viral replication. In non-HIV patients, such as organ transplant patients, immunosupression needs to be decreased or stopped [101]. At this stage, there is no specific antiviral agent for JC virus [97].

7. Respiratory viruses

Every year, the number of patients undergoing stem cell and solid organ transplantation to treat malignancy and end-organ failure increases. Despite advances in screening and prophylaxis strategies, infections remain a significant cause of morbidity and mortality among transplant recipients. From the available data, respiratory viruses remain common pathogens. The respiratory viruses, including Adenovirus, Influenza virus, Human Metapneumovirus (hMPV), Parainfluenza virus (PIV), Respiratory Syncytial virus (RSV), and Rhinovirus (HRV) are increasingly recognized as contributing to significant morbidity and mortality among hematpoietic stem cell transplant (HSCT) and solid organ transplant (SOT) recipients [102]. Iimmunocompromized patients often have atypical presentation of respiratory infections and viral shedding can be prolonged [103]. Not one virus is exclusively associated with one clinical syndrome and there is a high risk of infectious complications as viral pneumonia or bronchiolitis obliterans following acute respiratory infection. Lymphopenia is consistently a risk factor for more serious infections. Respiratory viral infections appear to be risk factors for acute and chronic rejection, especially in lung transplant patients [104]. There is increased risk of severe respiratory viral infections and its sequels among pediatric recipients, as compared to adult recipients (103).

All respiratory viruses are extremely dangerous for lung and HSCT cell recipients with high mortality rate [105, 106]. Adenoviruses induce respiratory and gastrointestinal diseases. Disseminated infections are characterized by fever, pneumonia, diarrhea, hemorrhagic cystitis, hepatitis, and CNS involvement in up to 10% of the cases. In some patients Adenoviruses can become a reason for organ rejection. Cases of death can occur if there is co-infection with CMV and different bacteria. Adenoviruses are usually in latent condition in the human body and the infection becomes clinically manifested after reactivation of the virus (107). HRV is probably the most common respiratory viral pathogen in the upper and lower respiratory tract in transplant recipients [108].

In general, all patients with presumed respiratory viral infections have a nasopharyngeal swab, wash, or brohoalbeolar aspirate performed. Diagnosis of the respiratory viruses can be achieved by the combination of serology, virus culture, antigen detection, nucleic acid testing, and histopathology. Serology is not useful for initial diagnosis and has reduced sensitivity in transplant recipients. Viral culture can be achieved for most viruses except hMPV and Coronaviruses because special cell lines are needed. Shell vial assays allow earlier detection of viruses with application of monoclonal and polyclonal antibodies. Recently, several fixed mixture of cells (R-Mix) has become commercially available [109]. Rapid antigen detection using several different techniques is available for Influenza, RSV, and Adenovirus. Direct fluorescent antibody (DFA) testing of primary patient specimens has documented sensitivity that approached PCR [110]. Nucleic acid amplification assay appears to be the most sensitive diagnostic tool available, and most allow for simultaneous detection of a broad range of respiratory pathogens from a simple sample [111].

Treatment depends on the etiological agent. Reduction of immune suppression, if possible, is recommended for all the transplanted recipients. For infections caused by RSV, combination therapy with aerosolized ribavirin and intravenous immunoglobulins appears to have the greatest benefit in reducing mortality [103, 112]. PIV and hMPV infections are treated with oral, aerosolized, or intravenous ribavirin in a combination with intravenous immunoglobulins [113]. Adenovirus infections are treated with cidofovir, vidarabin, and gancyclovir. Lymphocyte reconstitution plays a crucial role in the clearance of Adenovirus [114]. Treatment of Rhinovirus infections is done with pleconaril and 3C-protease inhibitors, but there is insufficient experience with them and this limits their application. Topical interferon might be efficacious in moderating viral shedding and symptoms [115, 116]. Prevention of Influenza depends on aider vaccination with Influenza vaccine [117] or antiviral therapy. Vaccination is not suitable for bone marrow transplant patients 6–12 months after the transplantation. Patients with severe Influenza should be treated with both M2 inhibitors (rimantadin and amantadin) and neuraminidase inhibitors (relenza and tamiflu [118].

8. Hepatitis B Virus (HBV)

Acute infection with HBV can result in fulminant hepatic failure, whereas chronic HBV infection can lead to end-stage liver disease, including cirrhosis and hepatocellular carcinoma. Understanding of the natural history and basic biology of HBV has increased greatly in recent years. HBV infection is by far the most common chronic viral infection affecting the liver [119]. Reactivation of HBV replication in patients undergoing immunosuppressive therapy is well recognized and is a frequently reported complication of considerable clinical importance [120, 121]. HBV reactivation following immunosuppression is defined by an abrupt rise in HBV replication followed by laboratory signs of hepatocellular injury in "silent" HBV-infected individuals (HBsAg carriers). Reactivation can also occur at a lower rate in patients with "occult" HBV infections. The clinical presentation of reactivation is variable, ranging from an asymptomatic course to severe hepatitis, liver failure, and death. It is most frequently observed in patients with lymphoma treated with rituximab and corticosteroids, as well as in patients undergoing stem cell and bone marrow transplantation. Others risk groups include patients with solid tumors, subjects infected with HIV, organ transplant recipients, and those with autoimmune diseases [122, 123]. It is believed that about 12% of patients with malignancy have chronic HBV infection. In transplanted patients, infection can also reactivate after immunosuppressive therapy. For these reasons, high-risk individuals should be identified and screened. Recommendation for screening for all three serologies, including HBcAb, HBsAg, and HBsAb in those planned for immunosuppression is available [124]. Despite advances in treatment of chronic HBV infection, liver transplantation remains the only hope for many HBV-related end-stage liver disease patients. The high rate of HBV reinfection or recurrence after liver transplantation is probably due to enhanced virus replication resulting from immunosuppression and other mechanisms. In the recent years, liver transplantation has shown encouraging results. The introduction of effective measures to prevent and treat reinfection or recurrence using strategies involving hepatitis B immune globulin (HBIG) and subsequently nucleos(t)ide analogues have significantly improved the outcome of liver transplantation [125, 126]. Overall HBsAg positive patients who are candidates for chemotherapy or treatment with biological agents, preemptive treatment with an antiviral agents such as lamivudine, and lately with the more potent tenofovir, entecavir, or adefovir, has become a standard of care, effectively preventing HBV reactivation. Patients with occult HBV should be monitored for alanine aminotransferase and HBV DNA (by real-time PCR) during the course of immunosuppression. Prompt administration of a potent antiviral agent upon diagnosis of reactivation may be lifesaving in such patients [122].

9. Hepatitis C Virus (HCV)

Infections with HCV can result in both acute and chronic hepatitis. Acute HCV typically leads to chronic infection in about 80% of cases. This condition leads to both extrahepatic and hepatic disorders, mainly chronic liver inflammation, cirrhosis and liver cancer [127, 128]. Chronic HCV infection is usually slowly progressive. Approximately 20% to 30% of chronic-infected individuals develop cirrhosis over a 20–30-year period of time. HCV-associated cirrhosis is the most common indication for orthotopic liver transplantation among adults. It is well documented, that recurrence of HCV and reinfection of the graft following liver transplantation more frequently occurs. The observations indicate that up to 40% of the patients experience recurrent hepatitis and cirrhosis 5 years later [129]. This progression depends on the age of the donor (below 40 years old), the gravity of the immunosuppression, viral status of the patient before transplantation and a month after it. Prevention and treatment of HCV reinfection and reactivation after liver transplantation remains an unsolved major clinical challenge. HCV-positive patients have poorer long-term outcomes after liver transplantation in comparison with patients with other underlying liver diseases. While treatment with pegilated interferon alpha and ribavirin can cure up to one-third of HCV-positive transplanted patients, there are many promising drugs in clinical and preclinical development targeting either the virion or essential host factors. New strategies to prevent HCV reinfection include neutralizing antibodies or drugs targeting cellular HCV entry factors. Unfortunately, it will take at least several years until most of these drugs will reach routine clinical practice.

The relationship between HCV infection and immunosuppression is complex. The complexity is further complicated by the intrinsic tendency of HCV infection in itself to lead to disorders of the immune system. After HCV discovery, it was shown that HCV is also a lymphotropic virus, and as a consequence of lymphatic infection, several lymphoproliferative disorders have been associated. Although HCV-related hepatocytolysis is classically interpreted as secondary to attack by cytotoxic T-lymphocytes against infected cells, the liver disease is usually exacerbated and more rapidly evolutive in immunosuppressed patients [130, 131]. Liver disease secondary to chronic HCV infection is an important cause of morbidity and mortality in dialysis patients and kidney transplant recipients. Eradication of infection before transplantation seems to reduce the risk for HCV-associated renal dysfunction after transplantation, and may reduce risk of HCV disease progression. For dialysis patients, ribavirtin is generally contraindicated and alternatives are needed to enhance antiviral effects of interferon. New therapies with taribavirin may offer specific advantage in this patient group [132, 133]. In individuals with defects in cell-mediated immunity, predominantly CD4Th1, occurring in HIV infection and in patients requiring multi-drug immunosuppression following solid organ transplantation, chronic liver disease caused by HCV progresses more rapidly than in immunocompetent individuals. The rate of progress seems to correlate with the degree of immunosuppression. The prolonged suppressive therapy aggravates liver function [134]. Liver-related mortality is higher in those patients who are co-infected with HCV and HIV. All immunosuppressed and HIV infected patients should be screened for HCV infection using sensitive immunoassay licensed for detection of antibodies to HCV. For laboratory tests, ELISA is most widely used from the serological methods. HCV seropositive patients should be tested for HCV RNA using a sensitive quantitative assay to confirm the presence of active infection by RT PCR. Patients with positive HCV-RNA test should be genotyped and should be evaluated for HCV therapy [134, 135]. Liver disease in an immunosuppressed patient is typically severe with unusual progression to cirrhosis. However, accurate screening and specialized advice is recommended as soon as possible in HCV-positive patients.

For the last few years, there has been great progress in the production and application of drugs for prophylaxis and treatment of latent and chronic viral infections in immunosuppressed and transplanted patients. Various schemes for drug usage have been developed and have been permanently completed. Immunosuppressed patients very often are affected with nosocomial infections in hospitals, and with infections in the society. For this reason, accurate screening and prompt and precise diagnosis can be performed to prevent exacerbation of diseases and provide appropriate treatment.

Author details

Liliya Ivanova*, Denitza Tsaneva, Zhivka Stoykova and Tcvetelina Kostadinova

*Address all correspondence to: liivanova@abv.bg

Medical University "Prof. d-r Paraskev Stoyanov" – Varna, Department of Microbiology and Virology, St. Marina University Hospital – Varna, Bulgaria

References

[1] Cohen LI. Epstein-Barr virus infection. N Engl J Med. 2000;343(7):481-492.

[2] Ivanova L. Herpesvirus infections in human population in Northeastern Bulgaria. Scr Sci Med (ISSN 0582-3250). 2007;39(2):1-6.

[3] Henle G, Henle W, Diehl V. Relation of Burkitt's tumor-associated herpes-type virus infectious mononucleosis. Proc Natl Acad Sci USA. 1968; 59(1):94-101.

[4] Hislop AD, Taylor GS, Sauce D, Rickinson AB. Cellular responses to viral infection in humans: Lessons from Epstein-Barr virus. Annu Rev Immunol. 2007;25:587-617.

[5] Zur Hausen H, Schulte-Holthausen H, Klein G, et al. EBV DNA in biopsies of Burkitt tumours and anaplastic carcinomas of the nasopharynx. Nature. 1970;228(276): 1056-1058.

[6] Cen H, Williams PA, McWilliams HP, et al. Evidence for restricted Epstein-Barr virus latent gene expression and anti-EBNA antibody response in solid organ transplant recipients with posttransplant lymphoproliferative disorders. Blood. 1993;81(5): 1393-1403.

[7] Dharnidharka VR, Lamb KE, Gregg JA, Meier-Kriesche HU. Association between EBV serostatus and organ transplant type in PTLPD risk: An analysis of the SRTR National Registry Data in the United States. Am J Transplant. 2012;12(4):976-983.

[8] Swimmer LJ, LeBlanc M, Grogan TM, Gordan LI, Stiff PL, Miller AM. Prospective study of sequential reduction in immunosuppression, interferon alpha-2B, and chemotherapy for posttransplantation lymphoproliferative disorder. Transplantation. 2008;86(2):215-222.

[9] Chubert S, Renner C, Hammer M, Abdul-Khaliq H, Lehmkuhl HB, Berger F. Relationship of imnmunosupression to Epstein Barr viral load and lymphoproliferative disease in pediatric heart transplant patients. J Heart Lung Transplant. 2008;27(1): 100-105.

[10] Capello D, Berra E, Cerri M, Gaidano G. Post-transplant lymphoproliferative disorders. Molecular analysis of histogenesis and pathogenesis. Minerva Med. Feb 2004;95(1):53-64.

[11] Caillard S, Lamy FX, Quelen C, Dantal J, Lebranchu Y, Lang P. Epidemiology of posttransplant lymphoproliferative disorders in adult kidney and kidney pancreas recipients: Report of the French registry and analysis of subgroups of lymphomas. Am J Transplant. 2012;12(3):682-693.

[12] Green M, Webber S. Post-transplantation lymphoproliferative disorders. Pediatr Clin North Am. 2003;50(6):1471-1491.

[13] Sampaio MS, Cho YW, Qazi Y, Bunnaparadist S, Hutchinson IV, Shah T. Posttransplant malignatcies in solid organ adult recipients: An analysis of the U.S. National Transplant Database. Transplantation. 2012;94(10):990-998.

[14] Cleper R, Ben Shalom E, Landau D, Weissman I, Krause I, Konen O. Post-transplantation lymphoproliferative disorders in pediatric kidney-transplant recipients – a national study. Pediatr Transplant. 2012;16(6):619-626.

[15] Kremer BE, Reshef R, Misleh JG, Christie JD, Ahya VN, Blumenthal NP. Pos-transplant lymphoproliferative disorder after lung transplantation: A review of 35 cases. J Heart Lung Transplant. 2012;31(3):296-304.

[16] Kremers WK, Devarbhavi HC, Wiesner RH, Krom RA, Mason WR, Habermann TM. Post-transplant lymphoproliferative disorders following liver transplantation: Incidence, risk factors and survival. Am J Transplant. 2006;6(5Pt1):1017-1024.

[17] Jagadeesh D, Woda BA, Draper J, Evens AM. Post-transplant lymphoproliferative disorders: Risk, classification, and therapeutic recommendations. Curr Treat Options Oncol. 2012;13(1):122-136.

[18] Tsai DE, Hardy CL, Tomaszewski JE, et al. Reduction in immunosuppression as initial therapy for posttransplant lymphoprolypherative disorder: Analysis of prognostic variables and long-term follow-up of 42 adult patients. Transplantation. 2001;71:1076-1088.

[19] Loren AW, Porter DL, Stadtmauer EA, Tsai DE. Post-transplant lymphoproliferative disorder: A review. Bone Marrow Transplantation. 2003;31:145-155.

[20] Heslop HE, How I treat EBV lymphoprolyferation. Blood. 2009;114(19):

[21] Cannon MJ, Scmid DS, Hyge TB. Review of cytomegalovirus seroprevalence and demographic characteristoics associated with infection. Rev Med Virol. 2010;20:202-210.

[22] Sinclair J, Sissons P. Latency and reactivation of human cytomegalovirus. J Gen Virol. 2006;87:1763-1779.

[23] Stratta RJ, Pietrangeli C, Baillie GM. Defining the risks for Cytomegalovirus infection and disease after solid organ transplantation. Pharmacotherapy. 2010;30:144-157.

[24] Manuel O, Pang XL, Humar A, Kumar D, Doucette K, Preiksaitis JK. An assessment of donor-to-recipient transmission patterns of human cytomegalovirus by analysis of viral genomic variants. J Infect Dis. 2009;199:1621-1628.

[25] Croen KD. Latency of human herpesvirus. Annu Rev Med. 1991;42:61-67.

[26] Razonable RR. Epidemiology of cytomegalovirus disease in solid organ and hematopoietic stem cell transplant recipients. Am J Health Syst Pharm. 2005;62:S7-13.

[27] Egli, A, Binggeli S, Bodaghi S, Dumoulin A, FunK GA, Khana N, Leuenberger D, Gosert R, Hirsch HH. Cytomegalovirus and Polyomsvirus BK post-transplant. Nephrol Dial Transplant. 2007;22(Suppl 8):viii72-vii82.

[28] Britt WJ. Infections associated with Human Cytomegalovirus. In: Glasser R and JE Jones (Edds), Herpesvirus Infection 1994 Marsel Dekker Ins. Pp 59-116.

[29] Razonable R. Direct and indirect effects of cytomegalovirus: Can we prevent them. Enferm Infecc Microbiol Clin. 2010;28:1-5.

[30] Eid AJ, Razonable RR. New developments in the management of cytomegalovirus infection after solid organ transplantation. Drugs. 2011;70:965-981.

[31] Brennan DC, Legendre C, Patel D et al. Cytomegalovirus incidence between everolimus versus mycophenolate in de novo renal transplants: Pooled analysis of three clinical trials. Am J Transplant. 2011;11:2453-2462.

[32] Portela D, Patel R, Larson-Keller JJ, et al. OKT3 treatment for allograft rejection is a risk factor for cytomegalovirus disease in liver transplantation. J Infect Dis. 1995;171:1014-1018.

[33] Ribin RH, Wolfson JS, Cosimi AB, et al. Infection in the renal transplant recipient. Am J Med. 1981;70:405-411.

[34] Eid AJ, Arthurs SK, Deziel PJ, Wilhelm MP, Razonable RR. Clinical predictors of relapse after treatment of primary gastrointestinal cytomegalovirus disease in solid organ transplant recipients. Am J Transplant. 2010;10:157-161.

[35] Razonable RR, Humar A, and the AST Infectious Disease Community of Practice. Cytomegalovirus in solid organ transplantation. Am J Transplant. 2013;13(s4):93-106.

[36] Lauttenschlager I, Loginov R, Makisalo H, Hockerstedt K. Prospective study on CMV-reactivations under preemptive strategy in CMV-seropositive adult liver transplant recipients. J Clin Virol. 2013;57:50-53.

[37] Donaldson PT, O'Grady J, Portmann B, et al. Evidence for an immune response to HLA class I antigens in the vanishing-bile duct syndrome after liver transplantation. Lancet. 1987;1:945-948.

[38] Smyth RL, Scott J, Borisiewicz LK, et al. Cytomegalovirus infection in heart-lung transplant recipients: Risk factors, clinical associations, and response treatment. J Infect Dis. 1991;164:1045-1050.

[39] Wingard JR, Mellitis ED, Sostrin MB, et al. Interstitial pneumonitis after allogeneic bone marrow transplantation. Medicine. 1988;67:175-186.

[40] Potena L, Valantine HA. Cytomegalovirus–associated allograft rejection in heart transplant recipients. Curr Opin Infect Dis. 2007;20:425-431.

[41] Eid AJ, Arthurs SK, Deziel PJ, Wilhelm MP, Razonable RR. Clinical predictors of relapse after treatment of primary gastrointestinal cytomegalovirus disease in solid organ transplant recipients. Am J Transplant. 2010;10:157-161.

[42] Paya CV, Hermans PE, Wiesner RH, et al. Cytomegalovirus hepatitis in liver transplantation: Prospective analysis of 93 consecutive orthotopic liver transplantations. J Infect Dis. 1989;160:752-758.

[43] Ljungman P, Griffiths P, Paya C. Definitions of cytomegalovirus infection and disease in transplant recipients. Clin Infect Dis. 2002;34:1094-1097.

[44] Humar A, Mazzulli T, Moussa G, et al. Clinical utility of cytomegalovirus (CMV) serology testing in high-risk CMV D+/R- transplant recipients. Am J Transplant. 2005;5:1065-1070.

[45] Razonable RR, Paya CV, Smith TF. Role of the laboratory in diagnosis and management of cytomegalovirus infection in hematopoietic stem cell and solid organ transplant recipients. J Clin Microbiol. 2002;40:746-752.

[46] Humar A, Limaye AP, Blumberg EA, et al. Extended valgancyclovir prophylaxis in D +/R- kidney transplant recipients is associated with long-term reduction in cytomegalovirus disease: Two-year results of the IMPACT study. Transplantation. 2010;90:1427-1431.

[47] Myhre HA, Haug Dorenberg D, Kristiansen KI, et al. Incidence and outcome of gancyclovir-resistent cytomegalovirus infection in 1244 kidney transplant recipients. Transplantation. 2011;92:217-223.

[48] Lurain NS, Choi S. Antiviral drug resistance of human cytomegaloirus. Clin Microbial Rev. 2010;23:689-712.

[49] Marty FM, Winston D, Rowley SD, Boeckh M, Vanse E, Papanicolaou G, Robertson A, Godkin S, Painter W. CMX001 for prevention and control of CMV infection in CMV-seropositive allogenic stem-cell transplant recipients: A phase 2 randomized, double-blind, placebo-controlled, dose-escalation trial of safety, tolerability and antviral activity. Biol Blood Marrow Transplant. 2012;18:S203-S204.

[50] Marcelin JR, Beam E, Razonable RR. Cytomegalovirus infection in liver transplant recipients: Updates on clinical management. World J Gastoenterology. 2014;20(31): 10658-10667.

[51] Griffiths, P, Plotkin S, Mocarski E, Pass R, Schleiss M, Krause P, Bialek S. Desirability and feasibility of a vaccine against cytomegalovirus. Vaccine. 2013;31(Suppl 2):B197-B203.

[52] Heininger U, Seward JE. Varicella. Lancet. 2006;368:1365-1376.

[53] Gilden DH, Kleinschmidt-DeMasters BK, LaGuardia JJ, Mahalingam R, Cohrs RJ. Neurological complications of the reactivation of varicella-zoster virus. N Engl J Med. 2000;342:635-645.

[54] Grose C. Varicella zoster virus infections: Chickenpox, shingles, and varicella vaccine. In; Glaser R, Jones JF (eds). Herpesvirus Infections 1994. Marsel Dekker Ins; 117-185.

[55] Howarth CB. Recurrent varicella-like illness in children with leukemia. Lancet. 1974;2:342.

[56] Rodriguez-Moreno A, Sanchez-Fructuolo AJ, Calvo N, Ridao N, Coneza J, Marques M, Prat SD, Barrientos A.Varicella infection in adult renal allograft recipients: Experience at one center. Transplant Proc. 2006;38:2416-2418.

[57] Levitsky J, Kalie AC, Meza JL, Hurst GE, Freifeld A. Chicken Pox after pediatric liver transplantation. Liver transplantation. 2005;11(12):1563-1566.

[58] Pacini-Edelstein SJ, Mehra M, Amen ME, Vargas JH, Martin MG, McDiarmid SV. Varicella in pediatric liver transplant patients: A retrospective analysis of treatment and outcome. J Pediatr Gastroenterol Nutr. 2003;37:183-186.

[59] Straus se, Ostrove JM, Inchauspe G, Felser JM, Freifeld A, Croen KD, Sawyer MH. NIH conference. Varicella-zoster virus infections. Biology, natural history, treatment, and prevention. Ann Intern Med. 1988;108:221-237.

[60] Blennow O, Fjaertoft G, Winiarski J, Ljungman P, Mattsson J, Remberger M. Varicella-zoster reactivation after allogeneic stem cell transplantation without routine prophylaxis the incidence remains high. Biol Blood Marrow Transplant. 2014;20(10): 1646-1649.

[61] Pergam SA, Forsberg CW, Boeckh MJ, et al. Herpes zoster incidence in a multicenter cohort of solid organ transplant recipients. Transplant Infect Dis. 2011;13:15-23.

[62] Locksley RM, Flounoy N, Sullivan KM, Meyers JD. Infection with varicella-zoster virus after marrow transplantation. J Infect Dis. 1985;152:1172-1181.

[63] Grose C, Giller RH. Varicella-zoster virus infection and immunization in the healthy and immunocompromized host. CRC Crit Rev Oncol/Hematol. 1988;8:27-64.

[64] Pergam SA, Limaye AP and the AST Infectious Diseases Community of Practice. Varicella zoster virus in solid organ transplantation. Am J Transplant. 2013;13:138-146.

[65] American Academy of Pediatrics. Varicella-Zoster Infections. In: Pickering LK, Baker CJ, Kimberlin DW, Long SS (eds). Red Book 2012: Report of the Committee on Infectious Diseases, 29th ed. Elk Grove Village, IL: American Academy of Pediatrics 2012; pages 774-789; 841-847.

[66] Coffin SE, Hodinka RL. Utility of direct immunofluorescence and virus culture to detection of varicella-zoster virus in skin lesions. J Clin Microbiol. 1995;33:2792-2795.

[67] Weinberg A, Horslen SP, Kaufman SS, et al. Safety and immunogenicity of varicella-zoster virus vaccine in pediatric liver and intestine transplant recipients. Am J Transplan 2006;6:565-568.

[68] Hata A, Asanuma H, Rinki M, et al. Use of an inactivated varicella vaccine in recipientas of hematopoietic-cell transplants. N Engl J Med. 2002;347:26-34.

[69] Smith JS, Robinson NJ. Age-specific prevalence of infection with herpes simplex type 2 and 1: A global review. J Infect Dis. 2002;186(Suppl 1):S3-S28.

[70] Corey L. Herpes Simplex Virus. In: Mandell GL, Bennett JE, Dolin R (eds). Mandell, Douglas and Bennett's Principles and Practice of Infectious Diseases. 6th ed. Philadelphia: Elsevier Churchill Livingstone 2005; p. 1762-1780.

[71] Xu F, Sternberg MR, Kottiri BJ, McQuillan GM, Lee FK, Nahmias AJ, Berman SM, Markowitz LE. Trends in herpes simplex virus type 1 and type 2 seroprevalence in the United States. JAMA. 2006;296(8):964-973.

[72] Kimberlin DW. Herpes simplex virus infections in neonates and early childhood. Semin Pediatr Infect Dis. 2005;16(4):271-281.

[73] Kimberlin DW, Rouse DJ. Genital herpes. New Engl J Med. 2004;350(19):1970-1977.

[74] Koelle DM, Corey L. Recent progress in herpes simplex virus immunobiology and vaccine research. Clin Microbiol Rev. 2003;16(1):96-113.

[75] Gnann JW. Herpes Simplex Virus and Varicella Zoster Virus Infections in Hematopoietic Stem Cell or Solid Organ Transplantation. In: Bowden RA, Ljungman P, Paya CV (eds). Transplant Infections. 2nd ed. Philadelphia: Lippincot, Williams, & Wilkins 2003; p. 350-366.

[76] Miller GG, Dummer JS. Herpes simplex and varicella zoster viruses: Forgotten but not gone. Am J Transplant. 2007;7(4):741-747.

[77] Patel R, Paya CV. Infections in solid-organ transplant recipients. Clin Microbiol Rev. 1997;10(1):86-124.

[78] Roizman B, Knipe DM, Whitley RJ. Herpes Simplex Viruses. In: Knipe DM, Howley PM (eds). Fields Virology. 5th ed. Philadelphia: Lippincot, Williams, & Wilkins 2007; p. 2501-2601.

[79] Wald A, Huang ML, Carrell D, Selke S, Corey L. Polymerase chain reaction for detection of herpes simplex virus (HSV) DNA on mucosal surfaces: Comparison with HSV isolation in cell culture. J Infect Dis. 2003;188(9):1345-1351.

[80] Hoshino Y, Dalai SK, Wang K, Pesnicak L, Lau TY, Knipe DM, Cohen JI, Straus SE. Comparative efficacy and immunogenicity of replication-defective, recombinant glycoprotein, and DNA vaccines for herpes simplex virus 2 infections in mice and guinea pigs. J Virol. 2005;79(1):410-418.

[81] Knowles MA, Pipkin P, Andrews N, et al. Population-based study of antibody to the human polyomavirises BKV and JCV and the simian polyomavirus SV40. J Med Virol. 2003;71:115-123.

[82] Flaegstad T, Ronne K, Filipe AR, Traavic T. Prevalence of BK virus antibody in Portugal and Norway. Scand J Infect Dis. 1989;21(2):145-147.

[83] Padgett BL, Walker DL. Prevalence of antibodies in human sera against JC virus, an isolate from the case of progressive multifocal leukoencephalopathy. J Infect Dis. 1973;127(4):467-470.

[84] Dolei A, Pietropaolo V, Gomes E, et al. Polyomavirus persistence in lymphocytes: Prevalence of lymphocytes from blood donors and healthy personnel of a blood transfusion center. J Gen Virol. 2000;81:21967-1973.

[85] Reploeg MD, Storch GE, Clifford DB. BK virus: A clinical review. Clin Infect Dis. 2001;33(2):191-202.

[86] Dropulic LK, Jones RJ. Poliomavirus BK infection in blood and marrow transplant recipients. Bone Marrow Transplant. 2008;41(1):11-18.

[87] Bressollette-Bodin C, Coste-Burel M, Hourmant M, Sebille V, Andre-Garnier E, Inbert-Marsille BM. A prospective longitudinal study of BK virus infection in 104 renal transplant recipients. Am J Transplant. 2005;5(8):1926-1933.

[88] Hirsch HH, Knowles W, Dickenmann M, et al. Prospective study of polyomavirus type BK replication and nephropathy in renal transplant recipients. N Engl J Med. 2002;347(7):488-496.

[89] Sood P, Senanayake S, Sujeet K, et al. Management and outcome of BK viremia in renal transplant recipients: A prospective single-center study. Transplantation. 2012;94(8):814-822.

[90] Hirsch HH, Randawa P; AST Infectious Disease Control. BK polyomavirus in solid organ transplantation. Am J Transplant. 2013;13(Suppl 4):179-188.

[91] Randhawa P, Bohl D, Brennan D, Ruppert K, Ramaswami B, Storch G, et al. Longitudinal analysis of levels of immunoglobulins against BK virus capsid proteins in kidney transplant recipients. Clin Vaccine Immunol. 2008;15(10):1564-1571.

[92] Wiseman AC. Polyomavirus nephropathy: A current perspective and clinical consideration. Am J Kidney Dis. 2009;54(1):131-142.

[93] Hirsch HH, Knowles W, Dickenmann M, Passweg J, Klimkait T, Mihatch MJ, et al. Polyomavirtus-associated nephropathy in renal transplantation: Interdisciplinary analysdis and recommendations. Transplantation. 2005;79(10)1277-1286.

[94] Hilton R and Tong CYW. Antiviral therapy for polyomavirus associated nephropathy after renal transplantation. J Antimicrobial Chemother. 2008;62(5):855-859.

[95] Sharma BN, Li R, Bernhoff E, Guttenberg TJ, Rinaldo CH. Fluoroquinolonesd inhibit human polyomavirus BK (BKV) replication in primary human kidney cells. Antiviral Res. 2011;92(1):115-123.

[96] Boothput R, Brennan DC. Human polyoma viruses and disease with emphasis on clinical BK and JC. J Clin Virol. 2010;47:306-312.

[97] Padgett BL, Walker DL, ZuRhein MG, Eckroade RJ, Dessel BH. Cultivation of papova-like virus from human brain with progressive multifocal leucoencephalopathy. Lancet. 1971;1(7712):1257-1260.

[98] Garsia-Suarez J, deMiguel D, Krsnik I, Banas H, Arribas I, Burgaleta C. Changes in the natural history of progressive multifocal leucoencephalopathy in HIV-negative lymphoproliferative disorders: Impact of novel therapies. Am J Hematol. 2005;80(4): 271-281.

[99] Engsig FN, Hansen AB, Omland LH, Kronborg G, Gerstoft J, Laursen AL, et al. Incidence, clinical presentation, and outcome of progressive multifocal leucoencephalopathy in HIV-infected patients during the highly active antiretroviral therapy era: A nationwide cohort study. J Infect Dis. 2009;199(1):77-83.

[100] Koralnic IJ, Boden D, Mai VX, Lord CI, Letvin NL. JC virus DNA load in patients with and without progressive multifocal leucoencephalopathy. Neurology. 1999;52:253-260.

[101] Crowder CD, Gyure KA, Drachenberg CB, Werner J, Morales RE, Hirsch HH, et al. Successful outcome of progressive multifocal leucoencephalopathy in a renal transplant patients. Am J Transplant. 2005;5:1151-1158.

[102] Ison MG. Respiratory viral infections in transplant recipients. Antiviral Therapy. 2007;12:627-638.

[103] Ison MG. Respiratory viral infections in transplant recipients. Curr Opin Organ Transplant. 2005;10:312-319.

[104] Billings JL, Hertz MI, Savik K, Wendt CH. Respiratory viruses and chronic rejection in lung transplant recipients. J Heart Lung Transplant. 2002;21:559-566.

[105] Anaissie EJ, Mahfouz TH, Aslan T, et al. The natural history of respiratory syncytial virus infection in cancer and transplant patients: Implication for management. Blood. 2004;103:1611-1617.

[106] Vilchez RA, McCurry K, Dauber J, et al. Influenza virus infection in adult solid organ transplant patients. Am J Transplant. 2002;2:287-291

[107] Ison MG. Adenovirus infections in transplant recipients. Clin Infect Dis. 2006;43:331-339.

[108] Martino R, Porras RP, Rabella N, et al. Prospective study of the incidence, clinical feature, and outcome of symptomatic upper and lower respiratory tract infections by

respiratory viruses in adult recipients of hematopoietic stem cells transplants for hematopoietic malignancies. Biol Blood Marrow Transplant. 2005;11:781-796.

[109] Weinberg A, Brewster L, Clark J, Simoes E. Evaluation of R-Mix shell vials for the diagnosis of viral respiratory tract infections. J Clin Virol. 2004;30:100-105.

[110] Rovida F, Percivalle E, Zavattoni M, et al. Monoclonal antibodies versus reverse transcription-PCR for detection of respiratory viruses in a patient population with respiratory tract infections admitted to hospital. J Med Virol. 2005;75:3369347.

[111] Brunstein J, Thomas E. Direct screening of clinical specimens for multiple respiratory pathogens using the Genaco Respiratory Panel 1 and 2. Diagn Mol Pathol. 2006;15:169-173.

[112] Boeckh M, Berrey MM, Bowden RA, Crawford SW, Balsley J, Corey I. Phase 1 evaluation of the respiratory syncytial virus-specific monoclonal antibody palivisumab in recipients of hematopoietic stem cell transplants. J Infect Dis. 2001;184:350-354

[113] Wyde PR, Chetty SN, Jewell AM, Boivin G, Piedra PA. Comparison of the inhibition of human metapneumovirus and respiratory syncytial virus by ribavirin and immune serum globulin in vitro. Antivir Res. 2003;60:51-59.

[114] Heemskerk B, Lankester AC, van Vreeswijk T, et al. Immune reconstitution and clearance of human adenovirus viremia in pediatric stem-cell recipients. J Infect Dis. 2005;191:520-530.

[115] Hayden FG, Herrington DT, Coats TL, et al. Efficacy and safety of oral pleconaril for treatment of colds due to picornavirus in adults: Results of 2 double-blind, randomized, placebo-controlled trials. Clin Infect Dis. 2003;36:1523-1532.

[116] Patick AK. Rhinovirus chemotherapy. Antivir Res. 2006;71:391-396.

[117] Center for Disease Control and Prevention. Prevention and control of influenza: Recommendation of the Advisory Committee on Immunization Practices (ACIP). MMWR Recomm Rep. 2006;55(RR-10):1-42.

[118] Moscona A. Neuraminidase inhibitors for influenza. N Engl J Med. 2005;353:1363-1373.

[119] Lai CL, Ratziu V, Yuen MF, Poynard T. Viral hepatitis B. Lancet. 2003;3622089-2094.2094.

[120] Vento S, Cainelli F, Longhi MS. Reactivation of replication of hepatitis B and hepatitis C viruses after immunosuppressive therapy: An unresolved issue. Lancet Oncol. 2002;3333-340.340.

[121] Calabrese LH, Zein NN, Vassilopoulos D. Hepatitis B virus (HBV) reactivation with immunosuppressive therapy in rheumatic diseases: Assessment and preventive strategies. Ann Rheum Dis. 2006;65(8):983-989.

[122] Shouval D, Shibolet O. Immunosuppression and HBV reactivation. Semmin Liver Dis. 2013;33(2):167-177.

[123] Berger A, Preiser W, Kachel HG, Stumer M, Doerr HW. HBV reactivation after kidney transplantation. J Clin Virol. 2005;32(2):162-165.

[124] Bhamidimarri KB, Pan C. Hepatitis B reactivation during immunosuppression: From pathogenesis to management strategy. N A J Med Sci. 2011;4(1):44-49.

[125] Terrault N, Roche B, Samuel D. Management of the hepatitis B virus in the liver transplantation setting: A European and American perspective. Liver Transpl. 2005;11:716.

[126] Burra P, Germani G, Adam R, et al. Liver transplantation for HBV-related cirrhosis in Europe: An ELTR study on evolution and outcomes. J Hepatol. 2013;58:287.

[127] Graxy A, Laffi G, Zignego AL. Hepatitis C virus (HCV) infection: A systematic disease. Mol Aspects Med. 2008;29:85-95

[128] Lauer GM, Walker BD. Hepatitis C virus infection. N Engl J Med. 2001;345:41-52.

[129] Watt K, Veldt B, Charlton M. A practical guide to the management of HCV infection following liver transplantation. Am J Transplant. 2009;9:1707-1713.

[130] Zignego AL, Giannini C, Ferri C. Hepatitis C virus-related lymphoproliferative disorders: An overview. World J Gastroenterol. 2007;13:2467-2478.

[131] Zignego AL, Ganini C, Gragnani L, Piluso A, Fognan E. Hepatitis C virus infection in the immunocompromised host: A complex scenario with variable clinical impact. J Translac Med. 2012;10:158.

[132] Benhamou Y, Pockros P, Rodriguez-Torres M, Gordon S, Shiffman M, Lirue Y, Afdhai N, Lamon K, Kim Y, Murphy B. The safety and efficacy of viramidine plus PegINF alpha-2b versus ribavirin plus PegINF alpha-2b in therapy-naïve patients infected with HCV: Phase 3 results (VISERI). J Hepatol. 2006;44(Suppl 2):S273.

[133] Terrault NA, Adey B. The kidney transplant recipients with hepatitis C infection; Pre- and posttransplantation treatment. CJASN. 2007;2(3):563-575.

[134] Firpi RJ, Nelson DR. Management of viral hepatitis in hematologic malignancies. Blood Rev. 2008;22:117-126.

[135] Centers for Disease control and Prevention. Testing for HCV infection: An update to guidance for clinicians and laboratorians. MMWR Morb Morta/Wkly Rep. 2013;62(18):362-365.

Chapter 7

Biological Concepts on Bisphosphonate Treated Patients in the Context of Increasing Patient Life Quality and the Need for Oral Surgical Procedures

Metodi Abadzhiev

Additional information is available at the end of the chapter

http://dx.doi.org/10.5772/61731

Abstract

Bisphosphonates are used for treatment of different bone conditions, most frequently for increasing bone density in osteoporosis patients and for treatment of primary or metastatic bone tumor as well as intake for osteoporosis patients.

The pharmacokinetics of bisphosphonates is well described in order to clarify mechanisms of action of each sub-group according to the classification of these drugs.

Bisphosphonate-induced avascular osteonecrosis is described as phenomenon in the human bones especially observed in human jaws. From pathophysiological point of view this process is studied describing the osteoclast activity inhibition. Several studies and results are stated.

Having in mind that this process occurs in cases that do not include bisphosphonates intake, the American Association of Oral and Maxillofacial surgeons accept a new diagnostic and treatment strategies as well as new name of the disease - Medicine related osteonecrosis of the jaw.

By comprehensive analysis of all studies by now and cases from our practice, several important and significant protocols are introduced in this chapter, effecting diagnosis, treatment preparation, treatment and post-surgical behavior.

Keywords: Bisphosphonate-induced osteonecrosis of the jaw, dental implantology, medicine related osteonecrosis of the jaw

1. Introduction

Since it was first identified in 2003, bisphosphonate-induced osteonecrosis has been under growing control by medical and dental specialist alike because it affects cancer patients receiving intra-venous bisphosphonate therapy and osteoporosis patients receiving oral bisphosphonate therapy.

It is of significant importance to introduce the mechanism of action of this type of medications, way of distribution and risk of complication during or after treatment with them. A strategy of preparation, medication support and techniques before, during and after dental surgery procedures and especially placement of dental implants must be clarified in order to avoid bisphosphonate-induced osteonecrosis.

2. Indications for bisphosphonates

Even though they were founded in the 18th century, their real clinical usage began only a hundred years ago with the synthesis of the first bisphosphonate (BP)–etidronate. The birthplace of these medicines is considered to be the scientific institute in Davos, Switzerland, where a team headed by Herbert Fleisch, Sylvia Bisaz, and Roman Muhlbauer proved the role of bisphosphonates in bone metabolism and their importance in bone disorders treatment in 1967.

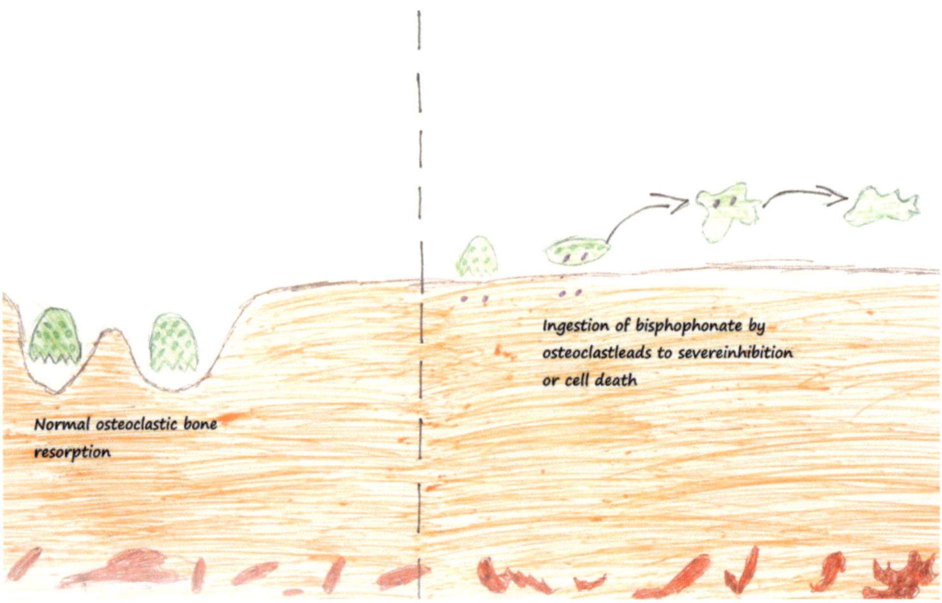

Figure 1. Normal osteoclast activity and osteoclasts death by bisphosphonate treatment (after R.E. Marx).

http://dx.doi.org/10.5772/61731

Data concerning pharmacokinetics of diphosphonates, later called bisphosphonates, were published for the first time in 1969. Forty-five years of experience, including researches, has significantly manifested the advantages and disadvantages of this drug group.

Inventing and developing bisphosphonates for treatment of different bone conditions is immense progress in solving fine mechanisms of bone formation and a significant development in medicine as a whole.

Bisphosphonates treatment indications are mainly for increasing bone density in osteoporosis patients (e.g. alendronate and rizedronate), and intravenous (IV) with mouth intake dosage for patients with primary or metastatic bone tumor (e.g. pamidronate and zoledronate). Intravenous intake is also recently tolerated in osteoporosis patients.

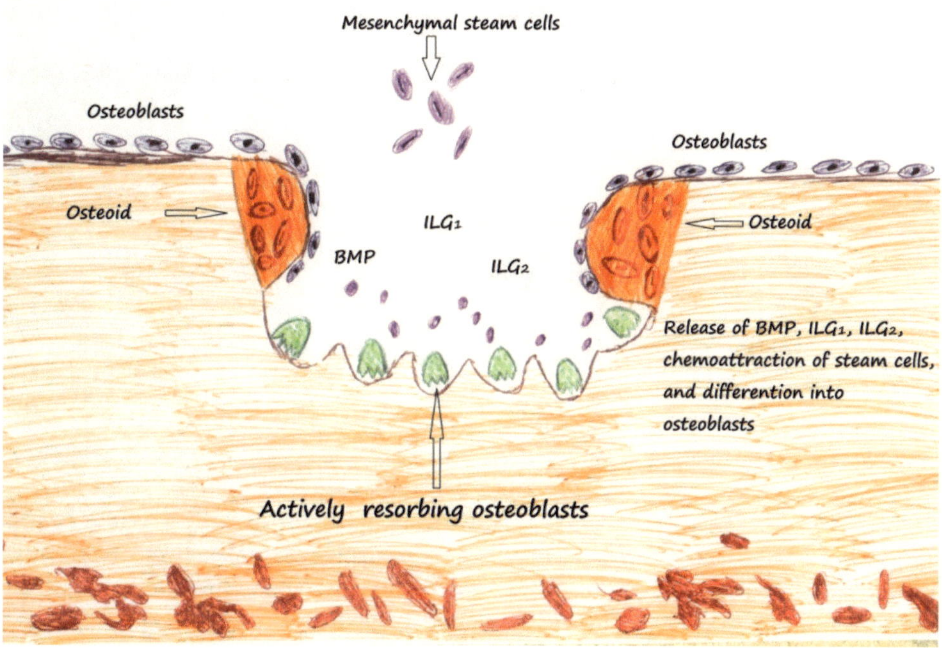

Figure 2. Scheme of bone metabolic unit (BMU) (after R.E. Marx).

3. Pharmacokinetics of the bisphosphonates

Bisphosphonates are chemically stable analogs of non-organic pyrophosphates (PPi) related to skeleton mineralization. Their development is related to inventing inhibitors of calcification in order to resist hydrolysis with alkaline phosphatase. PPi and BPs could not only slow down bone growth but also destroy hydroxyapatite crystals. BPs are remarkably efficient inhibitors to bone resorption during experiments in vitro and in vivo. During the process of their clinical application in the 1990s, it became clear that in order to clarify the chemical and physical reactions, and explain the variety of their biological effects, it is necessary to study the cell to cell interactions. Bisphosphonates suppress bone resorption by selective absorption to mineralized bone surface where they counteract to osteoclasts.

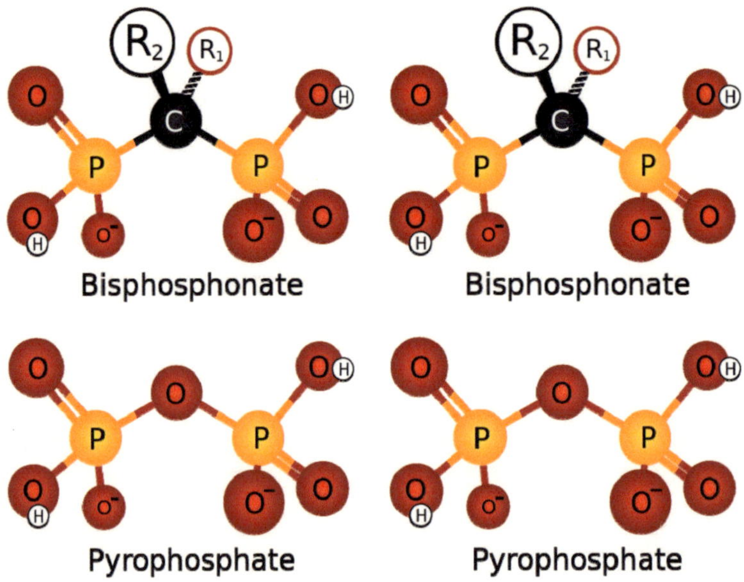

Figure 3. Basic molecular structure

Bisphosphonates couldcan be classified to at leastinto two groups with different molecular action mechanisms. The first one: is nitrogen free bisphosphonates (like etidronate and clodoronate) that interfere ATP-dependent intercellular ways. The second group is bisphosphonates with nitrogen, they that are more powerful (including pamidronate, alendronate, rizedronate, ibandronate, and zoledronate) they). They are metabolized differently, by inhibiting key enzymes of mevalonat/cholesterol biosynthetic way.

Precisely because of the obviously differentobvious biochemical and pharmacological differencedifferences and uneven intercellular interaction is important the division of, BPs in tohave been divided into separate groups and their specific usage according to a specific disease.

They are incorporated in skeletal bone without being degraded. Bisphosphonates are attached to Ca^{2+} in areas with increased bone resorption and stay integrated in the bone for 10 to 40 years – alendronate. For example, alendronate's half-life for example is 12 to 28 years. Once taken, BPs unlock cascade biochemical processes leading to loss of osteoclast ability to resorb bone or even to their apoptosis.

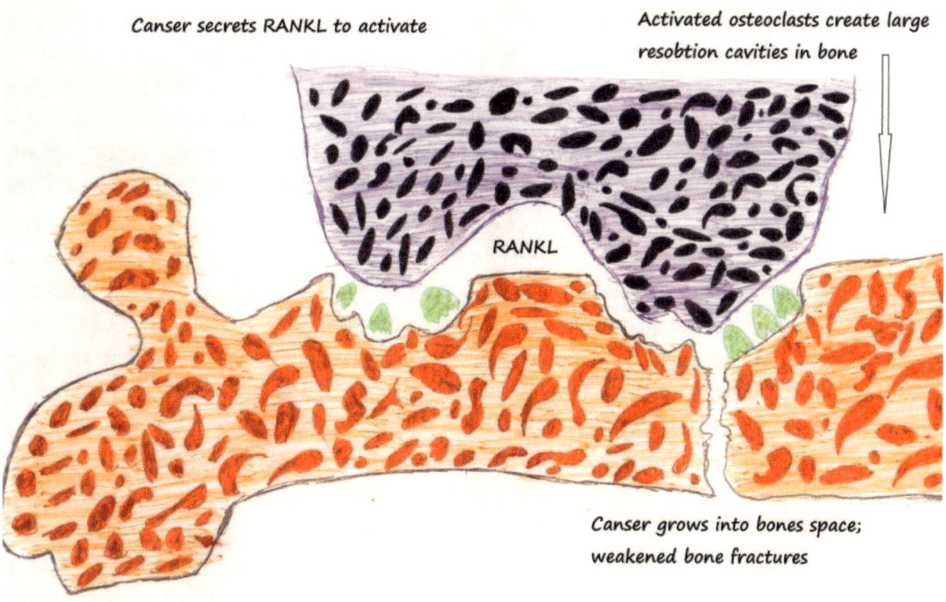

Figure 4. The way to bone fracture by solid bone tumors (after R.E. Marx).

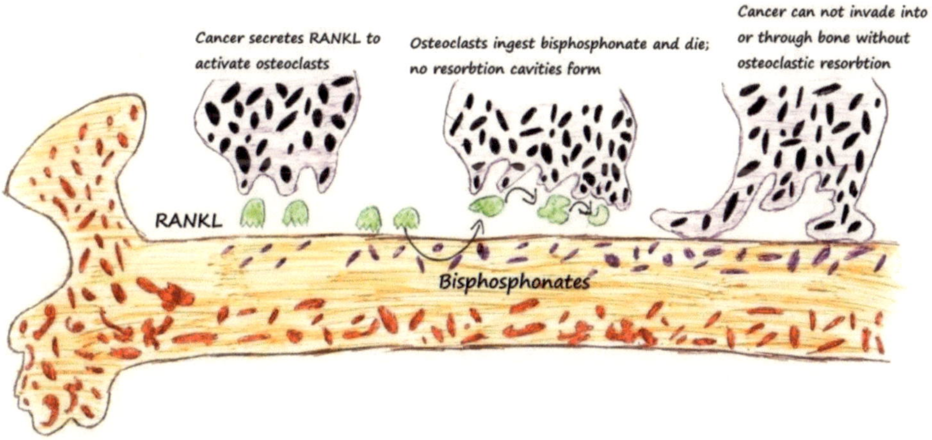

Figure 5. Prevention of bone resorption by bisphosphonate osteoclast inhibition (after R.E. Marx).

4. Bisphosphonate-induced osteonecrosis of the jaws

It is undoubtedly thatUndoubtedly, the intake increases the quality of life of the treated patients in general, but negative effecteffects should also be taken in tointo consideration. Stomach disorders, erosions of the esophagus, uveitis, flueflu-like conditions, muscle and joint pain, and severe necrosis in the maxillofacial area, known as BONJ – (bisphosphonate osteonecrosis of the jaw) could appear.

Recently inIn recent literature is found date for, a new type of complication associated with bisphosphonate intake –has been found, which is called avascular necrosis of the jaws. It is defined as necrosis associated with or without dental procedures, which could persist for more than 6-8 weeks with irresponsive to conservative treatment, found in patients without history of previous radiotherapy in the area affected but treated with nitrogen group bisphosphonates with nitrogen group, i.v. through IV for at least a year or per os for longer period, and associated with general condition withof bone resorption. Similar cases arewere published for the first time in 2003 by Marx with patients treated with pamidronate and zoledronate. Later, Carter and Gross, Ruggierro, Migliorati, and Wang reportalso reported similar cases. In 2005, Novartis (Aredia and Zometa48 producer) officially declaredeclared 475 cases of Bisphosphonate bisphosphonate-related osteonecrosis of the jaws. In nowadaysNowadays, the number of affected patients worldwide is unknown. Scientific literatures says the BONJ is from 1,.3% to 10%. More There are more than 5,.1 million patients are treated with bisphosphonates. More and more than 2 million acceptaccepted BPs as antimalignatanti-malignant therapy. The number of patients treated for osteoporosis with BPs is increasing rapidly. More than 10 million patients, mainly women in the USA has, have osteoporosis,. It and it is supposed that the number will increase to 12 million and 34. Thirty-four million patients older than 50 have decreased bone density and considered high risk for osteoporosis development. Oral BPs arewere prescribed to more than 70% of the patients diagnosed with osteoporosis in US during the USA in 2003- to 2006.((American association of Oral and Maxillofacial Surgeons)). More than 190 million prescriptions arewere issued in North America. In 2003 Alendronate, alendronate is 19th most prescribed medicine (17 million prescriptions) Risedronate), risedronate is 72nd (6 million prescriptions) zolendronate), while zoledronate is used from more than 300,000 sick people.

5. Pathophisiology of BONJ

Bisphosphonate-associated osteonecrosis of the jaws is a result of treatment with BPs, bone metabolism disorders and physiological micro damagemicrodamage of the jaws interferinginterfere their biomechanical properties. Oral cavity conditions, microtrauma, infections increase the efforts of the organism to bone recovery, exceeding the ability of the hipodynamic bone. Compared to all other bones maxilla and mandible are remodeled most frequently in the human body. This is the reason why BONJ is observed only in jaw-bones. Unlike to other bones in the human body, they are not enough protected enough. It is an important fact that only a thin mucosa and a periosteum are the only barriers protecting bone from injuries. From the other side teeth are prerequisite to easy microorganisms penetration and development of internal infections–caries and periodontal disease complications. It is interesting to mention that local factors like partial and full removable dentures are also factors that increase the risk of osteonecrosis. Smoking and continuous corticosteroid therapy are also risk factors.

According to Denn et al., all osteonecrosis cases describe todescribed in 2006 arewere associated with nitrogen containing bisphosphonates. In scientific literature, there is no single opinion which bisphosphonates exactly leads to more frequent BONJ development. The thought that Zoledroniczoledronic acid isis the most dangerous prevails. Most cases of BONJ are related with i.vIV intake.

In spite of the fact that for BONJ is has been here for a long period of time, factors that initiate the necrosis are still discussing.being discussed. It would be right to point out that for initiation of BONJ many factors are responsible with variable priority in different cases.

OnIn the first place, this is the inhibition of osteoclast activity and bone remodeling. But only this factor is not enough, because similar osteonecrosis would be observed in the other bones. Bacterial invasion with consequent inflammation is a factor that distinguish the condition in oral cavity compared to other body parts. The existence of various biofilm in oral cavity is dictated by different periodonatlperiodontal diseases, caries and its complications and periapical inflammation. This is a prerequisite for microorganism invasion to the left open bone left (after extraction, for example). In necroticNecrotic bone fragments after tooth extraction in BPs treated patients arehave isolated mainly Actinomyces species but also viruses and fungus. Angiogenesis suppression could also be initiator of jaw osteonecrosis. Medicines that disturb growth, migration, and differentiation of endothelial cells for new vessel formation playsplay an important role in avascular osteonecrosis. In addition to these basic factors to pathogenesis of medication-related osteonecrosis of the jaw (MRONJ could be added), microtrauma of the jaw during masticatory action and supposed harmful or acquired immune deficiency could also be added.

6. Prophylaxis and treatment of BONJ

In literature, there is no solidarity concerning bisphosphonate therapy suspension after the appearance of jaw-osteonecrosis. Marx suggests bisphosphonate therapy in onco-patients to be discussed with an oncologist in order to define positive effect/risk ratio, having in mind bisphosphonatebisphosphonate's half-life (10 years).

In literature thereThere is prevalence of BONJ with prior dental procedures compared to the so called spontaneous osteonecrosis and 33%–86% of the BONJ in literature are described after different dental procedures.

Prevailing opinion is that with ageas one gets older the danger from bisphosphonate osteonecrosis increases withby 9%.

Behavior inof diagnosed osteonecrosis patients is dependent on the disease stage. It should be mentioned that American Association of Oral and Maxillofacial Surgeons proposeproposed a change in the disease nomenclature formfrom BONJ to Medicine medication-related osteonecrosis of the jaws (MRONJ). The reason is an increasing number of patients with osteonecrosis of the jaws have been diagnosed after other drug intake (denosumab). Due to this reason Hence, the AAOMS changeschanged the name, which was accepted in 2009, on. On their consensus conference in 2014, with a Position Paper and in addition to the new name accepts, they accepted new diagnostic and treatment strategies corresponding to the contemporary researches., as follows:

1. I.v.IV bisphosphonates for treatment of primary bone tumors and bone metastasis, multiple myeloma, and severe osteoporosis but with lower dosage.

2. Oral bisphosphonates mainly for osteoporosis and osteopenia treatment, as well as PagetPaget's disease and osteogenesis imperfectimperfecta.

3. DenozumabDenosumab–RANK ligand inhibitor–it inhibits bone resorption by inhibition of the function of osteoclasts and as an advantage could be mentioned that it is not connected to the bone so within 6 months after treatment the risk of complications is slightly noticeable.

4. Antiangiogenetic medications–it is used in different tumor conditions and is useful due to the fact that preventsto prevent formation of new blood vessels. It connects to signal molecules responsible for blood vessels formation and interfereinterferes the angiogenesis signaling cascade.

According to AAOMSAAOMS's Position Paper, it is possible to think about MRONJ if several characteristics are present:

1. Antiresorptive or atiangiogenicantiangiogenic treatment conducted before or in the past.,

2. Bone that is exposed in the maxillofacial region through intraoral or extraoral fistula(e) persisting for more than 8 weeks, and

3. Lack of radiation therapy in the oro-facial region or metastatic disease to the jaws.

It should be mentioned that, according to the AAOMS, risk for osteonecrosis development in patients with bone tumors treated with zoledronate is 0% to 1%. It is similar in patients treated with denozumab.denosumab. A bit lower is the valuepercentage risk in patients treated with antiangiognetic drugs, like bevacizumab –, which is 0.2%. The risk for patients with osteoporosis treated with denozumabdenosumab and zoledoronate is 0.04%. It should be noted that with increasingthe longer the period of time for treatment is increasingthe higher the risk for jaw osteonecrosis form, from 0.5% for one year of treatment to 1.1% for three year years of treatment. After all it is a matter ofThese are based on retrospective studies of treated patients, which who have not been treated surgically in the oral cavity but has develophave developed spontaneous osteonecrosis. As aA trigger factor could be underlined tooth or even multiple teeth extraction and placement of dental implants. In differentDifferent retrospective studies are shown showed that 1.6% to 14.8% of patients treated i.v.through IV with BPs for longer than a year period of time and have developed osteonecrosis developed after tooth extraction. According to a research done by Carlos Pigrau ––Serralach et al since 2014, BONJ reachescases have reached 30.2% Viridance since 2014. Viridans group Streptococcistreptococci are isolated in 83.3% formfrom the cases and AcctinomycesActinomyces spp in 39.0% from all bone histological samples.

According to other studies, between 52% and 61% from all cases described of osteonecrosis of patientscases treated with bisphosphonates are triggered after surgical treatment – –a percentage that is extremely high. Retrospective research done by Kunchur R,., Need A,., Hughes T,., et al. in 2009, says stated that from0.5% out of 194 patients treated with oral bisphosphonates have developed osteonecrosis occurrence is 0.5% after tooth extraction. They assumeassumed that dental implant placement iswas with similar biological load as tooth extraction. Moreover, Donggeol Lee reportsreported that 77 patients treated with bisphosphonate undergounderwent implantology treatment, with 78 placed implants with 97.4% success equal to success in normal conditions. Sebastien Hoefert and Harald Eufinger report i.v.reported IV and per os antibiotic treatment in bisphosphonate treated patients before surgical treatment.

In 2009, P. Pechalova, A. Bakardjiev, B. Vladimirov, E. Poryazova, I. Angelova, and A. Jeleva publishpublished a case of a patient with bisphosphonate osteonecrosis of the mandible of a patient after consistent oral intake of 14 month consistent intake for fourteen months of FosamaxR (alendronate) (70mg per week dosage, taken once a week) and BonvivaR (ibadronate) (150mg month dosage, taken once a month) on the occasion ofdue to severe osteoporosis with pathological fractures of vertebras. The oddly think in the case published is bone sequester covered entirely with mucosa. Without fistula..

A group formfrom ITI (Bornstein, Cionca, Momblli)), based on a vast literature in 2009 differentiate, differentiated the surgeon behavior in patients with oral and i.v.IV bisphosphonate intake. They assumeassumed that, in addition to the way of intake there is, the duration of intake played an important role of the duration.. They saysaid that patients with osteoporosis/osteopenia take much lower dosage of bisphosphonate compared to cancer patients and, thus, the accumulation of the medicine should be several years. This is enough to conclude that In conclusion, patients who underwent oral surgical procedures are withhave significantly lower risk of necrosis in these patientscompared to those who had IV bisphosphonate intake.

Similar conclusions are were made by our team on the basis of 3 treatedthree patients in 3 yearswho underwent treatment for the period of three years. One of the patients were onhad an oral intake of bisphosphonates, one i.v.had IV, and one on DenozumabeDenosumabe (subcutaneous) As part of our). Our entire biological concept treatment include includes preliminary antibiotic treatment, irrigation with chlorxeidine solutions, general and local ozone therapy, hyperbaric chamber, PRGF usage, Er;Yag:YAG laser, photodynamic therapy, and minimally invasive surgical techniques.

7. Conclusions

During an surgical, respectively a surgery, such as implantology treatment, especially in bisphosphonate treated patients it is vital antibiotics preparation and is vital for the primary healing process to be guaranteed, especially in bisphosphonate treated patients. Usage of Clindamycin as osteotopicosteotropic antibiotics is a gold standard assuring lackto ensure absence of post-operation infection and prevention of complications. LackThe absence of dehiscence assureensures us smooth osteointegration process and lack of bone lose. That is whyFor this purpose, the common requirements for soft tissue management, include suitable implantology system, proper operation technique, atraumatic preparation, and last but not least proper suturing materials and technique. Implantology has extra sources like PRP, PRF,, PRGF, which could be applied with great success if it's needed. The high concentration of platelets rich in growth factors (PRGF) in the operation field contributecontributes to a light and with lack of troublestrouble-free post-operative process, guaranteeing perfect conditions for the osteointegration process. In cases of post-operative complications MethronidazoleMetronidazole is a matter of choice.

8. Clinical cases

8.1. Case 1

The patient has arrived at our clinic for the first time in 2009 with pain syndrome, periodontal abscess in the 47, 44, 31, 32, 41, and 42 area due to periodontitis developed formfrom the plaque with periodontal pockets form 6from 6mm to 8mm.,combined with chronic occlusal trauma from iatrogenic sharp edges of metal-ceramic constructions made years ago (X-ray, Fig. 1). Based on the anamnesis, a treatment with medicines was found–6 months treatment with Bonviva medicine–3mg once a month parenteral, associated with diagnosed osteopenia in 2007 with quantitative osteometry over tibia bone with T-score 2,9. It was considered that due to the short-term treatment with the bisphosphonate medicine and the 5five-year period after it by keepingto keep certain protocol for preparation and implantation, an implantology treatment could be initiated. A multiple extraction of 47, 44, 42, 41, 31, and 32 was undertaken after antibiotic protection, initial ultrasonic and sand-blasting therapy divided in tointo several appointments, high-intensity and low intensity laser therapy, local and general ozone therapy and hyperbaric therapy. Extraction sockets were filled with PRGF and sutured with PTFE. As an additional prophylaxis measure from bisphosphonates induced osteonecrosis, photodynamic therapy was used. The healing process was without any complications.

The treatment plane includesplan included the entire sanitation of the mouth, periodontal and endodontic preparation, and placement of 11 pieces titanium screwed implants. After uncovering of the implants, tooth 43 was planplanned for extraction despite the exact root-canal treatment, due theto long term prognosis and high risk of root fracture. TillUntil that time, this particular tooth was used for temporary fixed construction abutment. Because of the short clinical crowns, crown-lengthening was planplanned and performed with Er:YAG laser, based on the preliminary analysis of the size and shape of future prosthetic crowns and attached gingiva available. X-ray surgical guide was made, along with a prototype of the future prosthetic constructions, and was used for the CT. Due to the fact of previous bisphosphonate usage, a certain surgical protocol was used again including: antibiotic prophylaxis, high-intensity and low intensity laser therapy, local and general ozone therapy, hyperbaric therapy, PRGF, precise soft-tissue management and photodynamic therapy. One implant was placed in 15 area. Due to the lack of complications it was proceeded to, the placement of the rest of the planned implants proceeded. Bone type was D4 for the maxilla and D3 for the mandible. Bone spreaders were used for bone condensation. The primary stability of the implants was 15 up to 30 N/cm. Osteotomic implant beds were shaped by the usage of the existing surgical guide. Existing bone doesdid not demandeddemand additional augmentative procedures. Suture material was 4/0 PTFE. On the both jaws, fixed long-term temporary constructions

http://dx.doi.org/10.5772/61731

waswere provided. After longer than usual period of waiting (more than ana year)), implants were uncovered by half-thickness flaps moved apically. All 11 implants were osteointegrated. After open-tray, impression technique with transfers zirconium abutments with titanium base were made. CAD-CAM zirconium constructions were madmade directly on the same model. In the frontal area constructions were made by blend-ceramic and distally full anatomy zirconium.

Complete functional rehabilitation of the masticatory apparatus was achieved. Aesthetic demands of the patient was covered completely.

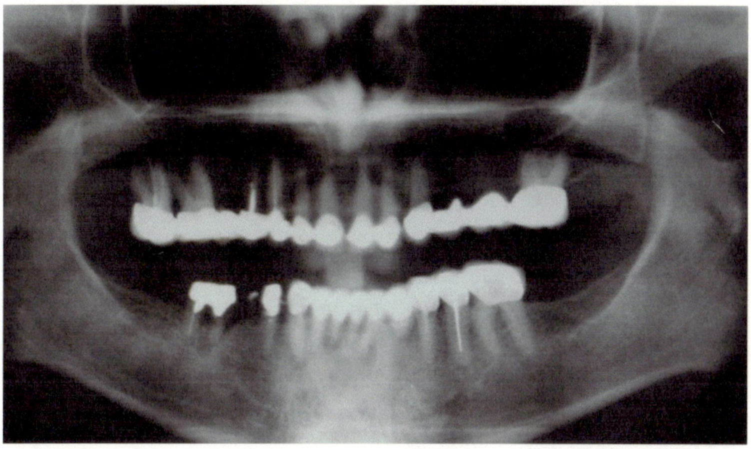

Figure 6. Basic X-ray

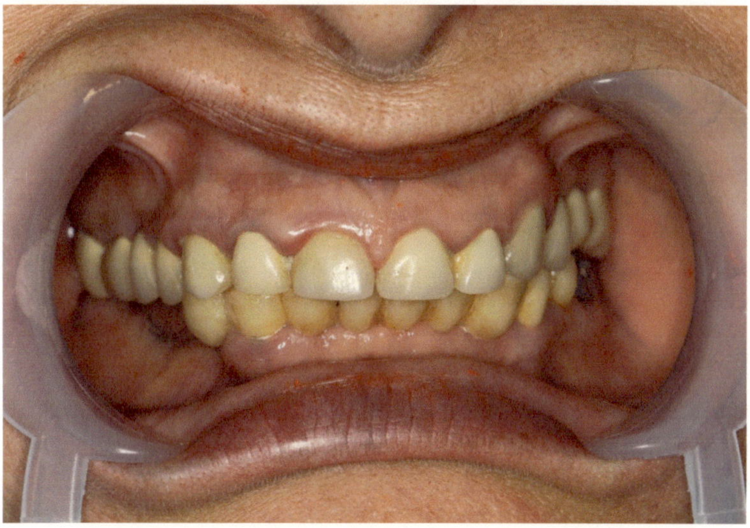

Figure 7. Intraoral situation after preliminary treatment

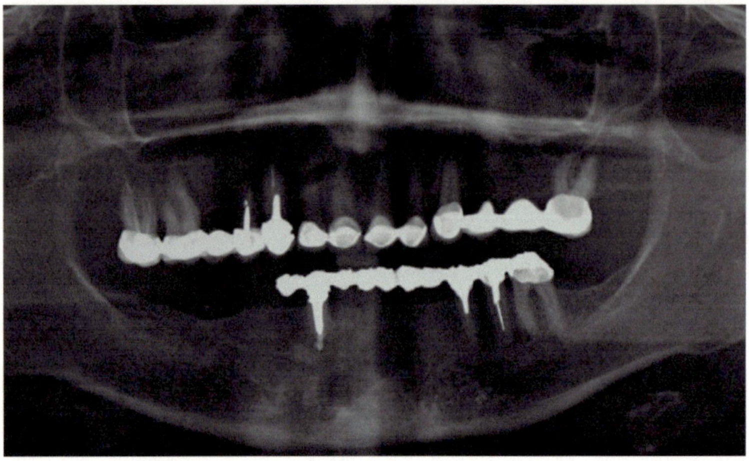

Figure 8. X-ray- before implant insertion

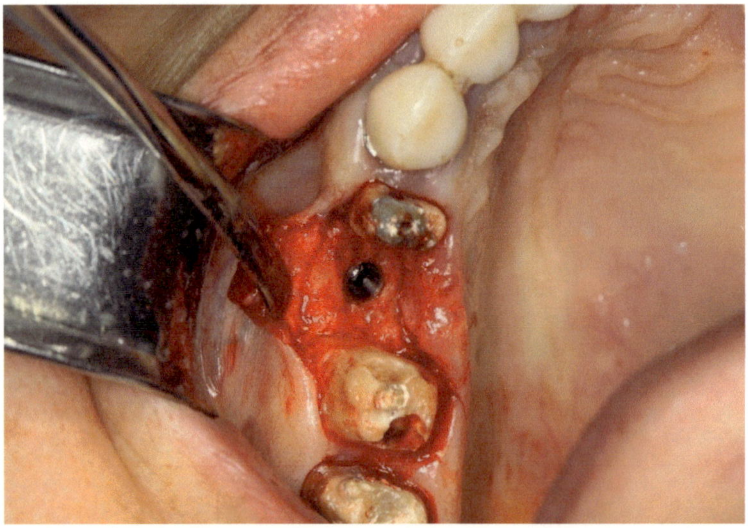

Figure 9. Minimal invasive insertion of the first implant

After preliminary treatment, the patient receivereceived one implnantimplant in the area of the second upper right premolar (15) accompanied with clindamycin prophylaxis, PRGF activation of the implant surface and covered by PRFG fibrin membrane, combined with postimplantationpost implantation photodynamic therapy using PhotoSan® for 4 minutes, two timetimes a day tilluntil the suture removal, and ozone therapy in the first three days combined with hyperbaric-chambers.

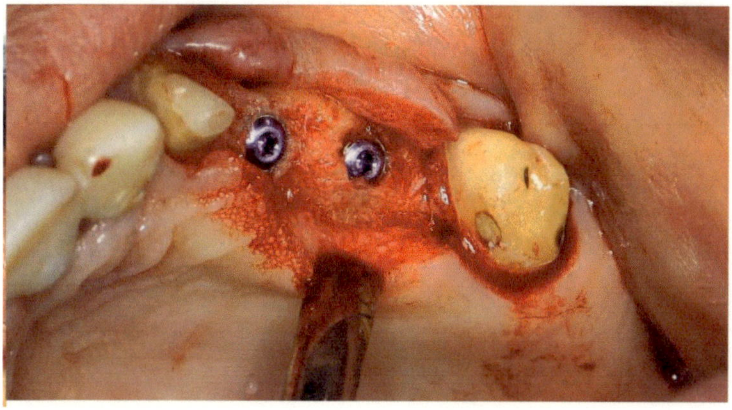

Figure 10. Implant insertion in second quadrant

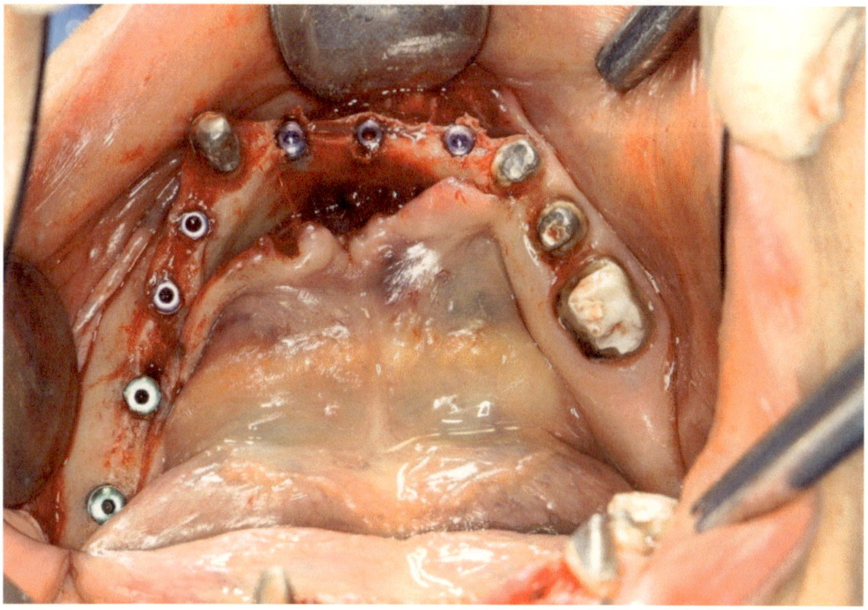

Figure 11. Implant insertion in lower jowjaw

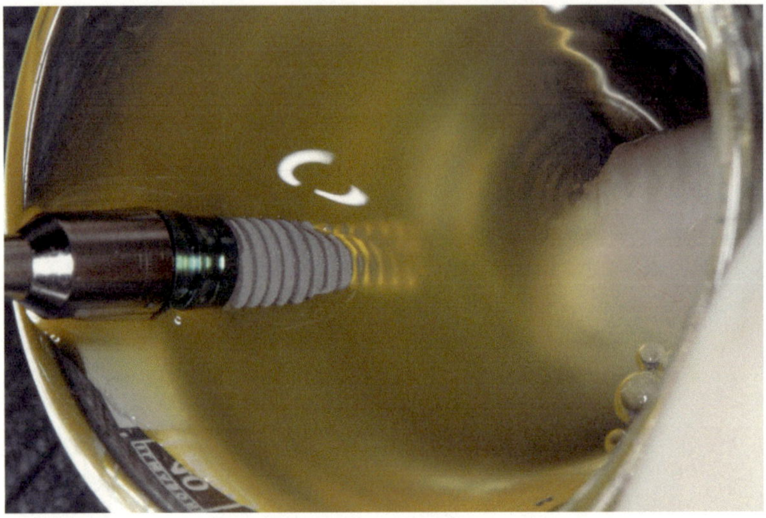

Figure 12. Activation of implant surface with PRGF

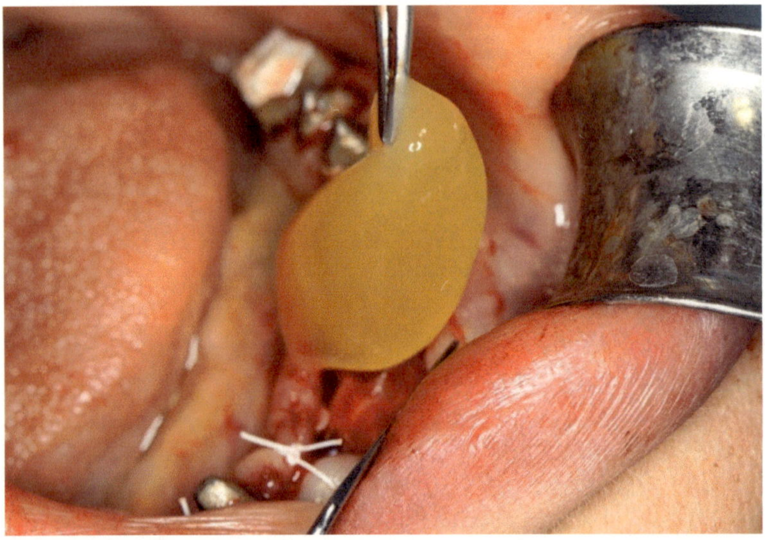

Figure 13. PRGF membrane for covering of the implants

The high concentration of platelets rich in growth factors (PRGF) in the operation field contributecontributes to a light and with lack of troubles trouble-free post-operative process, guaranteeing perfect conditions for the osteointegration process.

The process of tissue repair iswas based on a complex cascade of biological events controlled by a long list of biologically active growth factors and proteins. The spatial and temporal action of this family of mediators on the tissue-damaged area regulates the mechanisms and phases that govern tissue repair and regeneration

http://dx.doi.org/10.5772/61731

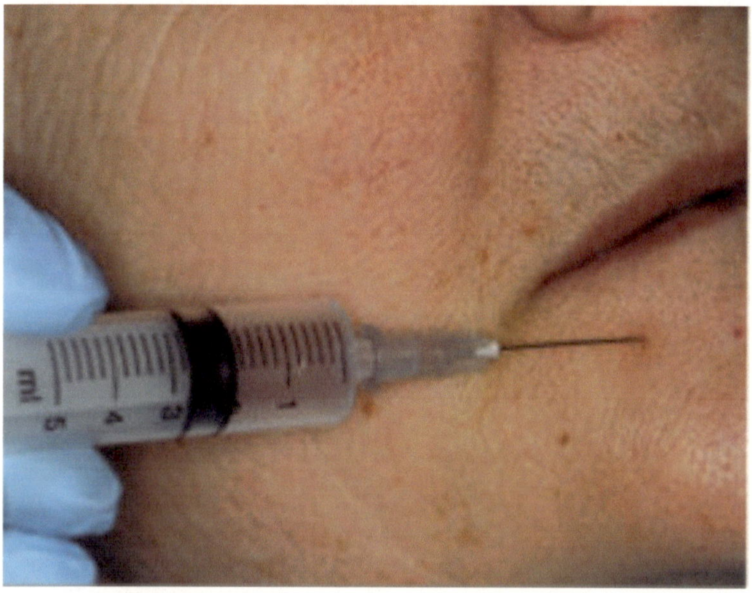

Figure 14. Pure ozone injected subcutaneously in the manipulation area

Another method used in our biological concept is ozone therapy. There are several known actions of ozone onin the human body, such as anti-microbial, immunostimulating, antihipoxyc, analgesic, detoxicating, bioenergetics and biosynthetic (activation of the metabolism of carbohydrates, proteins and lipids)), etc. Ozone is a relatively rare and unstable molecule composed of three oxygen atoms O_3. The normal oxygen molecule has two oxygen atoms O_2. Stratospheric ozone is important in the earth system because it absorbs ultraviolet radiation from the sun, protecting life on earth. The beneficial biological effects of ozone, is its antimicrobialantimicrobial activity. How we can derive ozon?the ozone? Using a simple electric arc, we can produce ozone. In case, for example, of bone regeneration, for example, the purpose of ozone using ozone is the initial local growth factor expression and stimulatetion stimulate the migration of osteoprogenitor cells to the wound site and subsequentlyand subsequently, in a controlled fashion, to direct their differentiation to the osteogenic cell line. Throughout this process, another set of factors will regulate the dynamic equilibrium between cell inhibition and proliferation, as well as angiogenesis and extracellular matrix formation. Ozone-generator can introduce pure ozone in saline. Ozone infusion is also precious for the fact that it generates a therapeutic effect on faster post op wound healing and preliminary preparation of the patient by avoiding further complications and assuring on 99% smooth primary closure. Anti-microbial effect of ozone asis a result of its action on cells by damaging its cytoplasmatic membrane due to ozonolysis of dual bonds and also ozone-induced modification of intercellular contents because of secondary oxidants effects. This action is non-specific and selective to microbial cells, it does not dameagedamage human cells because of their major antioxidative ability. Ozone is very efficient in antibiotics resistant strains. Its anti-microbial activity increases in liquid environment of acidic pH. In viral infections, the ozone action lies in the intolerance of infected cells to peroxides and change of activity of reverse transcriptase, which takes part in synthesis of viral proteins.

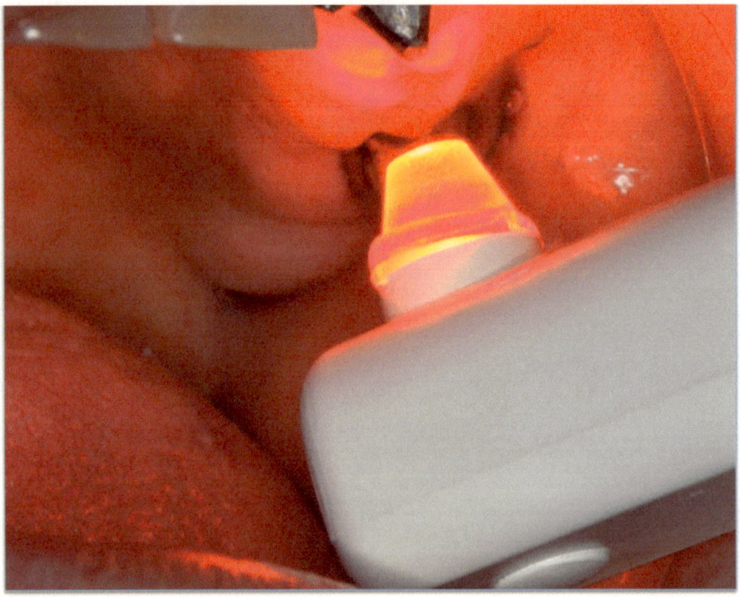

Figure 15. Usage of photodynamic therapy contributecontributes to cell destruction of the microorganisms and preventprevents complications and accelerateaccelerates wound healing

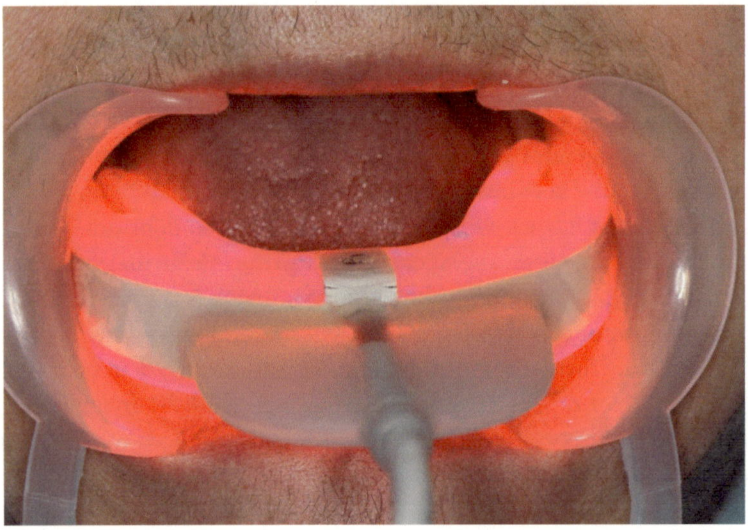

Figure 16. Photodynamic therapy with photodynamic intraoral tray

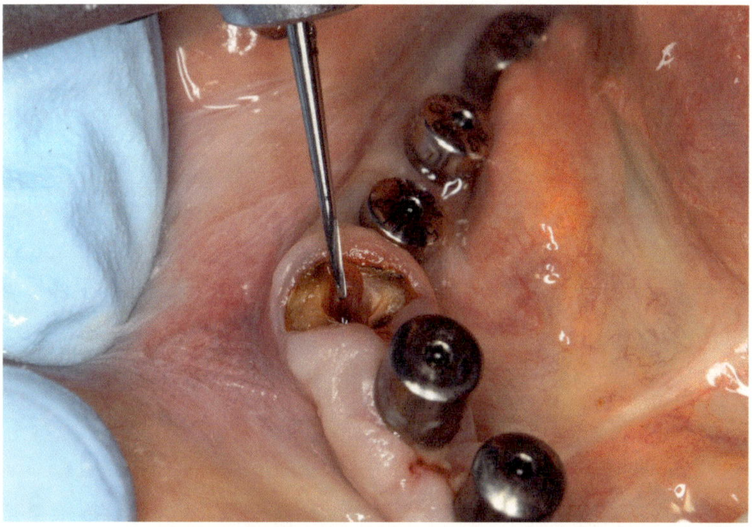

Figure 17. Minimal invasive extraction of 43- root separation

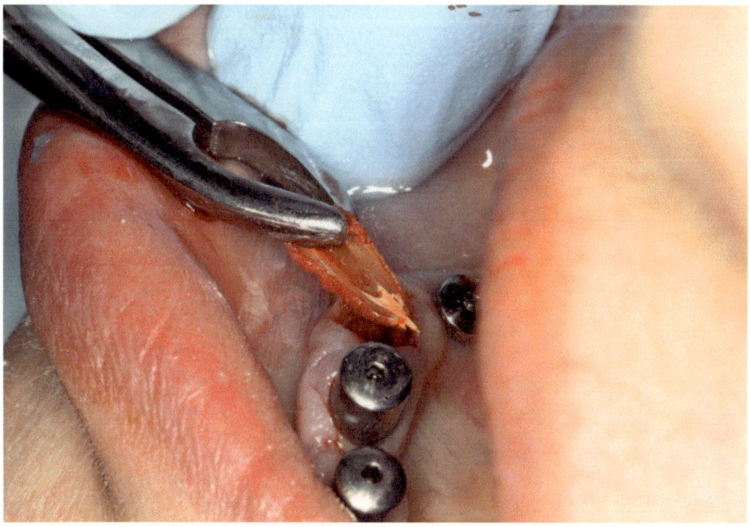

Figure 18. Minimal invasive extraction of 43

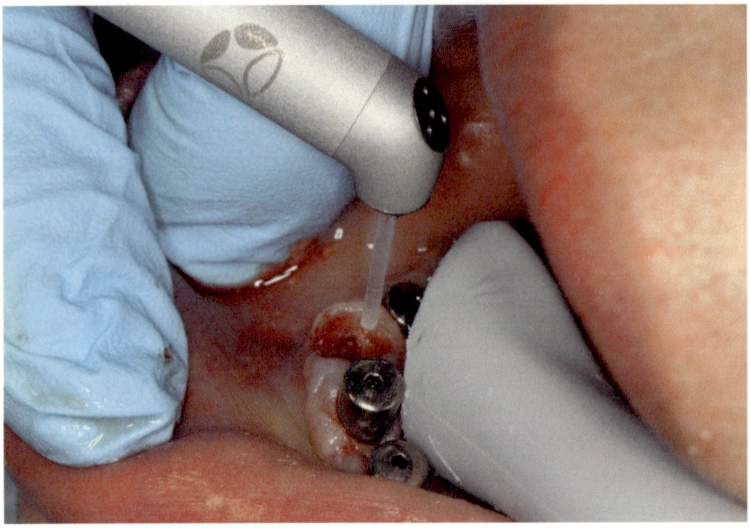

Figure 19. Granulation tissue ablation with Er:YagYAG laser

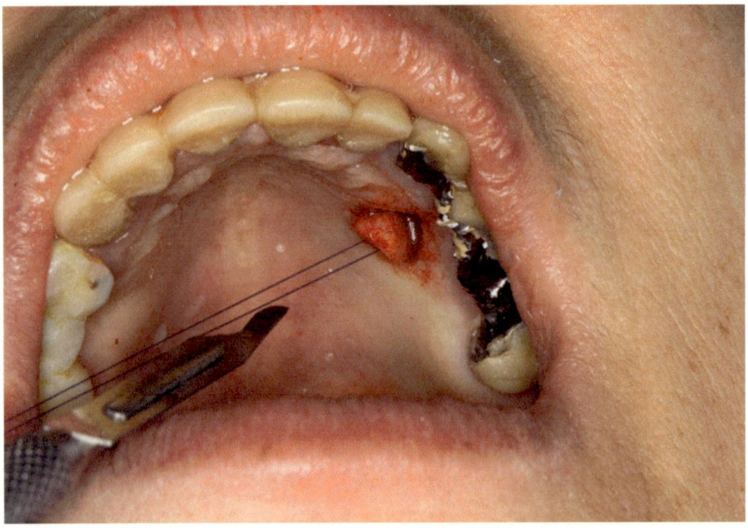

Figure 20. Palatal connective tissue graft

http://dx.doi.org/10.5772/61731

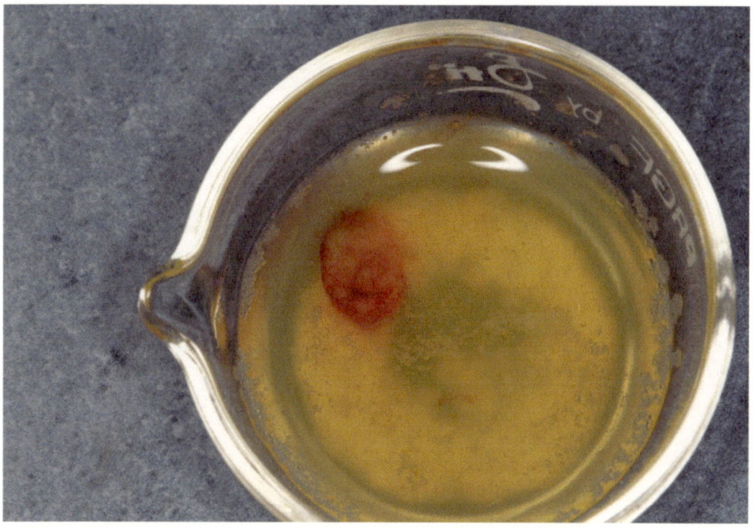

Figure 21. Palatal connective tissue graft in PRGF

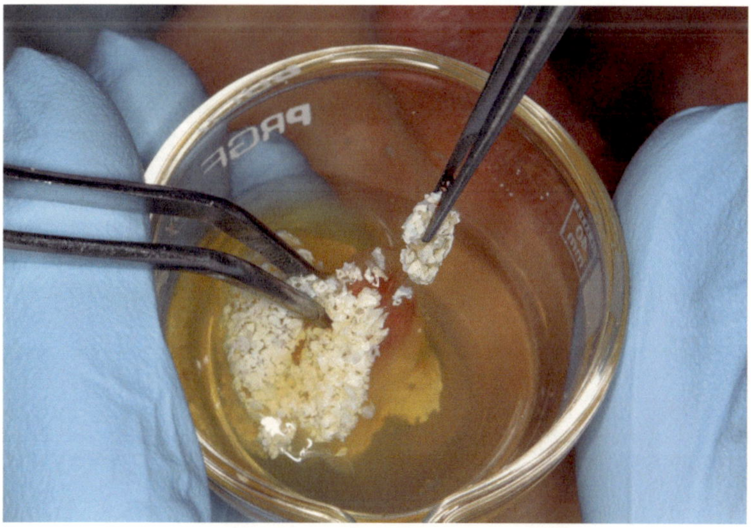

Figure 22. Bone graft material mixed with PRGF

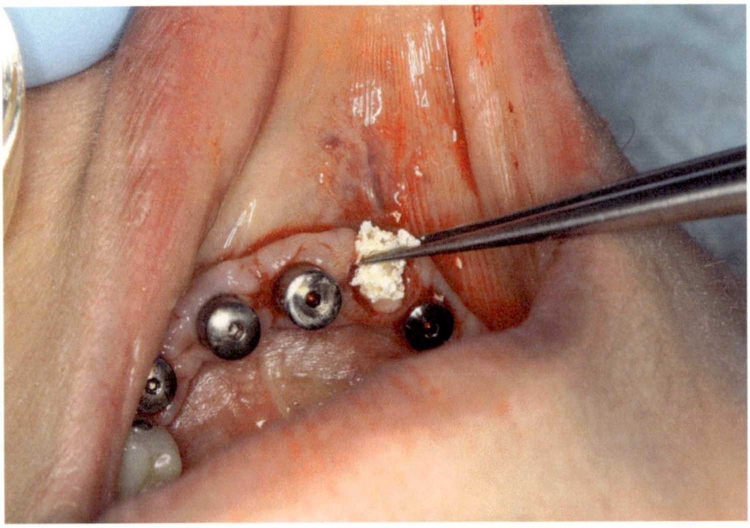

Figure 23. Bone graft material mixed with PRGF in postextractionpost-extraction socket

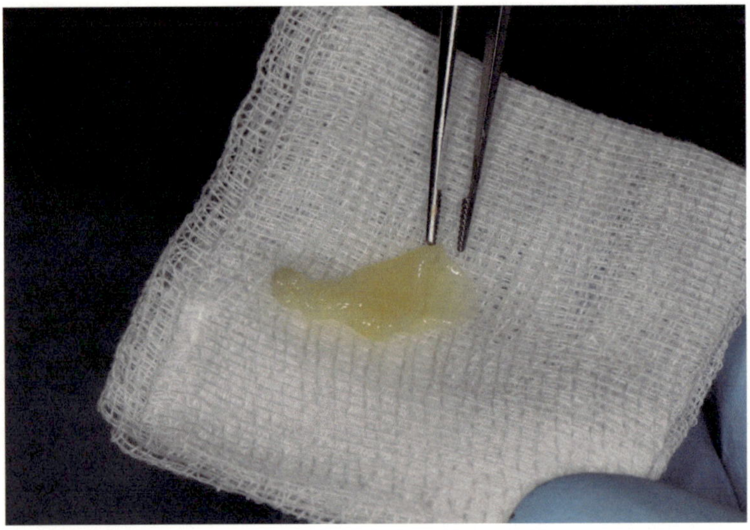

Figure 24. PRGF-clot cloth

http://dx.doi.org/10.5772/61731

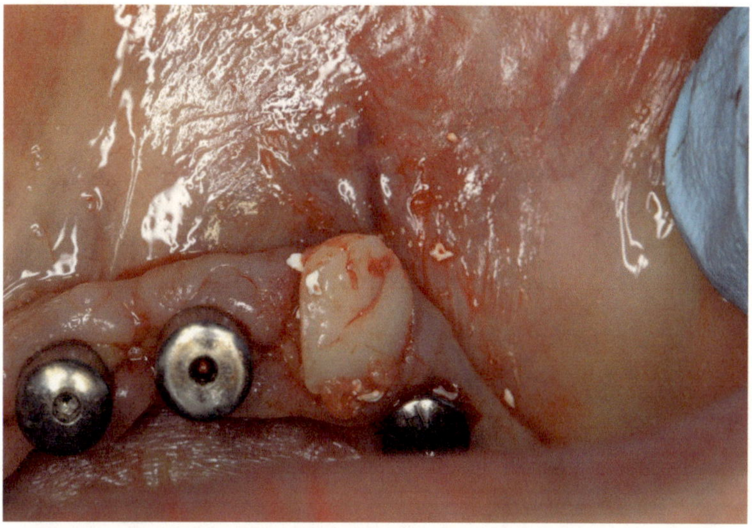

Figure 25. Covering of bone graft material with the PRGF clotcloth

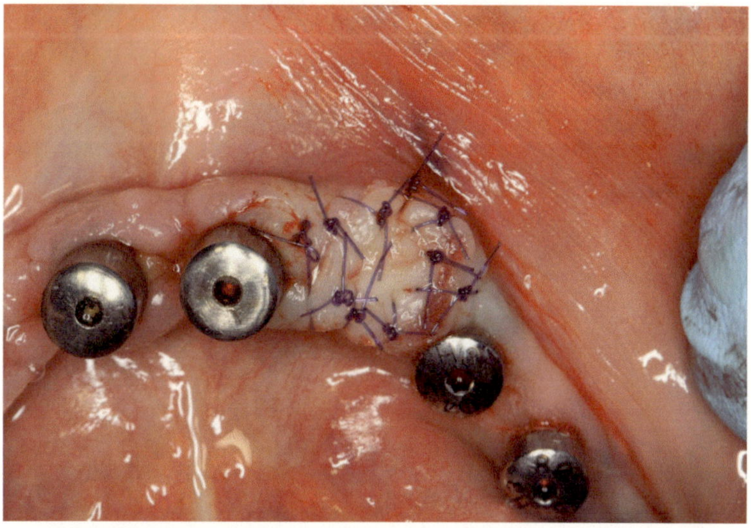

Figure 26. Suturing of the palatal connective tissue graft over the postextracted socetpost-extracted socket

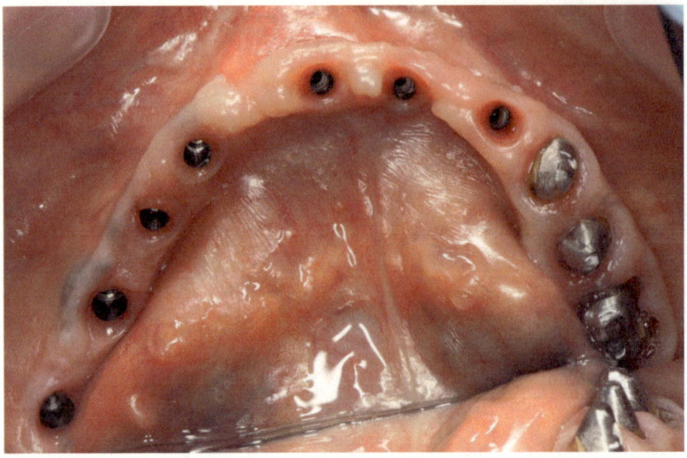

Figure 27. Soft healing process

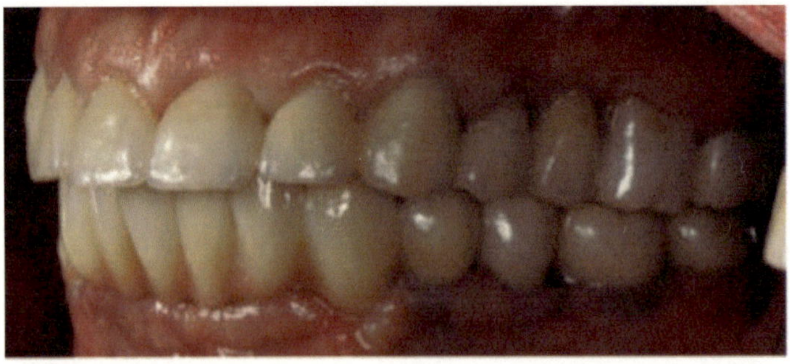

Figure 28. The end result

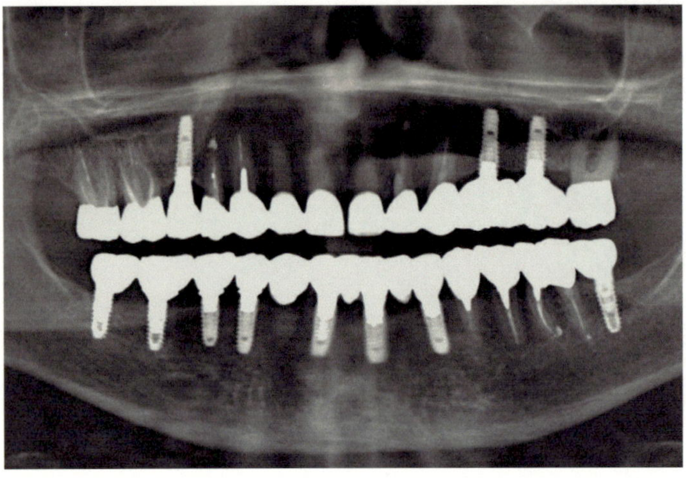

Figure 29. End result after treatment

8.2. Case 2

A female patient, 57 years old, S. H. in good general good health, non-smoker, was received at the clinic with complainscomplaints of mobility of the entire upper jaw prosthetic fixed construction, accompanied with pain and inability to eat, dating back to 3 months earlier. Clinical exam findfound out significant mobility (4th degree by Miller) of metal-ceramic fixed one-piece bridge prosthetic construction of the upper jaw. (Fig. 2). On the X-ray (Fig.1), 4 screwing dental implants arewere observed, "Tramonte design" and 4four residual roots were in terminal stage. There iswas a significant bone resorption around the implants visible on the x-ray (proven lack of osteointegration.). From the patient histori ispatient's history, it was known that these implants arewere placed 5five years ago. AnA year later, patient beginsbegan treatment with Fozamax per os once a week withfor the duration 2of two years because of osteoporosis diagnosediagnosis (T-scorscore-2.9%).

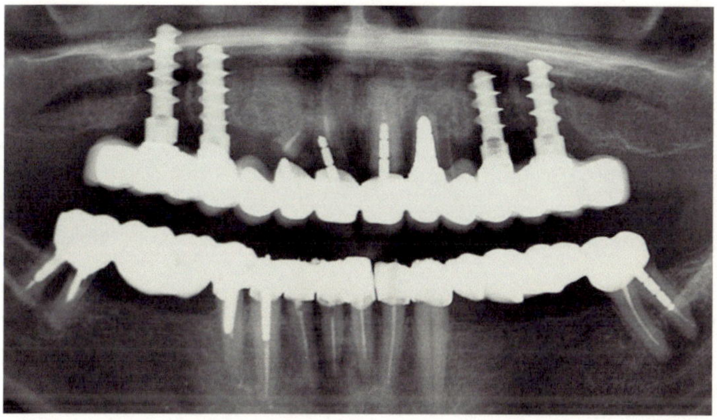

Figure 30. Initial X-ray

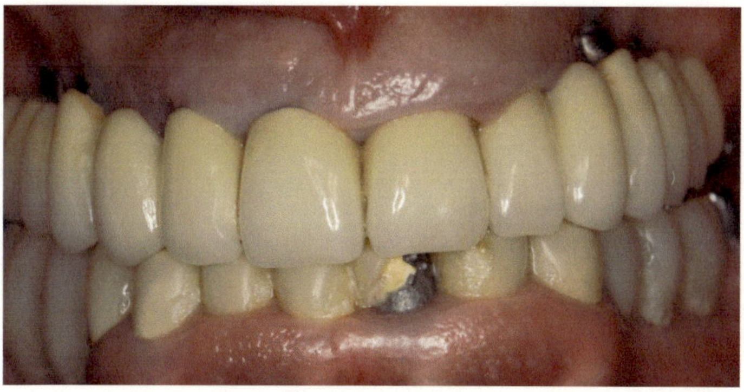

Figure 31. Intraoral view

After initial periodontal therapy, with ultrasonic device and highintensityhigh intensity laser, under antibiotic cover (clindamycin 600mg. /./8h per os), 2two times hyperbaric chamber before and three times after the dental procedures, saline enriched with ozone 9nine times and three were locally applied subcutaneously, photodynamic therapy tilluntil the 10th den after the dental procedure of removing all residual roots and implants. In the extraction sockets were placed PRGF cloth, collagen sponge and the wound were sutured. Post-operative period was smooth without any pain or complications. The patientspatient was given an immediate fabricated total removable dentures.

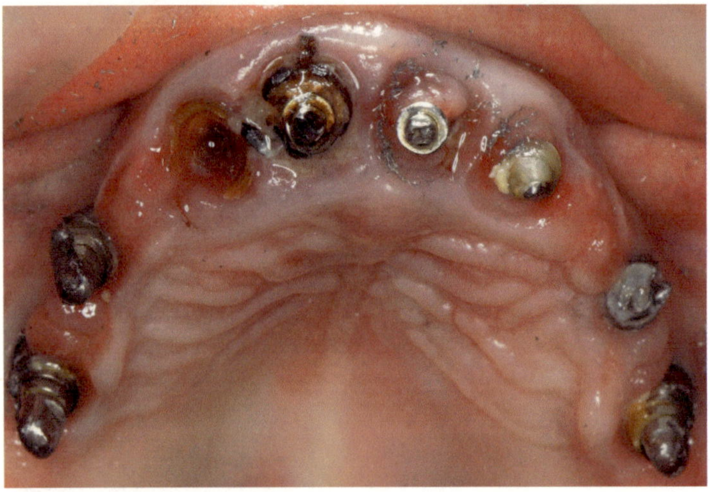

Figure 32. Intraoral view after bridge removal

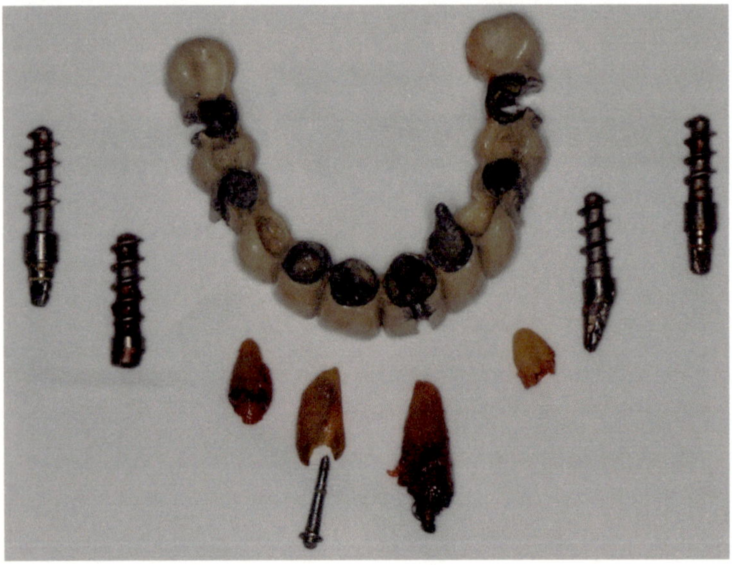

Figure 33. All implants, teeth and bridge after removal

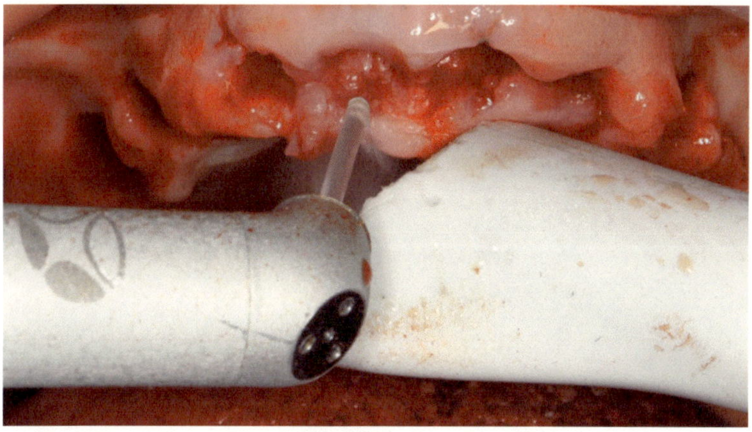

Figure 34. Granulation tissue ablation with Er:YagYAG laser

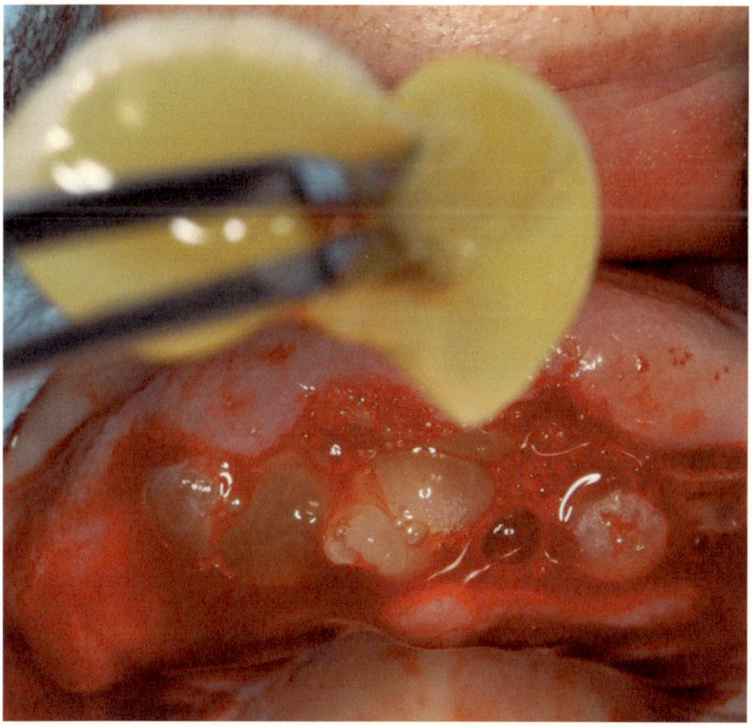

Figure 35. PRGF – cloth

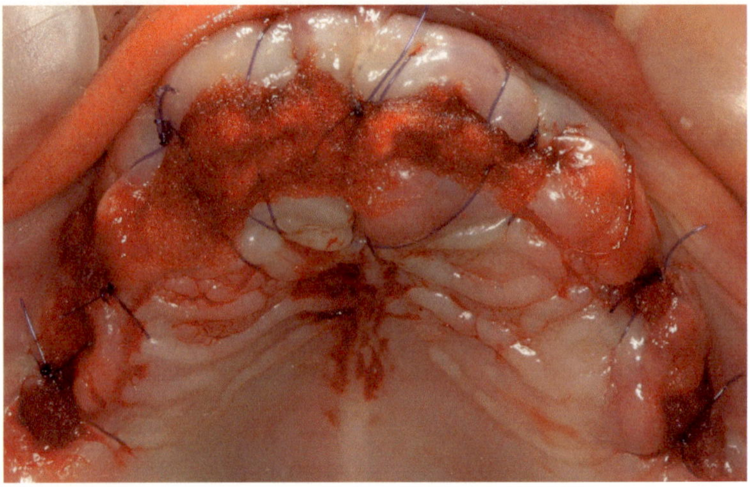

Figure 36. Covering with collagen sponge and suturing

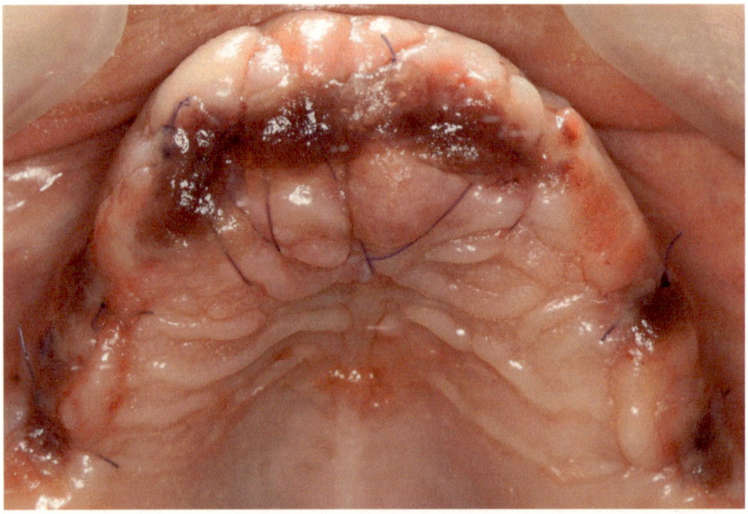

Figure 37. Day after surgery

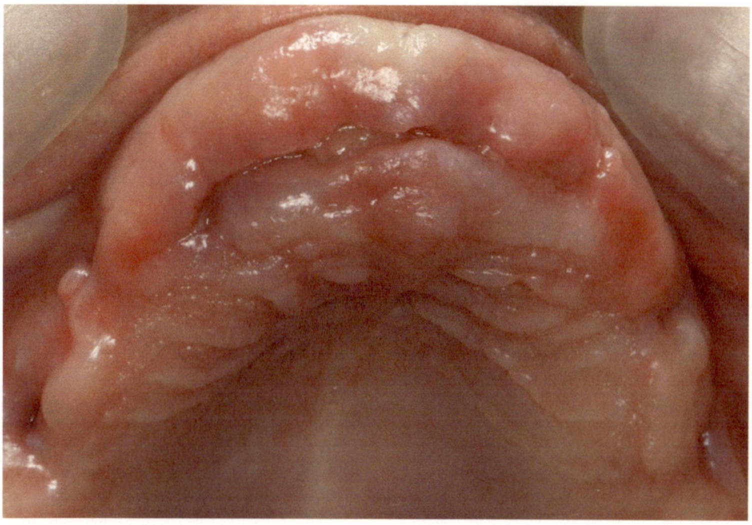

Figure 38. Ten days after surgery

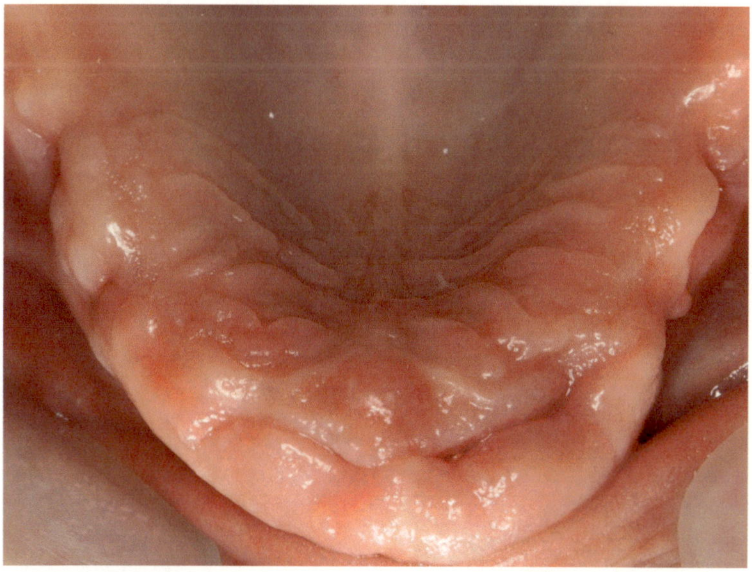

Figure 39. Three weeks after surgery

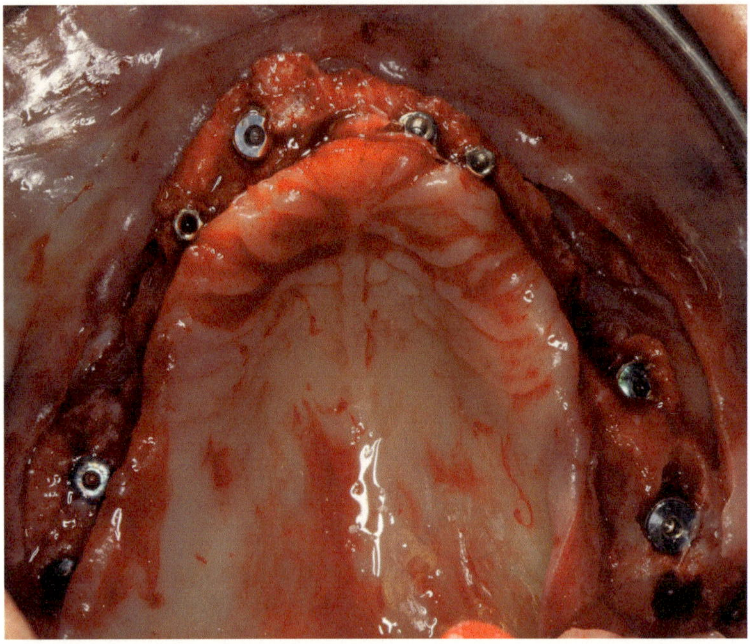

Figure 40. Intraoral view after implant insertion

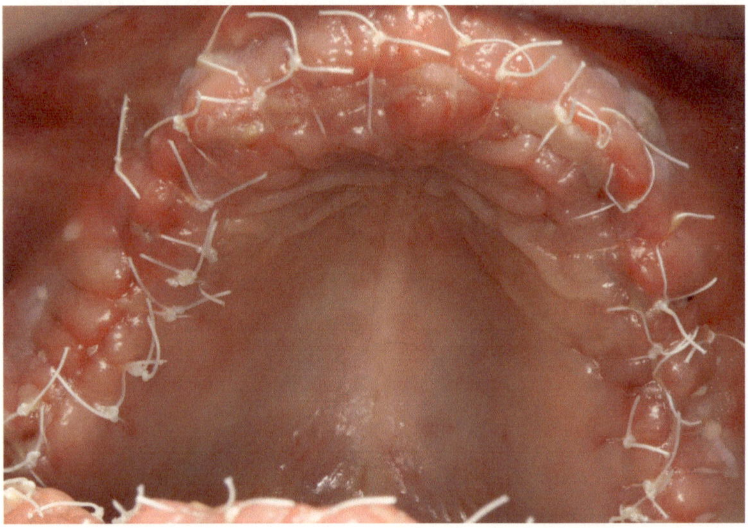

Figure 41. Intraoral view after suturing

http://dx.doi.org/10.5772/61731

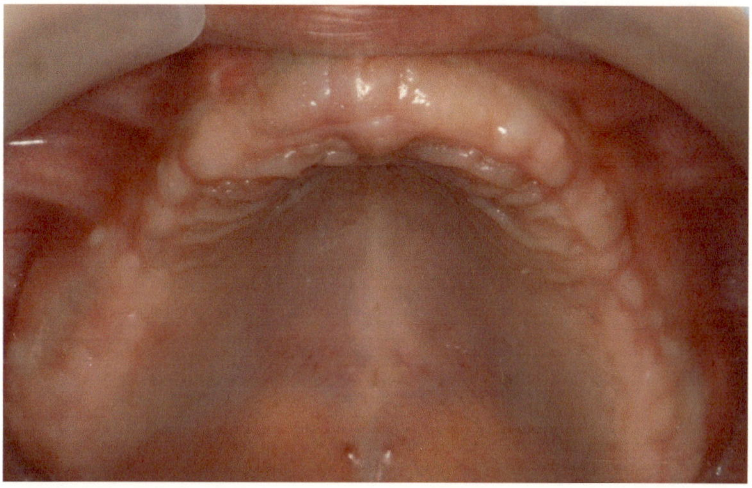

Figure 42. Two weeks after surgery

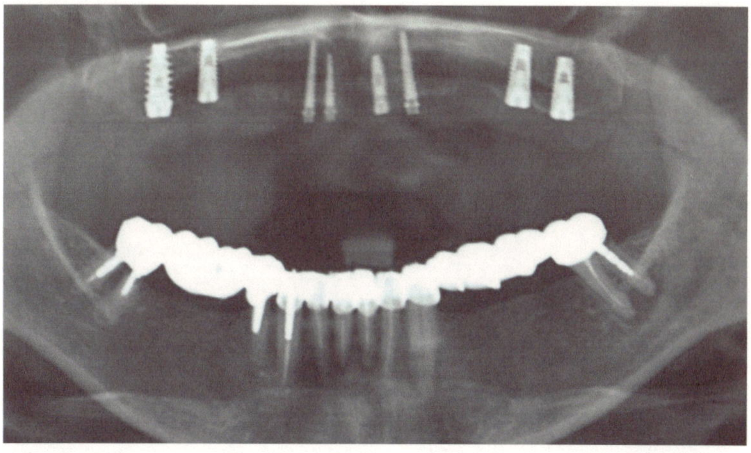

Figure 43. Panoramic X-ray after surgery

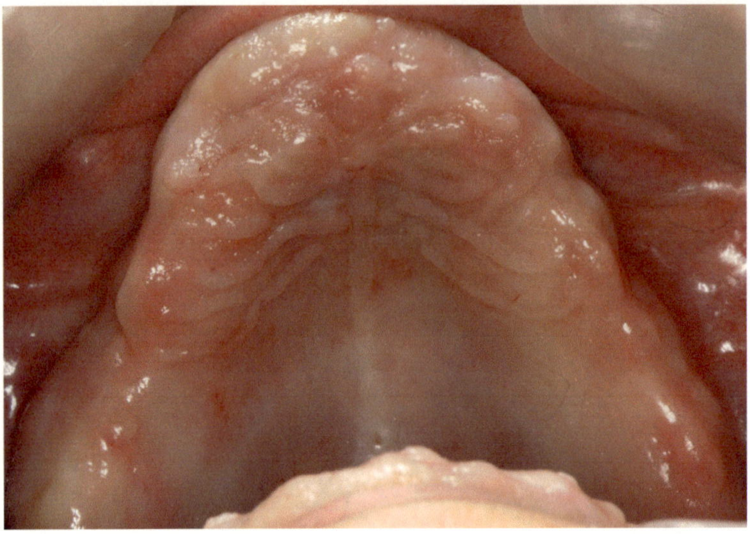

Figure 44. Four weeks after surgery

8.3. Case 3

A female patient, 54 years old, in good general health condition, smoker (over 10 cigarettes per day), was received at the clinic with complainscomplaints from fixed prosthetic construction mobility on the upper jaw, poor aesthetics, and inability to eat normally. X-ray proves anand aggressive periodntoalperiodontal disease with more than 9-10mm910mm bone resorption of interdental bone. PatientPatient's history sayssaid that she is was on Denosumabdenosumab (subcutaneously every 6 months) during for the last 3three years –in treatment for osteoporosis diagnose. The treatment plan was similar with case N2 and the healing process went smoothsmoothly.

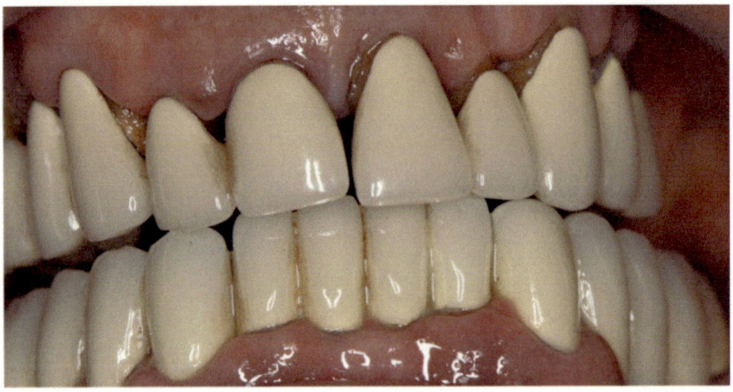

Figure 45. Intraoral view

http://dx.doi.org/10.5772/61731

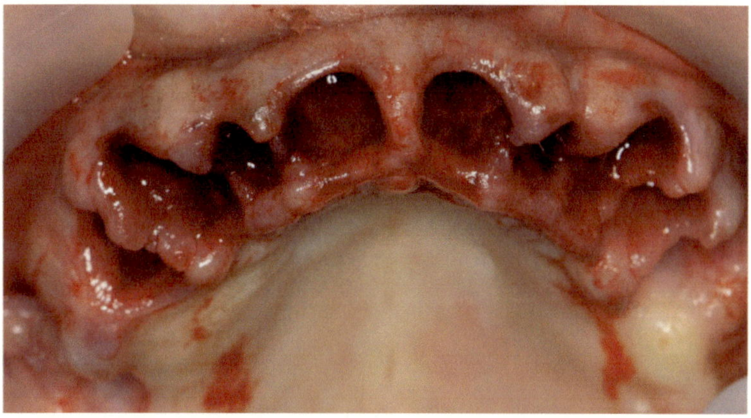

Figure 46. Postextracted sockets

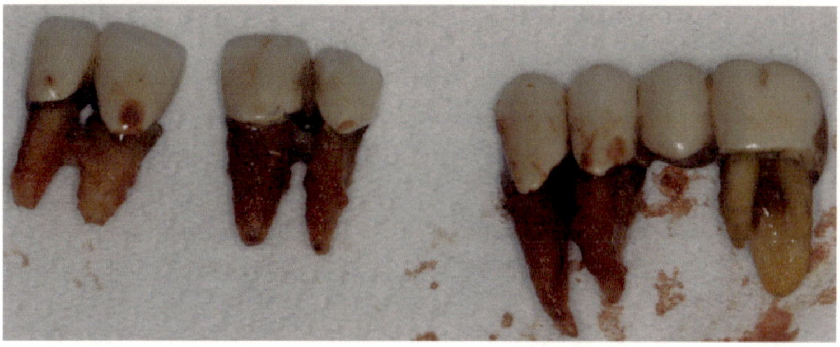

Figure 47. The extracted teeth

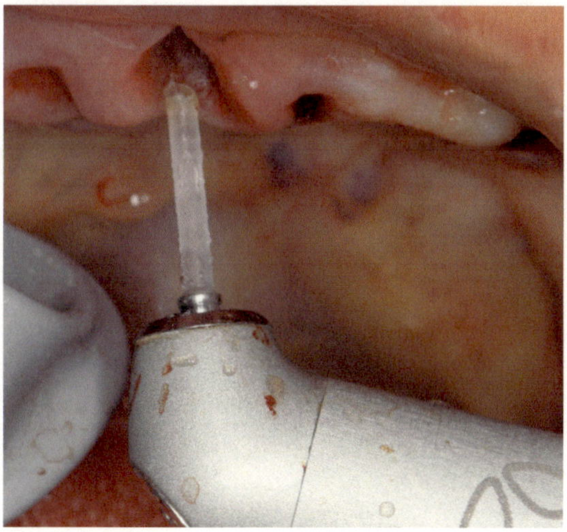

Figure 48. Granulation tissue ablation with Er:YagYAG laser

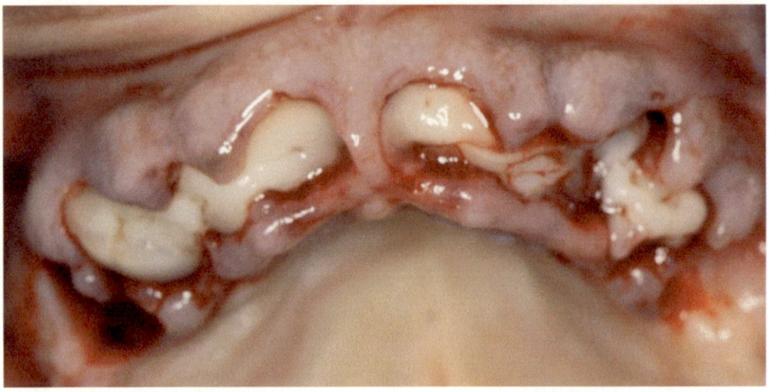

Figure 49. PRGF clotcloth

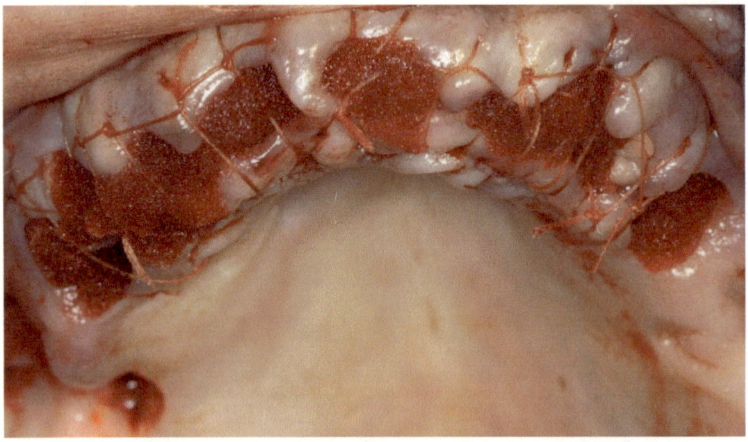

Figure 50. Covering with collagen sponge and suturing

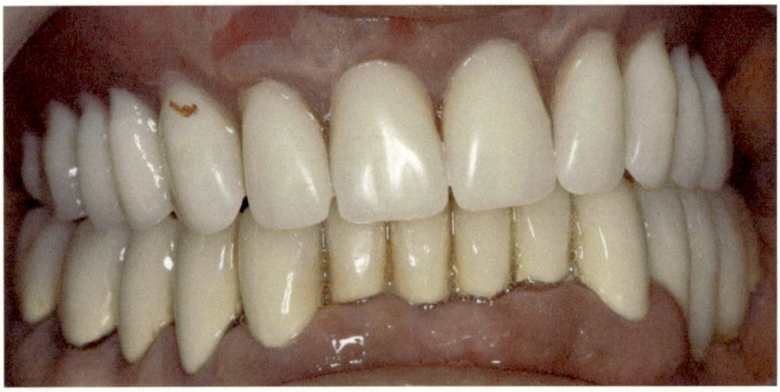

Figure 51. The immediate denture

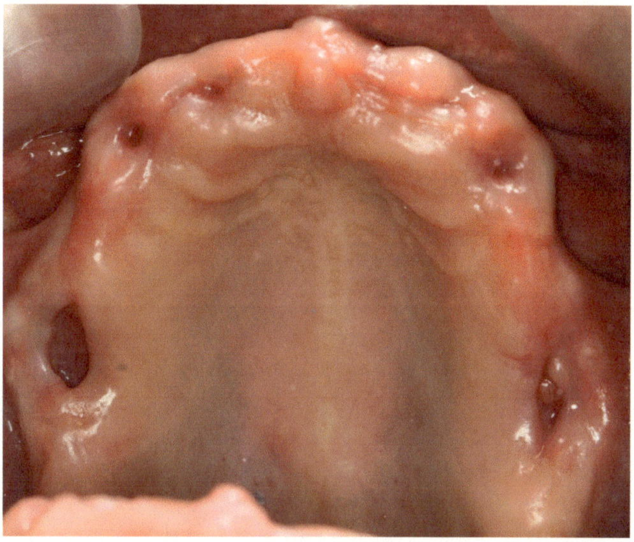

Figure 52. Three weeks after extraction

*All case-pictures are Dr. Abadzhiev's private practice patiens.

	Primary Indication	Nitrogen Containing	Dose	Route	Relative Potency**
Etidronate (Didronel)	Paget's Disease	No	300 -750 mg daily for 6 months	Oral	1
Tiludronate (Skelid)	Paget's Disease	No	400 mg daily for 3 months	Oral	50
Alendronate (Fosamax)	Osteoporosis	Yes	10 mg/day 70 mg/week	Oral	1,000
Risedronate (Actonel)	Osteoporosis	Yes	5 mg/day 35 mg/week	Oral	1,000
Ibandronate (Boniva)	Osteoporosis	Yes	2.5 mg/day 150 mg/month	Oral	1,000
Pamidronate (Aredia)	Bone Metastases	Yes	90 mg/3 weeks	IV	1,000 – 5,000
Zoledronate (Zometa)	Bone Metastases	Yes	4 mg/3 weeks	IV	10,000 +

Table 1. Usage and dosage of the bisphosphonates

After R.E. Marx

MRONJ† Staging	Treatment Strategies‡
At risk category No apparent necrotic bone in patients who have been treated with either oral or IV bisphosphonates	· No treatment indicated · Patient education
Stage 0 No clinical evidence of necrotic bone, but non-specific clinical findings, radiographic changes and symptoms	· Systemic management, including the use of pain medication and antibiotics
Stage 1 Exposed and necrotic bone, or fistulae that probes to bone, in patients who are asymptomatic and have no evidence of infection	· Antibacterial mouth rinse · Clinical follow-up on a quarterly basis · Patient education and review of indications for continued bisphosphonate therapy
Stage 2 Exposed and necrotic bone, or fistulae that probes to bone, associated with infection as evidenced by pain and ery- themaerythema in the region of the exposed bone with or without purulent drainage	· Symptomatic treatment with oral antibiotics · Oral antibacterial mouth rinse · Pain control · Debridement to relieve soft tissue irritation and infection control
Stage 3 Exposed and necrotic bone or a fistula that probes to bone in patients with pain, infection, and one or more of the fol- lowingfollowing: exposed and necrotic bone extending beyond the region of alveolar bone,(, (i.e.,. inferior border and ramus in the mandible, maxillary sinus and zygoma in the maxilla) resulting in pathologic fracture, extra-oral fistula, oral antral/oral nasal communication, or osteolysis extending to the inferior border of the mandible of sinus floor	· Antibacterial mouth rinse · Antibiotic therapy and pain control · Surgical debridement/resection for longer term palliation of infection and pain

Table 2. Staging and Treatment Strategies

Position Paper of American Association of Oral and Maxillofacial Surgeons (2014)

Author details

Metodi Abadzhiev*

Address all correspondence to: abaimplant@abv.bg

MU-Varna, Faculty of Dental Medicine, Bulgaria

References

[1] Alberto Bedogni, Stefano Fadele, Georgio Bedogni, Matteo Scoletta, Gianfranco Favia, Giordana Bettini, Olga Di Feda, Giacomo Oleri, Stephen Porter, M. Petrizzi, P. Arduino, S. DAmatoDamato, C. Ungari, P-L Fung Polly, G. Saia, et al. Standing of Osteonecrosisosteonecrosis of the jaw requires computed tomography for accurate definition of the extent of bony disease. British J Oral Maxillofac Surg, 52(7):603–608, 2014.

[2] Raj B. Lotwala, Geoffrey M. Greenlee, Susan M. Ott, Stanton H. Hall, Greg J. Huang. Bisphosphonates as a risk factor for adverse orthodontic outcomes; a retrospective cohort study Original Research Article. American J Orthodontics and Dentofacial Orthopedics, 142(5):625–634, e3, 2012.

[3] Ines Losada, Leonardo Sartoni, Elena di Gianantonio, Margherita Zen, Maurizio Clementi, Andrea Doria. Bisphosphonates in Patients with autoimmune rheumatic diseases: Can they be used in women of childbearing age? Review Article Autoimmunity Reviews, 9(8):547–552, 2010.

[4] Carlos Pigrau–Serrallach, Evelyn Carbal–Galeano, Benito Almirante-Gragera, Roger Sorde–Masip, Dolors Rodrigues–Pardo, Nuria Fernandez–Hidalgo, Niaves Larossa, Soccoro Bescos–Atin, Albert Pahissa–Berga. Long–term follow-up of jaw osteomyelitis associated with Bisphosphonatebisphosphonate use in a tertiary-care center. originalOriginal Research Article Entermadades infecciosas y Microbiologia Clinica, 32(1): 128–22, 2014.

[5] Atalay B, Yalcin S, Emes Y, et al: Bisphosphonate-related osteonecrosis: laser-assisted surgical treatment or conventional surgery? Lasers Med Sci 26:815, 2011.

[6] Ayllon J, Launay-Vacher V, Medioni J, et al: Osteonecrosis of the jaw under bisphosphonate and antiangiogenic therapies: cumulative toxicity profile? Ann Oncol 20:600, 2009.

[7] Ali-Erdem M, Burak-Cankaya A, Cemil-Isler S, et al: Extraction socket healing in rats treated with bisphosphonate: animal model for bisphosphonate related osteonecrosis of jaws in multiple myeloma patients. Med Oral Patol Oral Cir Bucal 16:e879, 2011.

[8] Aguirre JI, Akhter MP, Kimmel DB, et al: Oncologic doses of zoledronic acid induce osteonecrosis of the jaw-like lesions in rice rats (*Oryzomys palustris*) with periodontitis. J Bone Miner Res 27:2130, 2012.

[9] Aghaloo TL, Felsenfeld AL, Tetradis S: Osteonecrosis of the jaw in a patient on denosumab. J Oral Maxillofac Surg 68:959, 2010.

[10] Abu-Id MH, Warnke PH, Gottschalk J, et al: "Bis-phossy jaws" -high and low risk factors for bisphosphonate-induced osteonecro-sis of the jaw. J Craniomaxillofac Surg 36:95, 2008.

[11] Aghaloo TL, Kang B, Sung EC, et al: Periodontal disease and bisphosphonates induce osteonecrosis of the jaws in the rat. J Bone Miner Res 26:1871, 2011.

[12] Allen MR, Burr DB: The pathogenesis of bisphosphonate-related osteonecrosis of the jaw: so many hypotheses, so few data. J Oral Maxillofac Surg 67:61, 2009.

[13] Allen MR, Burr DB: Mandible matrix necrosis in beagle dogs after 3 years of daily oral bisphosphonate treatment. J Oral Maxillofac Surg 66:987, 2008.

[14] Aapro M, Saad F, Costa L: Optimizing clinical benefits of bisphosphonates in cancer patients with bone metastases. Oncologist 15:1147, 2010.

[15] Bagan JV, Jimenez Y, Gomez D, et al: Collagen telopeptide (serum CTX) and its relationship with the size and number of lesions in osteonecrosis of the jaws in cancer patients on intravenous bisphosphonates. Oral Oncol 44:1088, 2008.

[16] Black DM, Reid IR, Boonen S, et al: The effect of 3 versus 6 years of zoledronic acid treatment of osteoporosis: a randomized extension to the HORIZON-Pivotal Fracture Trial (PFT). J Bone Miner Res 27:243, 2012.

[17] Bedogni A, Fusco V, Agrillo A, et al: Learning from experience. Proposal of a refined definition and staging system for bisphosphonate-related osteonecrosis of the jaw (BRONJ). Oral Dis 18:621, 2012.

[18] Balmor GR, Yarom N, Weitzen R: Drug-induced palate osteonecrosis following nasal surgery. Isr Med Assoc J 14:193, 2012.

[19] Bonacina R, Mariani U, Villa F, et al: Preventive strategies and clinical implications for bisphosphonate-related osteonecrosis of the jaw: a review of 282 patients. J Can Dent Assoc 77:b147, 2011.

[20] Badros A, Weikel D, Salama A, et al: Osteonecrosis of the jaw in multiple myeloma patients: clinical features and risk factors. J Clin Oncol 24:945, 2006.

[21] Brown JJ, Ramalingam L, Zacharin MR: Bisphosphonate-associated osteonecrosis of the jaw: does it occur in children? Clin Endocrinol (Oxf) 68:863, 2008.

[22] Bozas G, Roy A, Ramasamy V, et al: Osteonecrosis of the jaw after a single bisphosphonate infusion in a patient with metastatic renal cancer treated with sunitinib. Onkologie 33:321, 2010.

[23] Boonyapakorn T, Schirmer I, Reichart PA, et al: Bisphosphonate-induced osteonecrosis of the jaws: prospective study of 80 patients with multiple myeloma and other malignancies. Oral Oncol 44:857, 2008.

[24] Bi Y, Gao Y, Ehirchiou D, et al: Bisphosphonates cause osteonecrosis of the jaw-like disease in mice. Am J Pathol 177:280, 2010.

[25] Briefing Information for the September 9, 2011 Joint Meeting of the Reproductive Health Drugs Advisory Committee and the Drug Safety and Risk Management Advisory Committee. Septemer 9, 2011;

[26] http://www.fda.gov/AdvisoryCommittees/CommitteesMeetingMaterials/Drugs/DrugSafetyandRiskManagementAdvisoryCommittee/ucm270957.htm. Accessed April 7, 2014.

[27] Bashutski JD, Eber RM, Kinney JS, et al: Teriparatide and osseous regeneration in the oral cavity. N Engl J Med 363:2396, 2010.

[28] Brunello A, Saia G, Bedogni A, et al: Worsening of osteonecrosis of the jaw during treatment with sunitinib in a patient with metastatic renal cell carcinoma. Bone 44:173, 2009.

[29] Bagan, J.V., Jimenez, Y., Murillo, J., Jaw osteonecrosis associated with bisphosphonates: Multiple exposed areas and its relationship to teeth extractions — Study of 20 cases, Oral Oncol, 42: 327–329, 2011.

[30] Background Document for Meeting of Advisory Committee for Reproductive Health Drugs and Drug Safety and Risk Management Advisory Committee. United States. Food and Drug Administration. September 9, 2011;

[31] Baron R, Ferrari S, Russell RG: Denosumab and bisphosphonates: different mechanisms of action and effects. Bone 48:677, 2011.

[32] Beuselinck B, Wolter P, Karadimou A, et al: Concomitant oral tyrosine kinase inhibitors and bisphosphonates in advanced renal cell carcinoma with bone metastases. Br J Cancer 107:1665, 2012.

[33] Carlson ER, Basile JD: The role of surgical resection in the management of bisphosphonate-related osteonecrosis of the jaws. J Oral Maxillofac Surg 67:85, 2009.

[34] Christodoulou C, Pervena A, Klouvas G, et al: Combination of bisphosphonates and antiangiogenic factors induces osteonecrosis of the jaw more frequently than bisphosphonates alone. Oncology 76:209, 2009.

[35] Cummings SR, San Martin J, McClung MR, et al: Denosumab for prevention of fractures in postmenopausal women with osteoporosis. N Engl J Med 361:756, 2009.

[36] Carlson ER, Fleisher KE, Ruggiero SL: Metastatic cancer identified in osteonecrosis specimens of the jaws in patients receiving intravenous bisphosphonate medications. J Oral Maxillofac Surg 71:2077, 2013.

[37] Coleman R, Woodward E, Brown J, et al: Safety of zoledronic acid and incidence of osteonecrosis of the jaw (ONJ) during adjuvant therapy in a randomised phase III trial (AZURE: BIG 01-04) for women with stage II/III breast cancer. Breast Cancer Res Treat 127:429, 2011.

[38] Dickinson M, Prince HM, Kirsa S, et al: Osteonecrosis of the jaw complicating bisphosphonate treatment for bone disease in multiple myeloma: an overview with recommendations for prevention and treatment. Intern Med J 39:304, 2009.

[39] Damm DD, Jones DM: Bisphosphonate-related osteonecrosis of the jaws: a potential alternative to drug holidays. Gen Dent 61:33, 2013.

[40] Engroff SL, Kim DD: Treating bisphosphonate osteonecrosis of the jaws: is there a role for resection and vascularized reconstruction? J Oral Maxillofac Surg 65:2374, 2007.

[41] Endodontic Implications of Bisphosphonate-Associated Osteonecrosis of the Jaws. Chicago, IL: American Association of Endodontists; 2010:4.

[42] Epstein MS, Epstein JB, Ephros HD: The effects of osteoclast modifiers on the oral cavity: a review for prescribers. Curr Opin Support Palliat Care 6:337, 2012.

[43] Eckardt AM, Lemound J, Lindhorst D, et al: Surgical management of bisphosphonate-related osteonecrosis of the jaw in oncologic patients: a challenging problem. Anticancer Res 31:2313, 2011.

[44] Edwards BJ, Hellstein JW, Jacobsen PL, et al: Updated recommendations for managing the care of patients receiving oral bisphosphonate therapy: an advisory statement from the American Dental Association Council on Scientific Affairs. J Am Dent Assoc 139:1674, 2008.

[45] Fleissig Y, Regev E, Lehman H: Sunitinib related osteonecrosis of jaw: a case report. Oral Surg Oral Med Oral Pathol Oral Radiol 113:e1, 2012.

[46] Ferrari S, Bianchi B, Savi A, et al: Fibula free flap with endosseous implants for reconstructing a resected mandible in bisphosphonate osteonecrosis. J Oral Maxillofac Surg 66:999, 2008

[47] Fedele S, S. Porter, F. Daiuto, N. Donos, H. Ireland, S. Humphries. P1.41. the GENVA-BO study (GENetic VAriants in Bisphosphonate–related Ostenecrosis of the jaws). A cooperation proposal. Oral Oncology Supplement, vol. 3. Issue 1. July 2009, p. 136.

[48] Ferlito S, Puzzo S, Palermo F, et al: Treatment of bisphosphonate-related osteonecrosis of the jaws: presentation of a protocol and an observational longitudinal study of an Italian series of cases. Br J Oral Maxillofac Surg 50:425, 2012.

[49] Fehm T, Felsenberg D, Krimmel M, et al: Bisphosphonate-associated osteonecrosis of the jaw in breast cancer patients: recommendations for prevention and treatment. Breast 18:213, 2009.

[50] Freiberger JJ: Utility of hyperbaric oxygen in treatment of bisphosphonate-related osteonecrosis of the jaws. J Oral Maxillofac Surg 67:96, 2009.

[51] Fizazi K, Carducci M, Smith M, et al: Denosumab versus zoledronic acid for treatment of bone metastases in men with castration-resistant prostate cancer: a randomised, double-blind study. Lancet 377:813, 2011.

[52] Fleisher KE, Welch G, Kottal S, et al: Predicting risk for bisphosphonate-related osteonecrosis of the jaws: CTX versus radiographic markers. Oral Surg Oral Med Oral Pathol Oral Radiol Endod 110:509, 2010.

[53] Freiberger JJ, Padilla-Burgos R, McGraw T, et al: What is the role of hyperbaric oxygen in the management of bisphosphonate-related osteonecrosis of the jaw: a randomized controlled trial of hyperbaric oxygen as an adjunct to surgery and antibiotics. J Oral Maxillofac Surg 70:1573, 2012.

[54] Fehm T, Beck V, Banys M, et al: Bisphosphonate-induced osteonecrosis of the jaw (ONJ): Incidence and risk factors in patients with breast cancer and gynecological malignancies. Gynecol Oncol 112:605, 2009.

[55] Fedele S, Porter SR, D'Aiuto F, et al: Nonexposed variant of bisphosphonate-associated osteonecrosis of the jaw: a case series. Am J Med 123:1060, 2010.

[56] Guarneri V, Miles D, Robert N, et al: Bevacizumab and osteonecrosis of the jaw: incidence and association with bisphosphonate therapy in three large prospective trials in advanced breast cancer. Breast Cancer Res Treat 122:181, 2010.

[57] Gerard DA, Carlson ER, Gotcher JE, et al: Early inhibitory effects of zoledronic acid in tooth extraction sockets in dogs are negated by recombinant human bone morphogenetic protein. J Oral Maxillofac Surg 72:61, 2014.

[58] Grbic JT, Black DM, Lyles KW, et al: The incidence of osteonecrosis of the jaw in patients receiving 5 milligrams of zoledronic acid: data from the health outcomes and reduced incidence with zoledronic acid once yearly clinical trials program. J Am Dent Assoc 141:1365, 2010.

[59] Graziani F, Vescovi P, Campisi G, et al: Resective surgical approach shows a high performance in the management of advanced cases of bisphosphonate-related osteonecrosis of the jaws: a retrospective survey of 347 cases. J Oral Maxillofac Surg 70:2501, 2012.

[60] Henry DH, Costa L, Goldwasser F, et al: Randomized, double-blind study of denosumab versus zoledronic acid in the treatment of bone metastases in patients with advanced cancer (excluding breast and prostate cancer) or multiple myeloma. J Clin Oncol 29:1125, 2011.

[61] Hellstein JW, Adler RA, Edwards B, et al: Managing the care of patients receiving antiresorptive therapy for prevention and treatment of osteoporosis: executive summary of recommendations from the American Dental Association Council on Scientific Affairs. J Am Dent Assoc 142:1243, 2011.

[62] Hoff AO, Toth BB, Altundag K, et al: Frequency and risk factors associated with osteonecrosis of the jaw in cancer patients treated with intravenous bisphosphonates. J Bone Miner Res 23:826, 2008.

[63] Hoefert S, Eufinger H: Sunitinib may raise the risk of bisphosphonate-related osteonecrosis of the jaw: presentation of three cases. Oral Surg Oral Med Oral Pathol Oral Radiol Endod 110:463, 2010.

[64] Hokugo A, Christensen R, Chung EM, et al: Increased prevalence of bisphosphonate-related osteonecrosis of the jaw with vitamin D deficiency in rats. J Bone Miner Res 25:1337, 2010.

[65] Hinchy NV, Jayaprakash V, Rossitto RA, et al: Osteonecrosis of the jaw-prevention and treatment strategies for oral health professionals. Oral Oncol 49:878, 2013.

[66] John W. Hellstein, Robert A. Adier, Beatrice Edwards, Peter L. Jacobsen, John R. Kalman, Sreenivas Koka, Cesar A. Migliorati, Helen Ristic. Managing the care of patients receiving antiresorptive for prevention and treatment of osteoporosis: Executive summery of recommendations from the American Dental Association Council on Scientific Affairs. J American Dent Assoc, vol. 142, issue 11, Nov.2011, p. 1243–1251.

[67] Khan AA, Sandor GK, Dore E, et al: Bisphosphonate associated osteonecrosis of the jaw. J Rheumatol 36:478, 2009.

[68] Kim I, Ki H, Lee W, et al: The effect of systemically administered bisphosphonates on bony healing after tooth extraction and osseointegration of dental implants in the rabbit maxilla. Int J Oral Maxillofac Implants 28:1194, 2013.

[69] Katz J, Gong Y, Salmasinia D, et al: Genetic polymorphisms and other risk factors associated with bisphosphonate induced osteonecrosis of the jaw. Int J Oral Maxillofac Surg 40:605, 2011.

[70] Koch FP, Walter C, Hansen T, et al: Osteonecrosis of the jaw related to sunitinib. Oral Maxillofac Surg 15:63, 2011.

[71] Kos M, Junka A, Smutnicka D, et al: Pamidronate enhances bacterial adhesion to bone hydroxyapatite. Another puzzle in the pathology of bisphosphonate-related osteonecrosis of the jaw? J Oral Maxillofac Surg 71:1010, 2013.

[72] Kumar SK, Gorur A, Schaudinn C, et al: The role of microbial biofilms in osteonecrosis of the jaw associated with bisphosphonate therapy. Curr Osteoporos Rep 8:40, 2010.

[73] Kyle RA, Yee GC, Somerfield MR, et al: American Society of Clinical Oncology Kang B, Cheong S, Chaichanasakul T, et al: Periapical disease and bisphosphonates induce osteonecrosis of the jaws in mice. J Bone Miner Res 28:1631, 2013.

[74] .Kwon YD, Kim DY, Ohe JY, et al: Correlation between serum C-terminal cross-linking telopeptide of type I collagen and staging of oral bisphosphonate-related osteonecrosis of the jaws. J Oral Maxillofac Surg 67:2644, 2009.

[75] Kyrgidis A, Vahtsevanos K, Koloutsos G, et al: Bisphosphonate-related osteonecrosis of the jaws: a case-control study of risk factors in breast cancer patients. J Clin Oncol 26:4634, 2008.

[76] Kim HK: Introduction to osteonecrosis of the femoral head (OFH) and osteonecrosis of the jaw (ONJ). J Musculoskelet Neuronal Interact 7:350, 2007.

[77] Kikuiri T, Kim I, Yamaza T, et al: Cell-based immunotherapy with mesenchymal stem cells cures bisphosphonate-related osteonecrosis of the jaw-like disease in mice. J Bone Miner Res 25:1668, 2010.

[78] Kunchur R, Need A, Hughes T, et al: Clinical investigation of C-terminal cross-linking telopeptide test in prevention and management of bisphosphonate-associated osteonecrosis of the jaws. J Oral Maxillofac Surg 67:1167, 2009.

[79] Kuroshima S, Kovacic BL, Kozloff KM, et al: Intra-oral PTH administration promotes tooth extraction socket healing. J Dent Res 92:553, 2013.

[80] Khan AA, Morrison A, Hanley DA, et al: International Consensus on Diagnosis and Management of Osteonecrosis of the Jaw. 2013:22.

[81] Lacey DL, Boyle WJ, Simonet WS, et al: Bench to bedside: elucidation of the OPG-RANK-RANKL pathway and the development of denosumab. Nat Rev Drug Discov 11:401, 2012.

[82] Lee CY, David T, Nishime M: Use of platelet-rich plasma in the management of oral biphosphonate-associated osteonecrosis of the jaw: a report of 2 cases. J Oral Implantol 33:371, 2007.

[83] Lane, N., Armitage, G.C., Loomer, P., Bisphosphonate therapy improves the outcome of conventional periodontal treatment: Results of a 12-month, randomized, placebo-controlled study J Periodontol, 2005: 76, 1113-1122.

[84] Lopez-Jornet P, Camacho-Alonso F, Martinez-Canovas A, et al: Perioperative antibiotic regimen in rats treated with pamidronate plus dexamethasone and subjected to dental extraction: a study of the changes in the jaws. J Oral Maxillofac Surg 69:2488, 2011.

[85] Lo JC, O'Ryan F, Yang J, et al: Oral health considerations in older women receiving oral bisphosphonate therapy. J Am Geriatr Soc 59:916, 2011.

[86] Lehrer S, Montazem A, Ramanathan L, et al: Normal serum bone markers in bisphosphonate-induced osteonecrosis of the jaws. Oral Surg Oral Med Oral Pathol Oral Radiol Endod 106:389, 2008.

[87] Landesberg R, Woo V, Cremers S, et al: Potential pathophysiological mechanisms in osteonecrosis of the jaw. Ann N Y Acad Sci 1218:62, 2011.

[88] Landesberg R, Cozin M, Cremers S, et al: Inhibition of oral mucosal cell wound healing by bisphosphonates. J Oral Maxillofac Surg 66:839, 2008.

[89] Lo JC, O'Ryan FS, Gordon NP, et al: Prevalence of osteonecrosis of the jaw in patients with oral bisphosphonate exposure. J Oral Maxillofac Surg 68:243, 2010.

[90] Lipton A, Fizazi K, Stopeck AT, et al: Superiority of denosumab to zoledronic acid for prevention of skeletal-related events: a combined analysis of 3 pivotal, randomised, phase 3 trials. Eur J Cancer 48:3082, 2012.

[91] Marini F, Tonelli P, Cavalli L, et al: Pharmacogenetics of bisphosphonate-associated osteonecrosis of the jaw. Front Biosci (Elite Ed) 3:364, 2011.

[92] Marx RE: Pamidronate (Aredia) and zoledronate (Zometa) induced avascular necrosis of the jaws: a growing epidemic. J Oral Maxillofac Surg 61:1115, 2003.

[93] Marx RE, Oral and Intravenous Bisphosphonata-Indiced Osteonecrosis of the Jaws. History, Etiology, Prevention and treatment, second edition, Quintessence, 2011

[94] Mehrotra B, Fantasia J, Ruggiero SL: Outcomes of bisphosphonate related osteonecrosis of the jaw. Importance of staging and management. A large single institution update. J Clin Oncol 26:20526, 2008.

[95] Marcelo Cunio Fonseca, Gabriela Tannus Branco de Araujo, Helder Etto, Alexandre Schiola, Natalia Santoni, Marko Machado. Economic Evalution of Clodronate and Zolesronatw in Patients Diagnosed with Metastatic Bone Disease From the Perspective of Public and III-rd Party Payors in Brazil. Clinical Therapeutics, 33 (11), 1769-1780, e2.

[96] Mucke T, Koschinski J, Deppe H, et al: Outcome of treatment and parameters influencing recurrence in patients with bisphosphonate-related osteonecrosis of the jaws. J Cancer Res Clin Oncol 137:907, 2011.

[97] Marx RE, Cillo JE, Jr., Ulloa JJ: Oral bisphosphonate-induced osteonecrosis: risk factors, prediction of risk using serum CTX testing, prevention, and treatment. J Oral Maxillofac Surg 65:2397, 2007.

[98] Mozzati M, Arata V, Gallesio G: Tooth extraction in patients on zoledronic acid therapy. Oral Oncol 48:817, 2012.

[99] Mauri D, Valachis A, Polyzos IP, et al: Osteonecrosis of the jaw and use of bisphosphonates in adjuvant breast cancer treatment: a meta-analysis. Breast Cancer Res Treat 116:433, 2009.

[100] Migliorati CA, Saunders D, Conlon MS, et al: Assessing the association between bisphosphonate exposure and delayed mucosal healing after tooth extraction. J Am Dent Assoc 144:406, 2013.

[101] Malden N, Lopes V: An epidemiological study of alendronate-related osteonecrosis of the jaws. A case series from the south-east of Scotland with attention given to case definition and prevalence. J Bone Miner Metab 30:171, 2012.

[102] Marx R: Oral and Intravenous Bisphosphonate Induced Osteonecrosis of the Jaws: History, etiology, prevention, and treatment. 2nd ed. Hanover Park, IL: Quintessence Publishing Co; 2011.

[103] Marx, R.E., Sawatari, Y., Fortin, M., Broumand, V., Bisphosphonate-induced exposed bone (osteonerosis/osteopetrosis) of the jaws: Risk factors, recognition, prevention, and treatment (2005) J Oral Maxillofac Surg, 63, pp. 1567-1575;

[104] Mortensen M, Lawson W, Montazem A: Osteonecrosis of the jaw associated with bisphosphonate use: Presentation of seven cases and literature review. Laryngoscope 117:30, 2007.

[105] Nicoletti P, Cartsos VM, Palaska PK, et al: Genomewide pharmacogenetics of bisphosphonate-induced osteonecrosis of the jaw: the role of RBMS3. Oncologist 17:279, 2012.

[106] Nicolatou-Galitis O, Migkou M, Psyrri A, et al: Gingival bleeding and jaw bone necrosis in patients with metastatic renal cell carcinoma receiving sunitinib: report of 2 cases with clinical implications. Oral Surg Oral Med Oral Pathol Oral Radiol 113:234, 2012.

[107] O'Ryan FS, Khoury S, Liao W, et al: Intravenous bisphosphonate-related osteonecrosis of the jaw: bone scintigraphy as an early indicator. J Oral Maxillofac Surg 67:1363, 2009.

[108] Qi WX, Tang LN, He AN, et al: Risk of osteonecrosis of the jaw in cancer patients receiving denosumab: a meta-analysis of seven randomized controlled trials. Int J Clin Oncol, 2013.

[109] Patel V, McLeod NM, Rogers SN, et al: Bisphosphonate osteonecrosis of the jaw—a literature review of UK policies versus international policies on bisphosphonates, risk factors and prevention. Br J Oral Maxillofac Surg 49:251, 2011.

[110] Papapoulos S, Chapurlat R, Libanati C, et al: Five years of denosumab exposure in women with postmenopausal osteoporosis: results from the first two years of the FREEDOM extension. J Bone Miner Res 27:694, 2012.

[111] Rosen LS, Gordon D, Tchekmedyian NS, et al: Long-term efficacy and safety of zoledronic acid in the treatment of skeletal metastases in patients with nonsmall cell lung carcinoma and other solid tumors: a randomized, Phase III, double-blind, placebo-controlled trial. Cancer 100:2613, 2004.

[112] Ruggiero, S., Gralow, J., Marx, R.E., Practical guidelines for the prevention, diagnosis, and treatment of osteonecrosis of the jaw in patients with cancer (2006) J Oncol Prac, 2, pp. 7-14;

[113] Ruggiero SL, Dodson TB, Assael LA, et al: American Association of Oral and Maxillofacial Surgeons position paper on bisphosphonate-related osteonecrosis of the jaws--2009 update. J Oral Maxillofac Surg 67:2, 2009.

[114] Ruggiero SL, Fantasia J, Carlson E: Bisphosphonate-related osteonecrosis of the jaw: background and guidelines for diagnosis, staging and management. Oral Surg Oral Med Oral Pathol Oral Radiol Endod 102:433, 2006.

[115] Ripamonti CI, Maniezzo M, Campa T, et al: Decreased occurrence of osteonecrosis of the jaw after implementation of dental preventive measures in solid tumour patients with bone metastases treated with bisphosphonates. The experience of the National Cancer Institute of Milan. Ann Oncol 20:137, 2009.

[116] Roelofs AJ, Thompson K, Gordon S, et al: Molecular mechanisms of action of bisphosphonates: current status. Clin Cancer Res 12:6222s, 2006.

[117] Reid IR, Cornish J: Epidemiology and pathogenesis of osteonecrosis of the jaw. Nat Rev Rheumatol 8:90, 2012.

[118] Reid IR, Bolland MJ, Grey AB: Is bisphosphonate-associated osteonecrosis of the jaw caused by soft tissue toxicity? Bone 41:318, 2007.

[119] Shannon J, Shannon J, Modelevsky S, et al: Bisphosphonates and osteonecrosis of the jaw. J Am Geriatr Soc 59:2350, 2011.

[120] Saad F, Brown JE, Van Poznak C, et al: Incidence, risk factors, and outcomes of osteonecrosis of the jaw: integrated analysis from three blinded active-controlled phase III trials in cancer patients with bone metastases. Ann Oncol 23:1341, 2012.

[121] Saussez S, Javadian R, Hupin C, et al: Bisphosphonate-related osteonecrosis of the jaw and its associated risk factors: a Belgian case series. Laryngoscope 119:323, 2009.

[122] Savoidelli C, F. le Page, J. Santini, G. Scortecci, G. Odin. Osteonecrose maxillaire sous Bisphosphonateset implants dentaires. Revue de Stomatologie et de Chirurgie Maxillo-faciale, vol. 108, issue 8, Dec. 2007, P. 555-558.

[123] Sedghizadeh PP, Kumar SK, Gorur A, et al: Identification of microbial biofilms in osteonecrosis of the jaws secondary to bisphosphonate therapy. J Oral Maxillofac Surg 66:767, 2008.

[124] Seth R, Futran ND, Alam DS, et al: Outcomes of vascularized bone graft reconstruction of the mandible in bisphosphonate-related osteonecrosis of the jaws. Laryngoscope 120:2165, 2010.

[125] Sinningen K, Tsourdi E, Rauner M, et al: Skeletal and extraskeletal actions of denosumab. Endocrine 42:52, 2012.

[126] Sedghizadeh PP, Kumar SK, Gorur A, et al: Microbial biofilms in osteomyelitis of the jaw and osteonecrosis of the jaw secondary to bisphosphonate therapy. J Am Dent Assoc 140:1259, 2009.

[127] Scoletta M, Arduino PG, Reggio L, et al: Effect of low-level laser irradiation on bisphosphonate-induced osteonecrosis of the jaws: preliminary results of a prospective study. Photomed Laser Surg 28:179, 2010.

[128] Scoletta M, Arata V, Arduino PG, et al: Tooth extractions in intravenous bisphosphonate-treated patients: a refined protocol. J Oral Maxillofac Surg 71:994, 2013.

[129] Scoletta M, Arduino PG, Dalmasso P, et al: Treatment outcomes in patients with bisphosphonate-related osteonecrosis of the jaws: a prospective study. Oral Surg Oral Med Oral Pathol Oral Radiol Endod 110:46, 2010.

[130] Smidt-Hansen T, Folkmar TB, Fode K, et al: Combination of zoledronic acid and targeted therapy is active but may induce osteonecrosis of the jaw in patients with metastatic renal cell carcinoma. J Oral Maxillofac Surg 71:1532, 2013.

[131] Scagliotti GV, Hirsh V, Siena S, et al: Overall survival improvement in patients with lung cancer and bone metastases treated with denosumab versus zoledronic acid: subgroup analysis from a randomized phase 3 study. J Thorac Oncol 7:1823, 2012.

[132] Soydan SS, Uckan S: Management of bisphosphonate-related osteonecrosis of the jaw with a platelet-rich fibrin membrane: technical report. J Oral Maxillofac Surg 72:322, 2014.

[133] Schubert M, Klatte I, Linek W, et al: The Saxon bisphosphonate register — therapy and prevention of bisphosphonate-related osteonecrosis of the jaws. Oral Oncol 48:349, 2012.

[134] Stopeck A, Body JJ, Fujiwara Y, et al: Denosumab versus zolendronic acid for the treatment of breast cancer patients with bone metastases: results of a randomized phase 3 study. Eur J Cancer Supplements [EJC supplements] 7:2, 2009.

[135] Sedghizadeh PP, Yooseph S, Fadrosh DW, et al: Metagenomic investigation of microbes and viruses in patients with jaw osteonecrosis associated with bisphosphonate therapy. Oral Surg Oral Med Oral Pathol Oral Radiol 114:764, 2012.

[136] Sivolella S, Lumachi F, Stellini E, et al: Denosumab and anti-angiogenetic drug-related osteonecrosis of the jaw: an uncommon but potentially severe disease. Anticancer Res 33:1793, 2013.

[137] Stockmann P, Vairaktaris E, Wehrhan F, et al: Osteotomy and primary wound closure in bisphosphonate-associated osteonecrosis of the jaw: a prospective clinical study with 12 months follow-up. Support Care Cancer 18:449, 2010.

[138] Stanton DC, Balasanian E: Outcome of surgical management of bisphosphonate-related osteonecrosis of the jaws: review of 33 surgical cases. J Oral Maxillofac Surg 67:943, 2009.

[139] Tsao C, Darby I, Ebeling PR, et al: Oral health risk factors for bisphosphonate-associated jaw osteonecrosis. J Oral Maxillofac Surg 71:1360, 2013.

[140] United States. Food and Drug Administration. Sutent (sunitinib malate) capsules Safety Information. http://www.fda.gov/safety/ medwatch/safetyinformation/ ucm224050.htm. Accessed March 13, 2014.

[141] United States. Food and Drug Administration. Office of Drug Safety. Postmarketing Safety Review. Bisphosphonates. http://www. fda.gov/ohrms/dockets/ac/05/briefing/ 2005-4095B2_03_04-FDATab3.pdf Accessed February 10, 2014.

[142] United States. Food and Drug Administration. Avastin (bevacizumab) Safety Information. http://www.fda.gov/Safety/MedWatch/ SafetyInformation/ucm275758.htm Accessed March 13, 2014.

[143] Vescovi P, Merigo E, Meleti M, et al: Bisphosphonates-related osteonecrosis of the jaws: a concise review of the literature and a report of a single-centre experience with 151 patients. J Oral Pathol Med 41:214, 2012.

[144] Vahtsevanos K, Kyrgidis A, Verrou E, et al: Longitudinal cohort study of risk factors in cancer patients of bisphosphonate-related osteonecrosis of the jaw. J Clin Oncol 27:5356, 2009.

[145] Van den Wyngaert T, Claeys T, Huizing MT, et al: Initial experience with conservative treatment in cancer patients with osteonecrosis of the jaw (ONJ) and predictors of outcome. Ann Oncol 20:331, 2009.

[146] Vandone AM, Donadio M, Mozzati M, et al: Impact of dental care in the prevention of bisphosphonate-associated osteonecrosis of the jaw: a single-center clinical experience. Ann Oncol 23:193, 2012.

[147] Wanger G, Gorby Y, El-Naggar MY, et al: Electrically conductive bacterial nanowires in bisphosphonate-related osteonecrosis of the jaw biofilms. Oral Surg Oral Med Oral Pathol Oral Radiol 115:71, 2013.

[148] Walter C, Al-Nawas B, du Bois A, et al: Incidence of bisphosphonate-associated osteonecrosis of the jaws in breast cancer patients. Cancer 115:1631, 2009.

[149] Yamazaki T, Yamori M, Ishizaki T, et al: Increased incidence of osteonecrosis of the jaw after tooth extraction in patients treated with bisphosphonates: a cohort study. Int J Oral Maxillofac Surg 41:1397, 2012.

[150] Yamashita J, McCauley LK: Antiresorptives and osteonecrosis of the jaw. J Evid Based Dent Pract 12:233, 2012.

Chapter 8

Platelet-rich Plasma (PRP) in Orthopedics and Traumatology — Review

Pencho Kossev and Tsvetan Sokolov

Additional information is available at the end of the chapter

http://dx.doi.org/10.5772/61326

Abstract

In the last few years various methods are being applied in the use of platelet-rich plasma (PRP) during treatment in different orthopedic disease and sports trauma. They allow improvement of local biological condition and regeneration of different types of tissues. PRP is a modern treatment strategy with worldwide recognition. There is a high concentration of platelet growth factors in small amounts of plasma. PRP and its various forms have become one of the best methods to support the healing process of various tissues. PRP is used in regenerative medicine, because it provides two of three components (growth factors and scaffolds) necessary for complete tissue regeneration. The particular reason for the appearance of lesions is important in order to select an appropriate treatment method and technical application. Main indications are acute and chronic wounds, pseudarthrosis, ligament and muscle injuries, some tendinopathies, osteoarthritis, chondral injuries.

Keywords: Platelet rich plasma, platelets, platelet growth factors, chronic skin wounds

1. Introduction

Platelet-rich plasma (PRP) is a modern treatment strategy with worldwide recognition. PRP was introduced in the 1950s and is currently used in multiple fields of medicine. There is high concentration of platelet growth factors in small amounts of plasma. This works for offering an "ideal environment" for tissue regeneration and is part of the so-called biological therapy. The PRP implementation is an autologous therapy, which eliminates the risk of blood-borne infections. PRP and its various forms has become one of the best methods to support the healing process of various tissues. The term „regenerative medicine" was introduced in the 1990s. Many studies related to stem cells, growth factors, and extracellular matrix support the development of this new treatment philosophy. It differs from classic tissue engineering, where tissue regenerates ex vivo. Here, the major idea is regeneration of fully functional tissue on the spot, while damaged tissue is provided for by cellular elements and the process is managed by local factors. PRP appears to be the main source of autologous products in regenerative medicine and a true precursor and foundation of the healing process along with scaffold and stem cells [1]. PRP is used in regenerative medicine, because it provides two of the three components (growth factors and scaffolds), necessary for complete tissue regeneration. This review discusses the state-of the-art-studies on PRP action mechanisms in surgical and non-surgical implementation (treatment of tendon injuries, cartilage damage, muscle trauma, cartilage and bone pathologies, and wound healing).

2. Platelet biology

Platelets are blood cells formed during hematopoiesis. They are built from cytoplasmic fragments of the long extensions of megakaryocytes and are small, discoid, and anucleate cells [2]. These extensions are interwoven through bone marrow sinusoids and are fragmented by shear forces, thus forming new platelets in the blood [3]. Their circulating lifespan is 5-9 days and their major clearance mechanism is via Kuppfer cells and hepatocytes. This became known after discovering the lectin receptor on the cell surface [4]. It is known that the functional activity of platelets changes depending on their size and age, as younger and larger platelets demonstrate better hemostatic function unlike smaller and older cells [5,6,7]. Platelets measure from 1 to 4 μm in diameter and apart from being anucleated, they contain different organelles. They are discoid or ellipsoid in shape and have three distinguishable zones: peripheral or outer zone, organelle zone, and cytosol zone.

Peripheral zone – This is the outermost section and it contains antigens, glycoproteins and various enzymes. This zone connects the platelets with other cells and blood vessel linings. Large quantities of plasma proteins and coagulation factors are firmly attached to this surface. Inside the membrane there are proteins (mostly glycoproteins and a small amount of carbohydrates). This membrane contains a double-layer of phospholipids, cholesterol and glycolipids. Glycoproteins have a number of specific receptors for certain coagulation factors, such as GPIb (thrombin receptors) and the von Willerband factor. The GPIIbIIIa complex is formed from glycoproteins IIb and IIIa and it acts as a fibrinogen receptor. Platelet adhesion and aggregation is affected by those glycoproteins [8].

Organelle zone – It is built from a variety of structures: dense granules, alpha granules, Golgi apparatus, dense tubular system and open canalicular system, lysosomes and mitochondria.

The dense granules (or dense bodies) are dense structures containing 65% of the total platelet adenosine-diphosphate and adenosintriphosphate. Serotonin, pyrophosphate, antiplasmin and large amounts of calcium, necessary for platelet aggregation are also stored there [8-10].

Alpha granules contain various growth factors (platelet-derived growth factor— PDGF, transforming growth factor beta—TGF-b, etc.), and clotting factors. Many of the 30 bioactive proteins, playing a key role for hemostasis are contained in these granules; hemostasis is considered to be the first stage of wound healing [11,12].

Upon platelet activation, internal membrane systems including the dense tubular system (DTS) and the open canalicular system (OCS) interact. By means of cellular membrane invaginations, the open canalicular system helps the communication between the endoplasm and the external milieu. The mitochondria synthesize ATP, which is functionally very important. Acid phosphatize enzymes, glucosamidase, and galactosidase are contained in the lysosomes. Many particles contain glycogen, thus storing energy for cells. The Golgi apparatus is part of the membrane system as well [8,13].

Cytosol zone - It contains microtubules and forms a circumferential zone around platelets. Microtubules are connected to microfilaments. This is how the platelet cytoskeleton is formed; it directs the cell's movement, eliminates secreted products, and retracts clots. Upon platelet activation microtubules could be seen in platelet pseudopods [8].

3. Functions of the platelets

Besides participation in hemostasis, platelets also have other functions. To obtain hemostasis, the interaction of three main mechanisms is necessary: vascular response, platelet activity, and clot formation. When platelets are not activated by various stimuli, they are present in blood circulation in a state of quiescence in disc-shape form. The variety of stimuli can comprise physical or chemical ones, or a combination of both. The sub-endothelial collagen forming in the wound as a result of trauma, along with the von Willebrand factor(vWF), are the main factors that activate blood platelets in vivo, as well as thrombin, adenosine diphosphate, or a combination of them.

In experimental conditions the major activators for the study of platelets are collagen, thrombin and adenosine diphosphate, as well as their synthetic substitutes and calcium ions. Integrin A2b1, glycoproteins complex Ib-V-IX (GPIb-V-IX), and glycoprotein VI (GPVI) are the main collagen receptors. The involvement of collagen by these receptors is done as follows: after the process of binding of von Willebrand factor to glycoprotein Ib (GPIb), the exposed collagen binds to glycoprotein V (GPV) in the same complex, thus slowing down the platelets for a time, sufficient to allow for the further binding of the integrin a2b1 and glycoprotein VI (GPVI) with collagen [7,14].

According to Mehta et al., tissue damage leads to vascular exposure. Thus activating platelets and forming platelet plugs and blood clots. This is how natural hemostasis is provided. This naturally occurring hematoms consists of 95% red blood cells, 4% platelets, and 1% white blood cells. An analysis of a platelet-rich clot shows significant differences in composition as compared to naturally occurring clot, with 95% platelets, 4% red blood cells and about 1% white blood cells [15].

Platelets also have non-hemostatic functions. In addition to their primary role in hemostasis, platelets participate in many non-hemostatic processes. Their secretion contains many different substances [16]. On their external layer, a number of surface receptors are arranged, including adhesion proteins, cytokines, and lipopolysaccharide [17]. Interesting is the fact that platelets also release various substances depending on the stimuli, by which they are activated [16,18]. Alpha granules contain many substances with directly opposing activities. This implies the existence of a mechanism for specific release of only a specific content of the granule, which is possible, but this is still not well studied [19,20]. Inflammation, immunity, and tissue recovery are some of the most characteristic features of platelets [7].

4. Platelet-Rich Plasma (PRP)

The PRP as a concept can be represented as the volume fraction of blood plasma, where the platelet concentration is increased compared to the baseline serum level. In platelet rich plasma, besides platelet concentrate, small amounts of white blood cells are also present and other blood components as well. Ideal is a concentration of 1,407,640 cells in microliter (with a standard deviation of 320.100) [21]. This value corresponds to a number of platelets, approximately five times higher than the normal, nomber in the blood, which is usually in the range of 150,000 to 350,000 cells in microliter (approximately an average value of about 200,000 cells in microliter) [22].

Marx et al. suggest that in order to obtain effective treatment with PRP, the approximate number of platelets should be about $1{,}000 \times 10^3$ platelets in microliter in volume of a 5 ml plasma [23,24]. Jacobson et al. studied the influence of higher than five times the platelet concentration and suggested that angiogenesis is initiated at concentrations of platelet rich plasma from $1{,}500 \times 10^3$ platelets in microliter and continues up to $3{,}000 \times 10^3$ platelets in microliter. Interestingly, at concentrations of $5{,}000 \times 10^3$ platelets in microliter, inhibition of angiogenesis is observed. They reached the conclusion that additional laboratory studies are necessary to elucidate the optimal concentration for use with a particular pathology. Concentration of the platelets less than 300×10^3 platelets in microliter is called "low", 300 -800×10^3 platelets in microliter is considered "moderate", and $>800 \times 10^3$ platelets in microliter is called "high" [7,25].

The presence of white blood cells in PRP may affect its use, independent of the concentration of the platelets [26]. The presence of the layer of leukocytes has led to the current classification, which distinguishes a clean (without leukocytes) PRP, identical to the platelet rich plasma of Anitua, and PRP with leukocytes. Also present in the classification the fibrin-rich gel known as a clean, without leukocytes, platelet-rich fibrin, and platelet-rich fibrin with leukocytes or Choukroun type [27,28].

Ehrenfest et al. categorized the kits based on their fibrin and leukocytes content.

- Pure platelet-rich plasma (P-PRP): cell separator PRP, Vivostat PRF, or Anitua's
- PRGF;
- Platelet-rich and leukocyte-rich plasma (L-PRP): Curasan, Regen, Plateltex,
- SmartPReP, PCCS, Magellan, or GPS PRP;
- Pure platelet-rich fibrin (P-PRF) Fibrinet;

- Platelet-rich and leukocyte-rich fibrin (L-PRF): Choukroun's PRF [27,29].

This classification, despite the various comments, is an important step towards the systematization of knowledge, which allows for more objective comparisons of the results of treatment. It is necessary in future therapy with PRP to choose the allegedly most appropriate kit for the particular pathology [29].

PRP is an autologous therapy, which stimulates the healing of tissues and positively influences the recovery processes. It ensures a high concentration of platelets in a small volume of plasma. Once platelets are activated, platelet aggregation occurs and the contents of their solid granules and alpha granules is released [30,31]. In order to release the growth factors of the platelets, PRP must be activated to start the clotting cascade. The activation of platelets in vivo is done in three ways: by adenosine diphosphate, via membrane phospholipids system (arachidonic acid), and by inducing the presence of thrombin [32]. In hospital and clinical conditions, the conversion of prothrombin to thrombin takes place by means of calcium dichloride and thus platelets are activated. Another way is by means of autologous or bovine thrombin [25].

In order for the platelets and the PRP to be sufficiently functional, they should be activated as with tissue injury. As a result platelets release their contents and a cascade of events is initiated. Normal collagen is repaired. Collagen repair consists of the following phases: inflammation, proliferation, and remodelling [33,34]. Each of these stages is needed to restore the normal function of the tissue.

The first phase may last up to three days. The growth factors are released during this phase. Then fibroblasts penetrate and initiate the second phase of wound healing. At this phase fibroblast differentiation and neovascularization are observed. During the third phase collagen matures and strengthens as this process may last over a year [33-35].

5. Cascade of wound healing

Wound healing is a complex process that comprises of a sequence of events, starting from the time of injury and lasting several months, which can be divided into three phases: inflammation, proliferation, and remodeling [10,36,37].

In the inflammatory phase is observed at the beginning of the cascade with the activation and aggregation of platelets and the formation of a fibrin matrix. With platelets degranulation, cytokines are released that guide the healing process. Leukocytes are attracted by the cytokines through hemostasis and migrate to the damaged area. The first leukocytes involved and responsible for the initial wound cleaning are the neutrophils, which eliminate the bacterial and cellular waste [36,38,39].

During the proliferative phase, which spans through the next few days, monocytes migrate to the wound area under the influence of chemical signals from growth factors. The differentiating of macrophages by circulating monocytes is observed. Platelet signaling and modulation function are also performed by the macrophages. Gradually, the damaged area is impoverished of platelets. The macrophages clean the area through phagocytosis and secrete factors responsible for the formation of granulation tissue from the fibroblasts. During this phase, angiogenesis also begins under the influence of growth factors and thrombin. With the recovery of vascular endothelial cells new vessels also develop. Endothelial cells are activated by thrombin, while a process of interaction is also ensured, which restricts the intensity of the formation of new vessels [40]. In this phase mesenchymal stem cells also emerge and their differentiation is performed in specific tissues such as bone, cartilage, or vascular tissues being determined by chemical signals [36,38,39].

At the time of the remodeling phase, contraction of the collagen and convergence of the edges of the wound is observed. Cell density and vascularization is reduced, excess matrix is removed, and the collagen fibrils are aligned along the stress lines, which increases the strength of the newly-formed tissue [10]. Accumulated granulation tissue remodels or slowly transforms into a specific tissue such as skin or bone [36,38,39].

6. Platelet growth factors

A number of growth factors are located in platelet alpha-granules. In order to be released into the injured tissue monocytes, neutrophils, fibroblasts, mesenchymal stem cells and osteoblasts need the chemotactic effect of an available growth factor. Platelet-derived growth factor (PDGF) produces such effect. This growth factor influences mitogenesis of fibroblasts and smooth muscle cells. PDGF improves the formation of fibrous tissue, assists in the three phases of the healing cascade, and also significantly affects angiogenesis and re-epithelialization. Another important growth factor is transforming growth factor beta (TGF-b). It impacts the connection between fibronectins. It influences cell migration, proliferation and replication, and is present during inflammation processes [41].

Chronic wounds' and endochondral ossification's healing processes are highly influenced by vascular endothelial growth factor (VEGF). It is active in angiogenesis, too [13,42]. The next factor taking part in the recovery of chronic wounds is epidermal growth factor (EGF). It also influences the mitogenesis of endothelial cells, fibroblasts, and keratinocytes [42]. Hepatocite growth factor (HGF) is located in various tissues (several types of epithelium, liver, lung, kidney and tumor). It affects tissue regeneration and possesses morphogenic, mitogenic, antiapoptotic, and neurotrophic qualities [38,43-46].

7. Application of PRP in the treatment of chronic wounds

The process of healing of skin wounds is very intense and includes a number of phenomena, such as hemostasis, inflammation, formation of granulation tissue, epithelialization, neovascularization, collagen synthesis, and wound contraction. Several studies demonstrate that the growth factors are depleted in chronic wounds. Platelets have a tendency to aggregate when activated, having a leading role in skin healing. Activated platelets release growth factors, adhesion molecules, and lipids through which migration, proliferation, and the function of keratinocytes, fibroblasts, and endothelial cells are regulated [47].

Skin wounds are defined as the absence of tissue, where epidermis and dermis are affected, while sometimes can reach the adipose tissue and muscle fascia. In this process, no natural regeneration is observed and tissue lesion is transformed into fibrotic scarring [48,49]. Skin wounds have a frequency of 0.78% and huge funts are spent for their treatment. Annually, 2% of the budget is used for health in the European Union (EU), £ 40 million in the UK, $-1.3 billion are used for the treatment of decubitus in the US [48].

According to Zhu et al., chronic cutaneous wounds are quite frequent in developing countries. They are difficult to treat due to insufficient amount of growth factors. Sometimes wound infections are observed. Conventional treatment with various known techniques and methods is not enough due to the insufficiency of growth factors. Dressing and surgical debridement is used for these patients, but these strategies do not lead to significant outcomes [50].

For the development of skin wounds facilitate various etiological factors such as: chronic venous disease, peripheral arterial disease, neuropathy, arterial hypertension, physical injury, hematologic disorders, skin infection, inflammatory diseases, neoplasms, iatrogenic changes, and those associated with nutrition [48,49,51].

PRP gel has been used for wound healing stimulation on molecular and cellular levels for the last two decades [48,52]. Martinez-Zapata et al. showed tissue regeneration in maxillofacial surgery, chronic ulcers, and surgical wounds in their systematic review [53]. Weglein et al. assessed studies dealing with diabetic wound healing and another study reviewed the healing of chronic wounds [24]. Carter et al. reviewed wound healing when PRP gel is applied and wound healing of control groups (conventional wound care) and reported on a number of indicators [48,52].

With these studies, it was observed that PRPs have effectively stimulated healing in wounds with delayed healing. In a study, Martinez-Zapata et al. reported that the percentage of full healing of wounds treated with PRP has increased compared to that of control wounds. Carter et al. performed a meta-analysis of articles for chronic wounds and support the idea that the use of platelet rich plasma favors full healing compared to control groups [9,19,43]. In a study by Villela et al., they reached similar conclusions, with one of their conclusions reaching so far as to conclude that PRP is the method of choice for the treatment of wounds [48,21].

Difficult to heal wounds are considered those that do not heal after the fourth week of their appearance after being treated with standard methods for the particular pathology. Chronic is a wound that is not healing for a period of three months. The evaluation of each wound is very important. For the purpose, a number of point scales suggested by Cancela et al. based on clinical and anatomical criteria for the size of the wound are used, while a patient variable is also taken into account. The points are randomly defined using clinical experience in wound healing. Common parameters are assessed such as the presence or absence of erythema and edema surrounding the wound, purulent discharge, presence of fibrin, swelling in pressure, swelling with ocher dermatitis, and granulation [48].

Anatomical features are noted and graded such as open bone or tendon, location of the wound, and quality of the pulse of artery dorsalis pedis and artery tibialis posterior (when related to wound location) [48]. Wounds are measured to determine their overall surface, depth, and distribution of undermining of the wound edges. The duration of the wound is determined by the history [48].

There are many studies relating to the pathophysiology of wounds. Skin wound healing is an intensive process and in it are observed a number of events such as hemostasis, inflammation, formation of granulation tissue, formation of new vessels, collagen synthesis, epithelialization, and contraction of the wound. The process of reduction of growth factors in chronic wounds is demonstrated in numerous reports as a result of their reduced production and release, sequestration, or degradation. These mechanisms can be combined [48,54].

Platelet aggregation has a clearly expressed effect in the process of skin wound healing. In this process, growth factors are released and, adhesion of molecules and lipids is observed, while they are responsible for the regulation of cellular migration, proliferation and function of keratinocytes, fibroblasts, and endothelial cells [11,55]. Platelets secrete several antimicrobial peptides when activated by thrombin. PRP has an important antimicrobial and immunoregulatory activity obtained from leukocytes [56,57]. A review of studies using different products rich in platelets demonstrates significant improvement in the treatment of chronic wounds.

Anitua et al. presented an open and randomized study to evaluate the effect of PRP in chronic ulcers of 14 patients. They reported good healing response in 80% of the cases after 8 weeks of treatment, compared with 20% in the control group. Leukocytes were not detected in the analyzed products. Their explanation for the good results lies in the high concentrations of growth factors [48,54].

Crovetti et al. monitored the evolution of chronic skin wounds in 24 patients treated with autologous or homologous gel (depending on the case) and observed a complete healing in 9 of them after an average of 10 applications, with a reduction of pain in all cases [48,49].

Marté-Mestre et al. reported the recovery of vascular chronic ulcers with the use of PRP in 12 of 14 patients for an average treatment period of 2.93 months (average of 0.5 - 7 months) [48,58].

Dellinger and Britton applied autologous platelet gel and reported positive results, with no complications and acceleration of the healing process (5 - 8 weeks) regardless of Pan size. A reduction of the risk of amputation and improvement of quality of life was observed [22,48]. PRP has the advantage of having no adverse effects [59].

Margolis et al. found in a retrospective group study with neuropathic wounds in diabetic feet greater efficiency in the use of PRP against the conventional therapies, with a more obvious effect in severe wounds [48,60].

PRP may be used for treatment of various chronic cutaneous wounds, especially when standard conventional therapy is not good enough and surgical treatment is not possible. It reduces the duration, cost of treatment and the hospital stay. These procedures may be performed in outpatient clinics. There is reduction of wound pain after starting the treatment, reduced risk of blood-borne disease transmission, wound healing is restored, and local immunity is activated [61,62].

8. PRP in osteoarthritis

Cartilage defects and the most common joint disease, osteoarthritis(OA), are characterized by degeneration of the articular cartilage that ultimately leads to joint destruction [50]. Several treatments for OA exist, including exercise, weight control, bracing, nonsteroidal anti-inflammatories, cortisone shots, and viscosupplementation. The biochemical environment of the disease process should be influenced in order to achieve better control of the symptoms. There is an imbalance between various cytokines resulting in the increased quantity of proteolytic enzymes leading to cartilage destruction [25,63 - 65]. The repair of damaged articular cartilage and bone defects represents a great challenge for the orthopedist because of the regenerative limitations of cartilage and the difficulty in obtaining an adequate bone substitute. Damages to the cartilage havess been treated by microfracture, debridement, and grafting procedures [42]. The results obtained by these techniques are so far unsatisfactory, and in most cases, these techniques result in deposition of fibrous connective tissue with low mechanical strength at the defect location [56,66]. Broad application of PRP is typical for oral, maxillofacial, and plastic surgery, while in the last few years there have been papers showing administrations in orthopedics and traumatology. When obtaining PRP, high concentration of growth factors in a volume unit is observed and acceleration of the regeneration process in the arthritic cartilage. Consecutively, PRP stimulates local cell activity. This technique is low-priced and has no side-effects or dangers for the patient [33,67].

The presence of concentrated growth factors modulates the phenotypic expression of chondrocytes. This improves their recovery. TGF-b plays a major role in the differentiation of stem cells into chondrocytes. Synthesis of cartilaginous matrix is improved, as well. PDGF and IGF are both key parts of the recovery process, as the first one stimulates proliferation of chondrocytes while the second one increases the synthesis of proteoglycan - macromolecules. Thus, the strength of cartilage is improved [30,56]. Not only does PRP stimulate cellular activity and the process of regeneration and repair, but it also improves bone and cartilage recovery when biomaterials are applied [68,69]. In order to recover cartilage defects, not only PRP is needed but also an adequate biomaterial that has similar characteristics as the natural tissue and promotes cellular adhesion, proliferation, and differentiation [56].

According to Hunziker et al., TGF-b increases chondrogenesis [24,70], while Kon et al. documented PRP amplification of chondrocyte proliferation with convincing clinical effects on degenerative knee OA [24,25,70,71]. Results of the Kon et al. publication on 115 arthritic knees treated with PRP showed improvement in the functional status and pain scores "which remained positive at 6 months, with only mild degradation of scores at 1 year". It was also mentioned that lower grades of arthritis and younger patients had better outcomes [25,72].

Qi et al. shared results on the treatment of osteochondral defects in rabbits with PRP and biodegradable collagen scaffolds. PRP was put into collagen scaffolds (0.05 ml PRP/structure) and then implanted in osteochondral defects (4 x 3 mm) produced in the patellar sulcus of rabbit femurs. Evaluation of tissues was completed after 6 and 12 weeks by histological analysis and a mechanical indentation test. The results in both follow-up times were improved and showed that PRP possesses the capacity to stimulate the regeneration of critical defects in cartilage [56,73].

According to Patel et al. in a study with level 1 evidence, PRP has a superior effect compared to placebo in patients with varying degrees of knee OA. They tested 78 patients (156 knees) and observed that PRP alleviated the symptoms of OA when compared with a saline injection used as control. Follow-up period was up to 6 months. The results showed that with the help of PRP, the homeostasis and function of the knee joint can be improved [74,75].

Wei et al. reported the effect of PRP on the regeneration of cartilage in vivo. Auricular cartilage chondrocytes from rabbits were added to PRP (5 x 10^7 cells/ml PRP), injected subcutaneously in the dorsum of the donor animal, and after 60 days the tissue was evaluated by magnetic resonance, histological, and histochemical analysis. The results exhibited cartilaginous tissue formation in those groups that were injected with chondrocytes and PRP. In the groups in which only PRP was injected, cartilaginous tissue formation was not

observed. The authors inferred that PRP is effective in stimulating regeneration of cartilage when associated with viable cells [56,76].

A level 1 study published in 2012 in the Journal of Arthroscopy by Sanchez et al. used PRP type 4A to observe the results of PRP injection compared with hyaluronic acid. In this study 176 patients, were randomized to receive three weekly applications of PRP (8 ml at weekly intervals) or hyaluronic acid injections. The study was well-conducted, but the results only focused on the short term (until 6 months of follow up). The study was awarded as the best randomized clinical trial (level 1) for 2012, which gives useful fundamental guidelines on how to study the effects of PRP [74,77,78].

In the light of orthopedic and trauma critical literature, there is no standardization of treatment methods, such that most of the works use 3–5 applications of PRP in intervals ranging from 1–3 weeks with no standardization of the amount of volume to be applied and the ideal platelet concentration method [74].

Important factors for results of PRP treatment are the amount of platelets, grade of chondrocyte damage, patient's physical activity, and medical history combined with psychosocial factors. It is good to investigate whether PRP balances anabolism-catabolism, and if there is, what effect of does the PRP have on the synovium. Given the patient's condition, appropriate PRP treatment in OA should use more anti-inflammatory cytokines instead of pro-inflammatory cytokines. The future of OA research aims at isolating cytokines contained in PRP termed as "autologous conditioned serum" to specifically inhibit IL-1 and TNF alpha and down regulate MMP-13 [25,79].

Early OA can be treated by implementing intra-articular PRP. Worse outcome is observed with patients of advanced age and disease process. Khoshbin et al. compared intra-articular administration of PRP to hyaluronic acid and non-setoroid injections and reported that sequential intra-articular PRP injections may have beneficial effects on adult patients with mild to moderate osteoarthritis for a period of 6 months [80].

Zhu et al. reported the fact that PRP contains growth factors, which may have a negative impact on the treatment of a joint with osteoarthritis. That is why those growth factors should be isolated. The following years may be focused on finding suitable and harmless growth factors to improve PRP outcome [50]. Dold et al. paid attention to the fact that there is insufficient data on PRP implementation on post-traumatic osteochondral defects. Further studies with long-term follow-up are necessary in order to illustrate the benefits of isolated PRP application or application in combination with surgical treatment when treating cartilage pathology [81].

9. Tendinopathies

Efficiency of PRP for treating tendinopathies has been vastly studied, and obtained results have been mostly positive (both in vitro and in vivo). Other research also supports the use of PRP for treating tendinopathies through testing cultures of equine and human cells [82,83]. An increase in the types of expression of collagen genes in tendon cell cultures with PRP was presented in a study by Schnabel et al [84]. Similar results were shown by Mishra and Pavelko in their study including an improvement in the pain felt by 15 patients with chronic elbow tendinosis after a single application of PRP [85]. In the PRP-treated group, 93% of the cases achieved pain reduction. Schepull et al. published the first randomized clinical study on the use of PRP in complete ruptures of the ankle tendon. Elasticity was evaluated after 7 weeks and functional assessments were completed after 1 year [86].

Creaney et al. in a recent study concluded that patients with resistant elbow tendinopathy were also considered appropriate for PRP treatment [87]. According to Peerbooms et al. in a double-blind study, with a level of evidence 1, the use of PRP in the treatment of chronic lateral epicondylitis was more favourable than injections of corticoids [88].

A significant statistic improvement at 1 year was observed in the group treated with PRP in comparison to the corticosteroid group that showed improvement only at the beginning. It can be inferred that in addition to conservative treatments, PRP provides a viable therapeutic alternative for refractory tendinopathies (as confirmed in a South Korean study in PRP treatment resulting in "increased cell proliferation, genic expression and synthesis of the tendon matrix in degenerative injuries of the rotatory cuff") [89].

Other findings include the successful use of PRP (alternatively to conservative therapies) in Achilles tendon injuries in conjunction with stem cells and with other various tendinopathies of 203 patients (epicondylitis, patellar tendonitis, hamstring origin (ischial tuberosity) tendonitis, plantar fasciitis, flexor carpi ulnarii tendonitis, pes anserinus tendonitis, biceps femoris tendonitis, iliopsoas tendonitis, athletic pubalgias, and biceps brachii tendonitis) whose status did not improve during conservative therapies [90]. Local infiltration with PRP was applied and 75% success ratio in patients was achieved. According to Virchenko and Aspenberg, and in another study by Eliasson et al. in Achilles tendon rupture patients, results are better with percutaneous suture, PRGF placement, and early load-bearing and mobilization [83,91,92].

10. Anterior Cruciate Ligament (ACL)

As a result of the growing popularity of growth factor treatment techniques, PRP treatment applications have increased for both soft and bone tissue therapies. Several studies include positive results from such treatments. Repair of ligament injuries was tested by Sánchez et al., resulted in better healing outcomes and fewer complications after applying PRP to 100 patients with ACL reconstruction [93]. Fixation of the PRPG graft was studied by Radice et al. and the results were evaluated using MRI images of the interior of the ACL graft and concluded a 48 % faster and completely homogenous repair of the PRPG graft in the experimental group [83, 94,95].

Controversial opinions are shared on the application of PRGF/PRP in the reconstruction of the ACL and posterior cruciate ligament (PCL), such as the degree of effectiveness in the integration of the graft into the bone tunnel and rates of graft maturation [29,94,96]. A statistically significant difference ($p = 0.023$) was found during stimulation of both ACL graft maturation and ACL graft-bone healing with PRP application [93]. After histological assessment of the ACL grafts with and without PRP, Sanchez et al. found "a significantly better maturity index for ACL grafts (12 pts vs. 14 pts, $p = 0.024$), and more newly developed synovial tissue enveloping the platelet treated grafts (77% of cases) compared to the control grafts without platelets (40%)" [93].

11. Muscle

The use of PRP in muscle injury treatment still hasn't been studied thoroughly in humans [74, 97]. There are a number of studies on the effects on muscle tissue. For instance, Shen et al. stated that the inflammatory phase of skeletal muscle healing was controlled by growth factors, macrophages, and COX-2 pathway products [90]. According to Sánchez et al. "the clinical benefits of the ultrasound-guided application of growth factor in physical therapy, electrotherapy, and isometric exercise" for athletes include "a decrease in pain and swelling, a complete recovery of functional capacities before the expected time, and regeneration of the muscle tissue according to ultrasound". No evidence of fibrosis and no recurrence of injuries were found in any of the treated athletes [65,98].

Nevertheless, there still have to be more studies necessary to define the efficiency of PRP in acute muscle injury treatment and to create adequate protocols for administration. The main reason is the insufficient number and low methodological quality of the current studies on the use of PRP in human muscle injuries [38].

12. Surgery and trauma (Autologous fibrin Glue)

The introduction of fibrin glue in repair techniques started in the beginning of the 20th century. Its main use remains within surgical interventions and undergoes constant modification for better results. Fibrin glue became the predecessor of contemporary PRP treatment [99].

A number of studies show the benefits of fibrin and platelet combined treatment. According to Everts et al., the application of autologous platelet gel and fibrin sealant in total knee arthroplasty lead to "significant postoperative increases in hemoglobin rates, required less allogeneic blood, and had fewer complications during wound treatment", thus showing high efficiency of treatment method [100]. Levy et al. evaluated the hemostatic efficiency of adhesive fibrin in 58 patients (a control group and a fibrin treated group) undergoing total knee arthroplasty. Outcomes were significantly higher blood loss for the control group (24 patients needed blood transfusion versus only six from the treated group) and no ostoperative adverse events in the treated group [101]. Sánchez et al.'s findings show the recovery of 12 athletes treated for total Achilles tendon rupture (six received an association of PRGF), during which repair was completed significantly faster than that of the control group, needed less time to recover range of motion and to resume training [102].

It is estimated that few studies have examined PRP action during treatment of orthopedic trauma [67,103], which shows that common treatment was the combination of PRP with bone graft, bone marrow and various bone substitutes (tricalcium phosphate, hydroxyapatite bio-ceramics), as well as treatment with human mesenchymal stem cells in an osteoconductive environment (platelet gel application used to increase formation of new bone tissue through modulating and stimulating the healing cell mediators) [67,103-105].

Other studies represent the effect of biological material in the hemostasis after total substitution of the articulation. According to the results of "98 total arthroplasties of the knee, 61 received application of PRP in the intraoperatory period on the exposed tissue and on the closure of the wound at the end of the procedure". Conclusions showed significant acceleration of recovery and better overall mobility and quality of life in PRP treated patients. The reasons for such fast recovery were attributed to the direct PRP application on knee surgery after arthroplasties. This seals the tissue and takes platelets directly to the wound, where the regeneration process starts immediately [106].

PRP may be used on patients with factures or in cases of total arthroplasies. With the introduction of new cement–free implants, the use of PRP between the implant and the bone might speed up the osteointegration process and improve the implant fixation [38].

13. Conclusion remarks

In the last few years various methods are applied in the use of PRP during treatment in different orthopedic disease and sports trauma. They allow improvement of local biological condition and regeneration of different types of tissues. Without doubt the use of PRP is absolutely a treatment option. According to Werner and Cramer the platelet is the most important cell for the repair processes of the body [74].

Recently, scientific research and technology have presented a new perspective concerning the understanding of "orthobiologic" treatments and the healing process of lesions [38].

PRP treatment is widely applied in the last ten years, especially for stimulating coagulation. A number of studies show that platelets demonstrate other functions, too. They are connected to liberating bioactive proteins and growth factors. The bioactive proteins as well as the growth factors improve tissue regeneration and the process of healing. PRP is the first true biologic therapy that has hit orthopedics by storm. Its ease of use and generally high safety profile has made it a preferred option for the most of the physicians and their patients worldwide. When trauma of musculoskeletal system injuries occur healing takes longer periods of time, and frequently they do not recover completely. Fast and effective recovery is of particular importance for athletes. That's why all healing methods that accelerate the recovery process are fundamentally important. Many different pathologies can be treated with PRP.

The administration of PRP in athletes has been gradually introduced in everyday patients. This has become another option for treatment in addition to conservative options. A number of surgical manipulations can influence results in PRP treatment, such as grafts, medication, and physical therapy.

"Following recommendations of the International Olympic Committee (IOC), the local applications of PRP have been used in the treatment of mild to moderate lesions with no surgical indication, or during surgery" [107].

Main indications are acute and chronic wounds, pseudarthrosis, ligament and muscle injuries, some tendinopathies, osteoarthritis, chondral injuries. Almost all the surgeries carried out since 2007 have used PRP, whether in gel or liquid form [108].

PRP represents an autologous biological material as its action is directly related to general clinical conditions of the patient. The particular reason for the appearance of lesions is important in order to select an appropriate treatment method and technical application. However, standardization in PRP protocols and long-term follow-up should clarify some of the questions regarding the durability of these procedures and any possible modification that should be done to achieve better results.

Various additional new studies are necessary to further improve the results of PRP application in different pathologies. This will help with understanding the different stages of the healing process and demonstrate the potential of PRP treatment in everyday patients.

Author details

Pencho Kossev and Tsvetan Sokolov*

*Address all correspondence to: sokolovi2001@abv.bg

Clinic of Orthopedics and Traumatology, MHAT – Rouse, Bulgaria

References

[1] Cugat R. Lecture Foreword I. In: Lana JF (ed), Platelet-Rich Plasma Regenerative Medicine: Sports Medicine, Orthopedic, and Recovery of Musculoskeletal Injuries, Springer. 2014;5-6. DOI: 10.1007/978-3-642-40117-6.

[2] Machlus KR, Italiano JE Jr. The incredible journey: From megakaryocyte development to platelet formation. J Cell Biol.10 Jun 2013;201(6):785-96. DOI: 10.1083/jcb.201304054.

[3] Thon JN, Macleod H, Begonja AJ, Zhu J, Lee KC, Mogilner A, Hartwig JH, Italiano JE Jr. Microtubule and cortical forces determine platelet size during vascular platelet production. Nat commun. 2012;3:852. DOI: 10.1038/ncomms1838.

[4] Grozovsky R, Hoffmeister KM, Falet H. Novel clearance mechanisms of platelets. Curr Opin Hematol. 2010;17(6):585–589. DOI: 10.1097/MOH.0b013e32833e7561.

[5] Hartley PS. Platelet senescence and death. Clinical laboratory. 2007;53(3–4):157–166.

[6] Karpatkin S. Heterogeneity of human platelets. VI. correlation of platelet function with platelet volume. Blood. 1978;51(2):307–316. DOI: http://dx.doi.org/.

[7] Textor J. Platelet-Rich Plasma (PRP) as a Therapeutic Agent: Platelet Biology,Growth Factors and a Review of the Literature. In: Lana JF(ed), Platelet-Rich Plasma, Platelet-Rich Plasma Regenerative Medicine: Sports Medicine, Orthopedic, and Recovery of Musculoskeletal Injuries, Springer. 2014;61-81. DOI: 10.1007/978-3-642-40117-6.

[8] Bittencourt CH, Bittencourt PB, Neto OAL, Arenas GCF.The Use of Platelet-Rich Plasma in Orthopaedic Injuries. In: Lana JF(ed), Platelet-Rich Plasma Regenerative Medicine: Sports Medicine, Orthopedic, and Recovery of Musculoskeletal Injuries, Springer. 2014;1-47. DOI: 10.1007/978-3-642-40117-6.

[9] Hanson SR, Harker LA. Blood coagulation and blood-materials interactions. In: Ratner BD, Hoffman AS, Schoen FJ, Lemons JE (eds) Biomaterials science. An introduction to materials in medicine. Academic Press, San Diego. 1996;193–199.

[10] Pietrzak WS, Eppley BL. Platelet-rich plasma: Biology and new technology. J Craniofac Surg. 2005;16(6):1043–1054.

[11] Anitua E, Andia I, Ardanza B, Nurden P, Nurden AT. Autologous platelets as a source of proteins for healing and tissue regeneration. Thromb Haemost. 2004;91(1): 4–15.

[12] Harrison P, Cramer EM. Platelet alpha-granules. Blood Rev. 1993;7(1):52–62.

[13] Maes C, Carmeliet P, Moermans K, et al. Impaired angiogenesis and endochondral bone formation in mice lacking the vascular endothelial growth factor isoforms VEGF164 and VEGF188. Mach Dev. 2002;111(1–2):61–73.

[14] Herr AB, Farndale RW. Structural insights into the interactions between platelet receptors and fibrillar collagen. J Biol Chem. 2009;284(30):19781–19785. DOI: 10.1074/jbc.R109.013219.

[15] Mehta S, Watson JT. Platelet-rich concentrate: Basic science and current clinical application J Orthop Trauma. 2008;22(6):433-438. DOI: 10.1097/BOT.0b013e31817e793f.

[16] Virchenko O, Aspenberg P. How can one platelet injection after tendon injury lead to a stronger tendon after 4 weeks? Interplay between early regeneration and mechanical stimulation. Acta Orthop Scand. 2006;77:806–812.

[17] Clemetson KJ, Clemetson JM. Platelet receptors. In: Michelson AD (ed) Platelets, 2nd edn. Academic Press, Elsevier, Burlington. 2007;117–134.

[18] Cognasse F, Hamzeh-Cognasse H, Lafarge S, Delezay O, Pozzetto B, McNicol A, Garraud O. Toll-like receptor 4 ligand can differentially modulate the release of cytokines by human platelets. Br J Haematol. 2008;141(1):84–91. DOI:10.1111/j.1365-2141.2008.06999.x. Epub 2008 Feb 12.

[19] Blair P, Flaumenhaft R. Platelet alpha-granules: Basic biology and clinical correlates. Blood Rev. 2009;23(4):177–189. DOI: 10.1016/j.blre.2009.04.001. Epub 2009 May 17.

[20] Nurden AT. Platelets, inflammation and tissue regeneration. Thromb Haemost. 2011;105(Suppl 1):13–33. DOI: 10.1160/THS10-11-0720. Epub 2011 Apr 11.

[21] Villela DL, et al. Topical therapy of chronic leg ulcers with platelet-rich plasma: A systematic review of the literature. Paper present at: WOCN 2010 Conference of the Wound Ostomy Continense Nurse Society, St Louis, Mo, June 2010.

[22] Dellinger R, Britton C. Autologous platelet grafting procedure—a new approach to healing chronic wounds and comparison between current therapies. Monograph White. 2001; Accessed 23 Mar 2013.

[23] Marx RE. Platelet-rich plasma (PRP): What is PRP and what is not PRP? Implant Dent. 2001;10(8):225–228.

[24] Weglein A, Sampson S,Aufiero D. Platelet-Rich Plasma Practical Use in Non-Surgical Musculoskeletal Pathology. In: Lana JF (ed), Platelet-Rich Plasma Regenerative Medicine: Sports Medicine, Orthopedic, and Recovery of Musculoskeletal Injuries, Springer. 2014;187-199. DOI: 10.1007/978-3-642-40117-6.

[25] Weibrich G, Kleis WKG, Hafner G, Hitzler WE. Growth factor levels in platelet-rich plasma and correlations with donor age, sex, and platelet count. J Cranio Maxillofacial Surg. 2002; 30(2):97–102.

[26] Everts PAM, Devilee RJJ, Brown-Mahoney C, Eeftinck SM, Box HAM, Knape JTA, Van Zundert A. Platelet gel and fibrin sealant reduce allogenic blood transfusions and in total knee arthroplasty. Acta Anaesth Scand. 2006;50:593–599.

[27] Ehrenfest DM, Rasmusson L, Albrektsson T. Classification of platelet concentrates: From pure platelet-rich plasma (P-PRP) to leucocyte- and platelet-rich fibrin (L-PRF).

Trends Biotechnol. 2009;27(3):158–167 DOI: 10.1016/j.tibtech.2008.11.009. Epub 2009 Jan 31.

[28] Perez AGM, Lana JF, Rodrigues AA, Luzo ACM, Belangero WD, Santana MHA. Challenges and a Feasible Strategy for Studies and Standardization of Platelet-Rich Plasma. In: Lana JF (ed), Platelet-Rich Plasma Regenerative Medicine: Sports Medicine, Orthopedic, and Recovery of Musculoskeletal Injuries, Springer. 2014;119-136. DOI: 10.1007/978-3-642-40117-6.

[29] Tarczynska M, Gaweda K. PRP in the Ambulatory Therapy of Tendinopathy of the Elbow, Knee and Foot. In: Lana JF(ed), Platelet-Rich Plasma Regenerative Medicine: Sports Medicine, Orthopedic, and Recovery of Musculoskeletal Injuries, Springer. 2014;237-247. DOI: 10.1007/978-3-642-40117-6.

[30] Cole BJ, Seroyer ST, Filardo G, et al. Platelet-rich plasma: Where are we now and where are we going? Sports Health Multi Approach. 2010;2(3):203–210. DOI: 10.1177/1941738110366385.

[31] Rodrigues AA, LanaJF, Luzo ACM, Santana MHA, Perez A, Lima-Silva DB, Belangero WD. Platelet-Rich Plasma and Tissue Engineering. In: Lana JF (ed), Platelet-Rich Plasma Regenerative Medicine: Sports Medicine, Orthopedic, and Recovery of Musculoskeletal Injuries, Springer. 2014;139-149. DOI: 10.1007/978-3-642-40117-6.

[32] Everts PA, Overdevest EP, Jakimowicz JJ, Oosterbos CJ, Schonberger JP, Knape JT, van Zundert A. The use of autologous platelet-leukocyte gels to enhance the healing process in surgery, a review. Surg Endosc. 2007;21(11):2063–2068. Epub 2007 Apr 13.

[33] Crane D, Oliver K. Platelet-Rich Plasma and Biocellular Grafts. In: Lana JF (ed), Platelet-Rich Plasma Regenerative Medicine: Sports Medicine, Orthopedic, and Recovery of Musculoskeletal Injuries, Springer. 2014;242-262. DOI: 10.1007/978-3-642-40117-6.

[34] Kumar V, et al. Acute and chronic inflammation. In: Robbins and cotran pathologic basis of disease, 7th edn. Saunders, Curtis Center 170 South Independece Mall W 300E, Philadelphia PA. 2005;103–116.

[35] Crane D, Everts PAM. Platelet-rich plasma (PRP) matrix grafts. PPM. 2008;8:12–27.

[36] Clark RAF. Overview and general considerations of wound repair. In: Clark RAF (ed) The molecular and cellular biology of wound repair. Plenum Press, New York. 1996;3–50.

[37] Marx RE. Platelet-rich plasma: A source of multiple autologous growth factors for bone grafts. In: Lynch SE, et al. (eds) Tissue engineering, applications in maxillofacial surgery and peiodontics. Quintessence Books, Carol Stream. 1999;71–82.

[38] Lana JF, Weglein A, Vicente E, Perez A, Rodrigues A, Luzo A, Santana N, Belangero W. Platelet Rich Plasma and Its Growth Factors: The State of the Art, In: Lana JF (ed), Platelet-rich Plasma Regenerative Medicine: Sports Medicine, Orthopedic, and Re-

covery of Musculoskeletal Injuries, Springer. 2014;1-47. DOI: 10.1007/978-3-642-40117-6.

[39] Lorenz HP, Longaker MT. Wounds: Biology, pathology, and management. In: Norton JA, Bollinger RR, Chang AE, et al (eds) Surgery: basic science and clinical evidence, Springer, New York. 2001;77–88.

[40] Minami T, Horiuchi K, Miura M, et al.Vascular endothelial growth factor- and thrombin-induced termination factor, Down syndrome critical region-1, attenuates endothelial cell proliferation and angiogenesis. J Biol Chem. 2004;279(48):50537–50554. DOI: 10.1074/jbc.M406454200.

[41] Molloy T, Wang Y, Murrell G. The roles of growth factors in tendon and ligament healing. Sports Med. 2003;33(5):381–394.

[42] Bennett SP, Griffiths GD, Schor AM, et al. Growth factors in the treatment of diabetic foot ulcers. Br J Surg. 2003;90(2):133–146.

[43] Boros P, Miller CM. Hepatocyte growth factor: A multifunctional cytokine. Lancet. 1995;345(8945):239–5.

[44] Kosai K, Matsumoto K, Fukanoshi H, et al. Hepatocyte growth factor prevents endotoxininduced lethal hepatic failure in mice. Hepatology. 1990;30(1):151–159.

[45] Matsumoto K, Nakamura T. Hepatocyte growth factor: Molecular structure, roles in liver regeneration, and other biological functions. Crit Ver Oncog. 1992;3(1–2):27–54.

[46] Miyazawa T, Matsumoto K, Ohmichi H, et al. Protection of hippocampal neurons from ischemia-induced delayed neuronal death by hepatocyte growth factor: A novel neurotrophic factor. J Cereb Blood Flow Metab. 1998;18(4):345–348.

[47] Yuan T, Zhang C-Q Tang M-J, Shang-Chun Guo S-C, Zeng B-F. Autologous platelet-rich plasma enchances healing of chronic wounds.Wounds. 2009;21(10):138-141.

[48] Cancela AM, Lana JF, Annichino-Bizzachi JM, Belangero WD,Luzo ACM. Use of Platelet-Rich Plasma (PRP) in Treating Chronic Wounds. In: Lana JF(ed), Platelet-Rich Plasma Regenerative Medicine: Sports Medicine, Orthopedic, and Recovery of Musculoskeletal Injuries, Springer. 2014;281-288. DOI: 10.1007/978-3-642-40117-6.

[49] Crovetti G, Martinelli G, Issi M, et al. Platelet gel for healing cutaneous chronic wounds. Transfus Apheres Sci. 2004;30:145–151.

[50] Zhu Y, Yuan M, Menq HY. Basic science and clinical application of platelet-rich plasma for cartilage defects and osteoarthritis: A review. Osteoarthritis Cartilage. 2013;21(11):1627-37. DOI: 10.1016/j.joca.2013.07.017. Epub 2013 Aug 7.

[51] Cieslik-Bielecka A, Gazdzik TS, Bielecki TM, et al. Why the platelet-rich gel has antimicrobial activity? Oral Surg Oral Med Oral Pathol Oral Radiol Endod. 2007; 103(3): 303–305.

[52] Carter MJ, et al. Use of platelet-rich plasma gel on wound healing: A systematic review and meta-analysis. J Plast Surg. 2011;15(11):382–410.

[53] Martinez-Zapata MJ, Marti-Carvajal A, Sola I, et al. Efficacy and safety of the use of autologous plasma rich in platelets for tissue regeneration: A systematic review. Transfusion. 2009;49(1):44–56. DOI: 10.1111/j.1537-2995.2008.01945.x. Epub 2008 Oct 14.

[54] Anitua E, Aguirre JJ, Algorta J, et al. Effectiveness of autologous preparation rich in growth factors for the treatment of chronic cutaneous ulcers. J Biomed Mater Res B Appl Biomater. 2008;84(2):415–421.

[55] Fu X, Li X, Cheng B, et al. Engineered growth factors and cutaneous wound healing: Success and possible questions in the past 10 years. Wound Rep Regen. 2005;13:122–130.

[56] El-Sharkawy H, Kantarci A, Deady J, et al. Platelet-rich plasma: Growth factors and pro- and anti-inflammatory properties. J Periodontol. 2007;78(4):661–669.

[57] Moojen DJ, Everts PA, Schure RM, et al. Antimicrobial activity of platelet-leukocyte gel against staphylococcus aureus. J Orthop Res. 2008;26:404–410.

[58] Marté-Mestre FX, Acosta-Gómez M, Bonell-Pascual A, et al. Resultados preliminares de la aplicación de factores de crecimiento en el tratamiento de las Úlceras vasculares. Angiologia. 2005;57:335–343.

[59] Ramos-Torrecillas J, De Luna-Bertos E, García-Martínez O, Ruiz C. Clinical Utility of Growth Factors and Platelet-Rich Plasma in Tissue Regeneration: A Review. Wounds. 2014; 26(7):207-213.

[60] Margolis DJ, Kantor J, Santanna J, et al. Effectiveness of platelet releasate for the treatment of diabetic neuropathic foot ulcers. Diabetes Care. 2001;24(3):483–488.

[61] Greenlagh DG. The role of growth factors in wound healing. J Trauma. 1996;41:159-167.

[62] Obolenskiy VN, Ermolova DA, Laberko LA, Semenova TV. Efficacy of platelet-rich plasma for the treatment of chronic wounds. EWMA Journal. 2014;14(1):37-40.

[63] Cook JL, Anderson CC, Kreeger JM et al. Effects of human recombinant interleukin-1 beta on canine articular chondrocytes in three-dimensional culture. Am J Vet Res. 2000; 61:766–770.

[64] Goldring MB. The role of the chondrocyte in osteoarthritis. Arthritis Rhuem. 2000;43:1916–1926.

[65] Sánchez M, Anitua E,Orive G, Mujika I, Andia I. Platelet-rich therapies in the treatment of orthopaedic sport injuries. Sports Med. 2009;39(5):345-54. DOI: 10.2165/00007256-200939050-00002.

[66] Hunziker EB. Articular cartilage repair: Basic science and clinical progress. A review of the current status and prospects. Osteoarthr Cartil. 2002;10(6):432–463.

[67] Biggi F, Caloprisco G, Scorrano A. Autologous platelet gel in orthopaedics and traumatology (3-year experience). J Bone Joint Surg. 2004;87(Suppl 2):173.

[68] Kasten P, Beverungen M, Lorenz H, Wieland J, Fehr M, Geiger F. Comparison of plateletrich plasma and VEGF-transfected mesenchymal stem cells on vascularization and bone formation in a critical-size bone defect. Cells Tissues Organs. 2012;196(6): 523–533. DOI: 10.1159/000337490. Epub 2012 Jul 10.

[69] Kasten P, Vogel J, Beyen I, et al. Effect of platelet-rich plasma on the in vitro proliferation and osteogenic differentiation of human mesenchymal stem cells on distinct calcium phosphate scaffolds: The specific surface area makes a difference. J Biomater Appl. 2008;21(4):386–389. DOI: 10.1177/0885328207088269

[70] Hunziker EB, Driesang IM, Morris EA. Chondrogenesis in cartilage repair is induced by members of the transforming growth factor-beta superfamily. Clin Orthop Relat Res. 2001; 391(suppl):171–181.

[71] Kon E, Filardo G, Presti ML et al. Utilization of platelet-derived growth factors for the treatment of cartilage degenerative pathology. Paper presented at the International Cartilage Repair Society Meeting, Electronic Poster Presentation 29.3. Warsaw, Poland, October 2007.

[72] Kon E, Buda R, Filardo G, et al. Platelet-rich plasma: Intra articular knee injections produced favorable results on degenerative cartilage lesions. Knee Surg Sports Traumatol Arthrosc. 2010;18:472–479. DOI: 10.1007/s00167-009-0940-8. Epub 2009 Oct 17.

[73] Qi YY, Chen X, Jiang YZ, et al. Local delivery of autologous platelet in collagen matrix simulated in situ articular cartilage repair. Cell Transplant. 2009;18(10):1161–1169. DOI: 10.3727/096368909X12483162197169. Epub 2009 Aug 5.

[74] Da Silva RT, Heidrich F. Therapy with Use of Platelet-Rich Plasma in Orthopedics and Sports Traumatology: Literature Review, Evidence and Personal Experience. In: Lana JF (ed), Platelet-Rich Plasma Regenerative Medicine: Sports Medicine, Orthopedic, and Recovery of Musculoskeletal Injuries, Springer. 2014;153-168. DOI: 10.1007/978-3-642-40117-6.

[75] Patel S, Dillon MS, Agarwall S, Marwaha M, Jain A. Treatment with platelet-rich plasma is more effective than placebo for knee osteoarthritis. Am J Sports Med. 2013;41(2):356-364. DOI: 10.1177/0363546512471299. Epub 2013 Jan 8.

[76] Weyrich AS, Lindemann S, Zimmerman GA.The evolving role of platelets in inflammation. J Thromb Haemost. 2003;1(9):1897–1905. DOI: 10.1046/j. 1538-7836.2003.00304.x.

[77] Sanchez M, Anitua E, Azofra J, Aguirre JJ, Andia I. Intraarticular injection of an autologous preparation rich in growth factors for the treatment of knee OA: A retrospective cohort study. Clin Exp Rheumatol. 2008;26(5):910–913.

[78] Sanchez M, Fiz N, Azofra J, Usabiaga J, Recalde EA, et al. A randomized clinical trial evaluating plasma rich in growth factors (PRGF-Endoret) versus hyaluronic acid in the shortterm treatment of symptomatic knee osteoarthritis. Arthroscopy. 2012;28(8): 1070–1078.

[79] Woodell-May J, Matuska A, Oyster M, Welch Z, O'Shaughnessey K, Hoeppner J. Autologous protein solution inhibits MMP-13 production by IL-1b and TNFa-stimulated human articular chondrocytes. J Orthop Res. 2011;29(9):1320–1326. DOI: 10.1002/jor.21384. Epub 2011 Mar 15.

[80] Khoshbin A, Leroux T, Wasserstein D, Theodoropoulos J. The efficacy of platelet-rich plasma in the treatment of symptomatic knee osteoarthritis: A systematic review with quantitative synthesis. Arthroscopy. 2013;29(12):2037-48. DOI: 10.1016/j.arthro.2013.09.006.

[81] Dold AP, Zywiel MG, Taylor DW, Dwyer T, Theodoropoulos J. Platelet-rich plasma in the management of articular cartilage pathology: A systematic review Clin J Sport Med. 2014; 24(1):31-43. DOI: 10.1097/01.jsm.0000432855.85143.e5.

[82] Mishra A, Woodall J, Vieira A. Treatment of tendon and muscle using platelet-rich plasma. Clin Sports Med. 2009;28(1):113–125. DOI: 10.1016/j.csm.2008.08.007.

[83] Silva R, Heidrich F. Therapy with Use of Platelet-Rich Plasma in Orthopedics and Sports Traumatology: Literature Review, Evidence and Personal Experience. In: Lana JF (ed), Platelet-Rich Plasma Regenerative Medicine: Sports Medicine, Orthopedic, and Recovery of Musculoskeletal Injuries, Springer. 2014;153-170. DOI: 10.1007/978-3-642-40117-6.

[84] Schnabel LV, Mohammed HO, Miller BJ, et al. Platelet-rich plasma (PRP) enhances anabolic gene expression patterns in flexor digitorum superficialis tendons. J Orthop Res. 2007;25(2):230–240.

[85] Mishra A, Pavelko T. Treatment of chronic elbow tendinosis with buffered platelet-rich plasma. Am J Sports Med. 2006;34(11):1774–1778. DOI: 10.1177/0363546506288850.

[86] Schepull T, Kvist J, Norrman H, et al. Autologous platelets have no effect on the healing of human Achilles tendon ruptures: A randomized single-blind study. Am J Sports Med. 2011;39(1):38–47. DOI: 10.1177/0363546510383515. Epub 2010 Nov 3.

[87] Creaney L, Hamilton B. Growth factor delivery methods in the management of sports injuries: The state of play. Br J Sports Med. 2008;42(5):314–320. Epub 2007 Nov 5.

[88] Peerbooms JC, Sluimer J, Bruijn DJ, Gosens T. Positive effect of an autologous platelet concentrate in lateral epicondylitis in a double-blind. randomized controlled trial:

Platelet-rich plasma versus corticosteroid injection with a 1-year. Am J Sports Med. 2010;38:255. DOI: 10.1177/0363546509355445.

[89] Jo CH, Kim JE, Yoon KS, Shin S. Platelet-rich plasma stimulates cell proliferation and enhances matrix gene expression and synthesis in tenocytes from human rotator cuff tendons with degenerative tears. Am J Sports Med. 2012;40(5):1035–1045. DOI: 10.1177/0363546512437525. Epub 2012 Feb 23.

[90] Chen L, Dong SW, Liu JP, Tao X, Tang KL, Xu JZ. Synergy of tendon stem cells and platelet-rich plasma in tendon healing. J Orthop Res. 2012;30(6):991–997. DOI: 10.1002/jor.22033. Epub 2011 Dec 12.

[91] Eliasson P, Fahlgren A, Pasternak B. Unloaded rat Achilles tendons continue to grow, but lose viscoelasticity. J Appl Physiol. 2007;103:459–463. Epub 2007 Apr 5.

[92] Wei W, Chen F, Liu Y, et al. Autologous injectable tissue-engineered cartilage by using platelet-rich plasma: Experimental study in a rabbit model. J Oral Maxillofac Surg. 2007; 65:1951–1957. DOI:/10.1016/j.joms.2006.11.044.

[93] Sánchez M, Azofra J, Aizpurua B, et al. Use of autologous plasma rich in growth factors in arthroscopic surgery. Cuader Artroscopia. 2003;10:12–19.

[94] Radice F, Yánez R, Gutiérrez V, et al. Comparison of magnetic resonance imaging findings in anterior cruciate ligament grafts with and without autologous platelet-derived growthfactors. Arthroscopy. 2010;26(1):50–57. DOI: 10.1016/j.arthro. 2009.06.030.

[95] Mei-Dan O, Mann G, Maffulli N. Platelet-rich plasma: Any substance into it? Br J Sports Med. 2010;44(9):618–619. DOI:10.1136/bjsm.2009.067108.

[96] Orrego M, Larrain C, Rosales J, et al. Effects of platelet concentrate and a bone plug on the healing of hamstring tendons in a bone tunnel. Arthroscopy. 2008;24:1373–1380.

[97] Sampson S, Gerhardt M, Mandelaum B. Platelet-rich plasma injection grafts for musculoskeletal injuries: A review. Curr Rev Musculoskelet Med. 2008;1:165–174. DOI: 10.1007/s12178-008-9032-5.

[98] Shen W, Li Y, Zhu J, Huard J. Interaction between macrophages, TGFbeta1, and the COX-2 pathway during inflammatory phase of skeletal muscle healing after injury. J Cell Physiol. 2008;214(2):405–412.

[99] Silva A, Sampaio R. Anatomic ACL reconstruction: Does the platelet-rich plasma accelerate tendon healing? Knee Surg Sports Traumatol Arthrosc. 2009;17(6):676–682. DOI: 10.1007/s00167-009-0762-8. Epub 2009 Mar 14.

[100] Everts PAM, Knape JTA, et al. Platelet-rich plasma and platelet gel, a review. J Extra Corpor Techn. 2006;38:174–187.

[101] Levy O, Martinowitz U, Oran A, et al. The use of fibrin tissue adhesive to reduce blood loss and the need for blood transfusion after total knee arthroplasty. A pro-

spective, randomized, multicenter study. J Bone Joint Surg Am. 1999;81(11):1580–1588.

[102] Sánchez M, Anitua E, Azofra J, et al. Comparison of surgically repaired achilles tendon tears using platelet-rich fibrin matrices. Am J Sports Med. 2007;February;35(2): 245–251.

[103] Alsousou J, Thompson M, Hulley P, Noble A, Willett K. The biology of platelet-rich plasma and its application in trauma and orthopaedic surgery. J Bone Joint Surg Br. 2009;91(8):987–996. DOI: 10.1302/0301-620X.91B8.22546.

[104] Drengk A, Zapf A, Stürmer EK, et al. Influence of platelet-rich plasma on chondrogenic differentiation and proliferation of chondrocytes and mesenchymal stem cells. Cells Tissues Organs.2009;189(5):317–326.

[105] Lin SS, Landesberg R, Chin HS, et al. Controlled release of PRP-derived growth factors promotes osteogenic differentiation of human mesenchymal stem cells. Conf Proc IEEE Eng Med Biol Soc. 2006;1:4358–4361.

[106] Gardner MJ, Demetrakopoulos D, Klepchick PR, et al. The efficacy of autologous platelet gel in pain control and blood loss in total knee arthroplasty: An analysis of the haemoglobin, narcotic requirement and range of motion. Int Orthop. 2007;31(3):309–313.

[107] Engebretsen L, Steffen K, Alsousou J, et al. IOC consensus paper on the use of platelet-rich plasma in sports medicine. Br J Sports Med. 2010;44:1072–1081.

[108] Eppley BL, Woodell JE, Higgins J. Platelet quantification and growth factor analysis from platelet-rich plasma: Implications for wound healing. Plast Reconstr Surg. 2004; 114(6):1502–1508.

Chapter 9

Probiotics and Immunity

Marieta Georgieva, Kaloyan Georgiev and Peter Dobromirov

Additional information is available at the end of the chapter

http://dx.doi.org/10.5772/61337

Abstract

Probiotics are "living microorganisms" which exert a prophylactic and therapeutic effect by improving the internal microbial balance. Probiotics play a role in defining and maintaining the delicate balance between necessary and excessive defence mechanisms including innate and adaptive immune responses. The beneficial effects of probiotics have been demonstrated in many diseases.

New therapeutic approaches toward several inflammatory diseases are being developed by affecting the microbial composition of the gut immune system. They are based on the fact that this part of immune system is influenced by many factors, including dietary components and commensal bacteria. An understanding of the molecular mechanisms behind the direct and indirect effects on the gut immune response will facilitate better and possibly more efficient therapy for diseases, although probiotics (live microorganisms) have already shown promise as treatments for several diseases in both clinical and animal studies.

Further, the concept of probiotics and the direct and indirect mechanisms by which they can influence gut immunity are described. Emphasis will be placed on the relationship of microbiota and the gut immune system.

A review of the history of *Lactobacillus bulgaricus*, probiotics, and probiotic functional foods is made and legislation and modern challenges are discussed.

Keywords: Probiotics, immunity, probiotic genomic, history, legislation

1. Introduction

Probiotics are defined by the World Health Organization as "live microorganisms, which when administered in adequate amounts, confer a health benefit upon the host." The main benefit of probiotics is that they help restore balance in the intestinal microbiota. Probiotics play a role in defining and maintaining the delicate balance between necessary and excessive defence mechanisms including innate and adaptive immune responses. The immunological mechanisms supporting probiotics and prebiotics effects continue to be better defined with novel mechanisms being described for dendritic cells, epithelial cells, T regulatory cells, effector lymphocytes, natural killer T cells, and B cells [1].

Looking to probiotics to support immune health is nothing new; the idea has existed for more than 100 years [2]. For millennia, humans have consumed microorganisms via fermented foods. Human beings and gut microbiota are in a symbiotic relationship, and the hypothesis of a "super organism" composed of the human organism and microbes has been recently proposed. The gut microbiota performs important metabolic and immunological tasks, and the impairment of its composition might alter homeostasis and lead to the development of microbiota-related diseases [3].

The most common illnesses associated with alterations of the gut microbiota include inflammatory bowel disease, gastrointestinal infections, irritable bowel syndrome and other gastrointestinal functional diseases, colorectal cancer, metabolic syndrome and obesity, liver disorders, allergy, and neurological diseases [4,5].

Neural pathways and central nervous system (CNS) signalling systems, according to new studies, can be activated by bacteria in the gastrointestinal (GI) tract, including commensal, probiotic, and pathogenic bacteria. Novel approaches for prevention and treatment of mental illness, including anxiety and depression [6], may be provided by actual and future animal and clinical studies, aimed at understanding the microbiota–gut–brain axis. In theory, every disease associated with the impairment of intestinal microflora might benefit from the therapeutic modulation of the gut microbiota.

The purpose of this review is to address the most recent findings regarding probiotic regulation of immune health. Probiotic genes and probiotic-derived factors involved in the regulation of host immunity, molecular targets of probiotic action responsible for the host immune responses, and roles and mechanisms of probiotics in prevention and treatment of diseases [7], which are included in clinical applications and mechanisms of action, are of special interest.

The role of specific microorganisms and the overall diversity of the microbiota in many human diseases can be understood to a great extent owing to the rapid growth of metagenomics strategies. Therapies focused on specific effects of different probiotics and prebiotics on the gut microbiota [8] can be helped by the development of this knowledge.

2. Probiotics and immune health

Hippocrates (460-370 EC) stated, "All diseases begin in the gut." Both microbial diversity and abundance in the gut play an important role in maintaining human health. The attachment, growth, and penetration of pathogenic microorganisms on the gut surface can essentially be prevented by microbiota. Pathogen resistance, both by direct interaction with pathogenic bacteria and by influencing the immune system, is influenced greatly by the intestinal microbiota [9, 10]. Many diseases start with an initial imbalance of human resident microflora and the related immunobiological reactivity [11]. One key player in immune health is the gut, a part of the body that is constantly exposed to toxins and foreign antigens, such as those from food and microbes. According to nutrition and immune expert Meydani, "The gut is the largest immune organ in the body, accounting for 25% of the immune cells in the body that provide 50% of the body's immune response." Meydani called intestinal flora "forgotten organ" because of their vital but still underestimated health functions [12]. There are more than 400 species of bacteria residing in the gut, and they have symbiotic relationships with the body. There are 100 trillion bacteria in our intestines. They form an ecosystem like a "flower garden", reported Haruji Sawada, director of the Yakult Central Institute, at the Yakult International Nutrition and Health Conference on May 17, 2010, in Tokyo. The mammalian gut immune system should be viewed as a complex interplay between physical, chemical, and cellular barriers, a vast community of bacteria, and a plethora of host immune cells which mediate innate and adaptive immunity. The intestinal microbiota helps in proper development of the host immune system, which in turn regulates the homeostasis of the microbiota [13]. Accumulating evidence over the last decade indicates that the immune system and microbiota interaction should be finely balanced and any perturbations of this interaction would result in microbiota and immune dysbiosis, leading to inflammatory disorders The rapid surge in the emerging new-age disorders such as inflammatory bowel disease (IBD), rheumatoid arthritis, cardiovascular disease, and metabolic syndrome has driven investigators to explore their etiology in multiple directions such as genetics, diet, and environmental factors, as well as immune system/microbiota interactions. In addition, the practice of strict hygienic and sanitary conditions and consumption of highly processed foods containing high fat, high carbohydrate, and low fiber with numerous food additives and preservatives may account for altered microbial composition, metabolism, and interaction with host immunity. Nearly all the above diseases are characterized by local as well as systemic low-grade chronic or subclinical inflammation in which the inflammation originated in the intestine via the interaction between host immune system and microbiota.

Several beneficial effects of probiotics on the host intestinal mucosal defense system, including blocking pathogenic bacterial effects by producing bactericidal substances and competing with pathogens and toxins for adherence to the intestinal epithelium, have been identified. Probiotics promote intestinal epithelial cell survival, enhance barrier function, and stimulate protective responses from intestinal epithelial cells [14-16] in the case of intestinal epithelial homeostasis. What matters most is that the modulation of the immune system is one of the most reasonable mechanisms underlying the beneficial effects of probiotics on human health. Enhancement of the innate and adaptive immunity and modulation of pathogen-induced inflammation are the discovered effects of probiotics.

Strictly defined strains using genetic, serological, microbiological, and biochemical analyses; lack of pathogenicity, lack of cancerogenicity, presence of beneficial factors; possibility for colonization of the large intestine; viable cultures; acid and bile resistance; proved clinical efficacy are among the requirements for the organisms to be used as probiotics [17].

The established probiotics that meet these criteria are generally lactic acid bacteria (LAB), most commonly *Lactobacillus* and *Bifidobacterium* species, but also *Lactococcus, Streptococcus,* and

Enterococcus species and certain yeast strains. Numerous other LAB have shown probiotic potential in animal studies. For the treatment of IBD, several probiotics have been shown to be efficacious: *Lactobacillus casei, Lactobacillus plantarum, Lactobacillus bulgaricus,* and *Lactobacillus acidophilus*; three strains of *Bifidobacteria* and *S. thermophilus.* In recent years, evidence has accumulated that probiotic strains can exhibit the same activities as commensal bacteria, including immunomodulation [5,11].

Lactic acid bacteria are present in many feeds such as yogurt and are frequently used as probiotics to improve some biological functions of the host. Beneficial effects of the lactobacilli on the body have been identified in the treatment or prevention of acute viral gastroenteritis, after antibiotic-associated diarrhea, certain pediatric allergic diseases, necrotizing enterocolitis, and inflammatory bowel disease such as Crohn's disease and postoperative hernias. Probiotics have been long reported to aid in the treatment of many dysfunctions of the GI tract, and the mechanisms by which probiotics work have recently been elucidated. There are experimental and clinical data [18-24]. Probiotics are described as useful also in combating oxidative stress, improvement in mucosal immunity [25], and general immunity [26]. The desirable changes of the intestinal microbiota were achieved as yogurt was able to attenuate the symptoms of acute inflammation by reducing inflammatory cytokines and increasing regulatory cytokine IL-10-producing cells. The use of murine models demonstrated that the consumption of fermented milks can modulate the immune system and can maintain it in a state of surveillance, which could affront different pathologies such as cancer and intestinal inflammation on its part.

3. Gut's role in immune function

The contributions of the gut microbiota to the development of the immune system have been extensively characterized. One of these characterizations suggests that the host is able to tolerate the large amount of antigens present in the gut [27], owing to the coordinated cross talk between the gut microbiota and the immune system.

Progress in the current knowledge on biodiversity of the intestinal microbiota allows us to understand the mechanisms of how different microorganisms affect the function of the body and the impact of these mechanisms. Altered microflora (dysbiosis) is generally associated with gastrointestinal disorders, but rather a microbial imbalance is associated with common diseases, which are not limited to the gastrointestinal tract [28, 29]. Studies in germ-free (GF) mice give much of the evidence about how microflora forms immune system as GF mice are completely lacking microflora. These mice show profound immune defects, such as fewer and smaller Peyer plaques and mesenteric lymph nodes and also reduced B and T cell immune response [30-32]. Therefore, the serum immunoglobulin (Ig) G and IgA levels in the gut GF mice were reduced [33, 34]. Moreover, many studies in mice and humans show that certain inflammatory diseases are associated with an altered microflora [9, 35, 36].

Inflammatory diseases are often caused by microbial dysbiosis. It was found in a prospective study of children with a high risk of developing asthma that changes in the microbiota occur before the development of the disease [37]. Regulation of immune responses requires certain species of gut commensal microbiota and perturbations in the microbiota could lead to a lack of immune regulation, the outgrowth of more pathogenic microbes, and the promotion of inflammation. The microbial composition of the microbiota in the adult human gut is mainly determined by the microorganism to which the newborn child is exposed during the first years of life. Strategies to manipulate the microbiota during infancy have been shown to prevent development of allergic and atopic diseases later in adult life [38-40]. Thus, the use of probiotics and prebiotics during the early postnatal period has been proposed for the intentional modulation of the microbiota composition. In addition, diet and exposure to microbes during pregnancy may affect the metabolic and immunological profiles of the pregnant uterus and the risk of developing the disease in the offspring [41]. The application of probiotics and prebiotics during pregnancy has been also proposed [42-44]. Differences in this composition are related lo colonization; host factors, such as sex and age; genetic factors; and health state. The dynamic state of the microbe's ecology is increasingly being associated with an expanding number of disorders. New high throughput methodologies such as metagenomics, transcriptomics, proteomics, and metabolomics in the post-genomic era have greatly helped the understanding of the mechanisms, by which the microbiota contributes to host physiology in healthy and ill individuals. Metagenomic studies of the human gut microbiota, for example, have suggested that host metabolism is affected by low bacterial diversity, which is also related to obesity and other diseases [45, 46J.

4. Probiotic modulation of the gastrointestinal mucosal immune system

Perhaps one of the most important aspects of probiotic bacteria is the ability to modulate the host GIT mucosal immune system locally and systemically The interaction between the probiotic microbe with the resident microbiota, gastrointestinal epithelia and gut immune cells to produce an immunomodulatory response is quite complex, and has been reviewed exhaustively [34, 47- 49].

The expression of cytokines and chemokine genes was carried out by activated nuclear factor kappa-B (NF-κB) and mitogen-activated protein kinase signalling cascades, mediated of MAMPs, PRRS (including NOD-like receptor, Toll-like receptors, and C-type lectin receptors). Lipoteichoic acids (DMA), peptidoglycan and S-layer proteins are mostly found MAMPs from probiotic microorganisms. [48, 50] [Figure 1].

Multiple studies have explored the immunomodulatory effect of these MAMPs using functional genomic techniques. Various studies have demonstrated a significant reduction in product ion of proinflammatory cytokines with a simultaneous increase in anti-inflammatory IL-10 and the down regulation of pro-inflammatory IL-12 and TJMF-H. [23, 51J. Microflora in the intestine promotes mucosal barrier function, and also improves the immunity of the host to enteric infection. During the active infection a cytokine normally produced is IL-1β, which is critical for neutrophil restoration and eradication of the pathogen. Microflora play a vital role in the production of homeostatic levels of pro-IL-1β in local intestinal macrophages. The

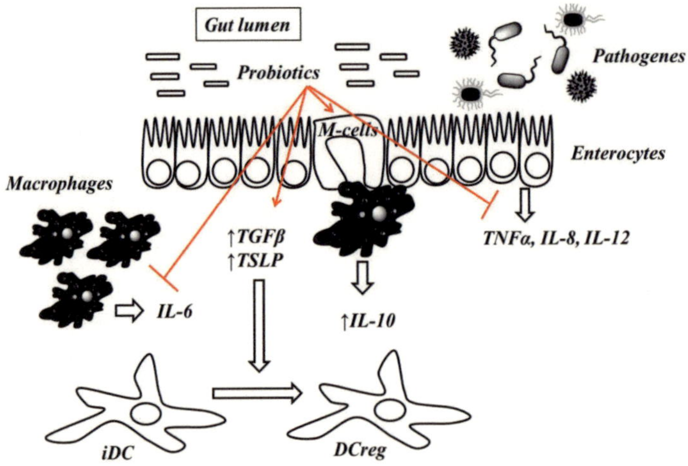

Figure 1. Probiotic modulation of the gastrointestinal mucosal immune system. While intestinal epithelial cells (IECs) exposed to pathogenic microbes or related stimuli produce proinflammatory mediators such as interleukin 8 (IL-8) and tumour necrosis factor a (TNF-a), probiotics suppress the production of these cytokines and instead induce anti-inflammatory mediators such as transforming growth factor b (TGF-b) and thymic stromal lymphopoietin (TSLP), which can promote the differentiation of immature dendritic cells (iDCs) to regulatory dendritic cells (DCregs). Macrophages in the inflamed mucosa produce high amounts of IL-6, and probiotics can decrease their IL-6 production and increase IL-10 production.

gut microbiota can also enhance host immunity through MyD88-independent mechanisms (MyD88 – Myeloid differentiation primary response gene 88). Notably, colonization of GF mice by commensal bacteria induces development of Th-17 cells in the intestine, which is important for protection against *Citrobacter rodentium* infection [52].

5. Immune cells

Probiotics regulate host innate and adaptive immune responses by modulating the functions of dendritic cells, macrophages, and T and B lymphocytes. Probiotics regulate immunomodulalory functions through the activation of toll-like receptors, which is one of the mechanisms of regulation. Recent studies indicate that probiotics activate innate immunity by enhancing adaptive immune response [20, 53]. One of the proposed mechanisms is by activation of toll-like receptors.

Regulatory dendritic cells are the primary professional antigen presenting cells (APCs) modulating adaptive immune responses. Probiotics containing *L. acidophilus, L. casei, L. reuteri, E. bifidium,* and *Streptococcus thermophilus*, stimulate dendritic cells to produce IL-10, TGF-β, COX-2, and indoleamine 2,3-dioxygenase, which in turn increase the formation of CD4 Foxp3 regulatory T cells (Tregs) and the suppressor activity of naturally occurring CD4 CD25 Tregs. They also decrease responsiveness of T and B lymphocytes and the number of T helper (Th) 1, Th2, and Th17 cytokines without inducing apoptosis. This mixture suppressed 2,4,6-

trinitrobenzenesulfonic acid-induced intestinal inflammation, which was associated with enrichment of CD4 Foxp3 Tregs in the inflamed regions, as was found by in vivo studies. Thus, probiotics that enhance the generation of regulatory dendritic cells to induce Tregs, represent a potential therapeutic approach for inflammatory disorders [50, 54].

Nowadays, the exact mechanism of interaction between probiotic microorganisms and host cells remains elusive. Nevertheless, there is enough gathered information that microbiota in the gut could affect the immune response at both systemic and mucosal levels. Some putative mechanisms include: influence of the microflora itself, amelioration of membrane barrier function, and direct effects of probiotic microorganisms on different epithelial and immune cell types. Many patients with inflammatory bowel disease (IBD) use probiotics to manage this intestinal condition. Downregulation of production of proinflammatory cytokines and other inflammatory mediators seems to constitute important mechanisms for the partial amelioration of colitis, seen with numerous LAB strains in various models. It must also be noted that TNF-α blocking agents are also quite successful in the treatment of patients with CD (Crohn's disease) [55]. However, it should be taken into account that different probiotic bacterial species and strains have various beneficial effects and therefore need to be selected in a more rational manner to treat human diseases.

6. *Lactobacillus bulgaricus* – The contribution to modern healthy nutrition

Lactobacillus bulgaricus is the only probiotic microorganism named after a certain territory and nation. It only multiplies in the region of modern Bulgaria, coinciding with ancient Thrace. It mutates and stops its multiplication after 1-2 fermentations in other regions of the world. Bulgarian traditional food comprises *Lactobacillus bulgaricus. Lactobacillus bulgaricus* is included in the production of Bulgarian food products based on lactic acid, such as yogurt, feta yogurt, white brine cheese, other cheeses and cream, humanized baby food, probiotic functional foods, and whole food supplements [56-58].

Lactobacillus bulgaricus was known to the Thracians – the ancient population that lived in what is at present Bulgarian land, more than 7–8 thousand years ago. The word yogurt is Thracian and means hard, solid milk. During his tour in Thrace, the Greek scientist Herodotus (484–425 BC) wrote that the Thracians prepare special fermented dairy food, which is a gift from their Gods [59].

The father of probiotics and Nobelist – Ilya Metchnikoff (the Russian scientist) attributes the long and healthy life of Bulgarians largely to the yogurt consumption and in particular to the local bacterium in yogurt in his work "Prolongation of Life" [Figure 2].

In 1905 in Geneva, the Bulgarian student Stamen Grigorov isolated *Lactobacillus bulgaricus* from yogurt, brought from Bulgaria [Figure 3].

BSS (Bulgarian State Standard) for yogurt was established in Bulgaria in compliance with European standards of origin. Responding to this standard, the lactic acid fermentation should be accomplished using only *Lactobacillus bulgaricus* and *Streptococcus thermophilus*. Yogurt is a

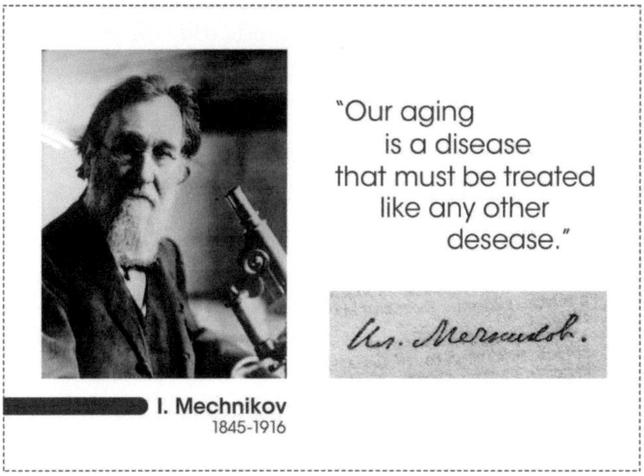

Figure 2. Prof. I. Metchnikoff

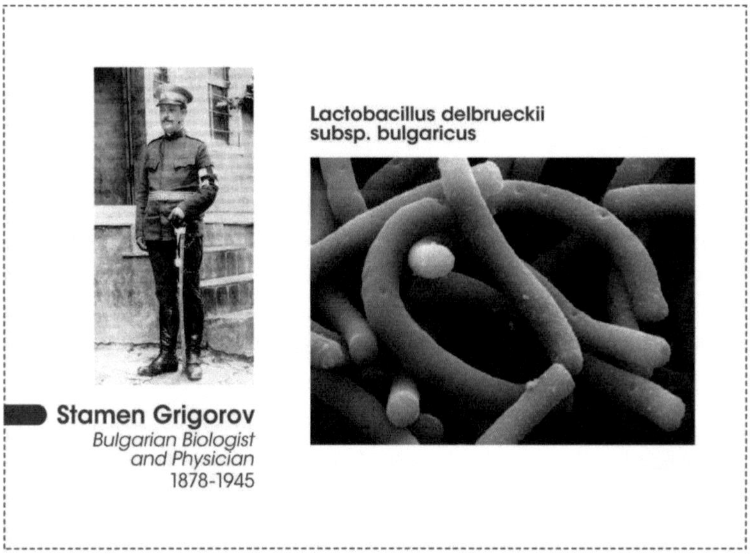

Figure 3. Dr Stamen Grigorov

fermented milk product with the typical bacterial cultures *Lactobacillus bulgaricus* and *Streptococcus thermophilus* (the standards of identity, published in the US Code of Federal Regulations).

In Commission Regulation (Elf) No 432/2012 in the list of the permitted health claims made on foods, the only probiotic microorganisms included are *Lactobacillus bulgaricus* and *Streptococcus thermophilus*. According to the claim, in doses over 10^8 colony forming units, they improve lactose digestion [60].

In the 1990s, *Lactobacillus bulgaricus* was used in the production of probiotic functional food for astronauts, which was tested during the flight of the second Bulgarian astronaut in Space [61],

Until recently it was considered that *Lactobacillus bulgaricus* can be isolated from plants – dogwood, rose cup, etc. Bulgarian scientists, N. Alexandrov and D. Petrova have isolated *Lactobacillus bulgaricus* and other fermented milk probiotic microorganisms from spring water in Bulgaria [62, 63]. There is experimental and clinical scientific evidence from around the world of the beneficial effects of *Lactobacillus bulgaricus* in stimulating the immune system, regulating functions and microbial flora of the gastrointestinal tract, including diarrhea and dysbacteriosis, reducing the risk of cancer, radiotherapy protecting effect, regulating cholesterol levels, competitive inhibition of pathogenic strains causing infections, alleviating lactose intolerance, and anti-mutagenic effect. *Lactobacillus bulgaricus* has a beneficial effect on the health of women because of its similarity to the Doederlein flora in the vagina of the woman [64]. *Lactobacillus bulgaricus*, unlike other probiotic microorganisms, which secrete only L (+) lactic acid, secretes L (+) and D (-) lactic acid during fermentation. This determines its powerful antioxidant and anticancer effect. *Lactobacillus bulgaricus* produces antimicrobial substance, known as Bulgariacan, which is resistant to heat and active against highly virulent (pathogenic) strains of microorganisms [56, 57]. It has been shown that *Lactobacillus bulgaricus* adheres best on the colonic mucosa, followed by a rapid reproduction in the body. This is crucial for its more powerful treatment and detoxic effect than other lactic acid bacteria probiotics.

Lactobacillus bulgaricus is reproduced best with *Streptococcus thermophilus*. To gain rapid biomass and biologically active substances and to potentiate their effect, joint cultivation of *Lactobacillus bulgaricus* and *Streptococcus thermophilus* is needed. Lots of scientific studies of yeasts, containing *Lactobacillus bulgaricus* and *Streptococcus thermophilus*, used in yogurt production, were carried out in Bulgaria. The results show that these specific bacteria of yogurt are stable and survive after passage through the human gastrointestinal tract.

Certain Bulgarian companies are using modern biotechnology, and wrap strains of *Lactobacillus bulgaricus* and other probiotic microorganisms with a natural coating, consisting of components of the growing medium, during fermentation. This helps the production of probiotics and the isolation of the new probiotic strains from spring water, which normally survives under changing climatic conditions. Theses probiotic microorganisms should retain their stability and vitality when passing through the gastrointestinal tract, as well as when stored in shops at temperatures of up to 24° C for the entire shelf life.

Lactobacillus bulgaricus is the ancient contribution of mankind to modern science and to the creation of the first healthy foods in the world.

7. Probiotics and probiotic functional foods – Legislation and modern challenges

According to the World Health Organization (WHO) and the Food and Agriculture Organization (FAO), probiotics are live microorganisms which, when administered in adequate amounts, confer a health benefit on the host [65].

For the last decades, there has been a rapid growth in the application of probiotics among both people and animals. They are used in the production of fermented products (milk, cheese), as ingredients in adapted milk for babies and children, in bakery products or confectionery, or as material for the production of food additives. Another modern trend in agricultural science is the use of probiotics in animal breeding and poultry farming to reduce the disease rates with young animals, for maximum utilization of nutrition ingredients of fodder, and fast accumulation of muscle mass without treatment with hormonal preparations and antibiotics, as well as to increase the volume of additional products that animals and poultry give – eggs, milk, etc.

Probiotic microorganisms belong to the *Lactobacillus, Lactococcus, Bifidobacterium, Pediococcus,* or *Bacillus* family, with the microorganisms from Lactobacillus family being most frequently used as probiotics.

According to Claire M. Hassler from the Illinois University, the probiotics from the Lactobacillus family are functional ingredients contained in yogurt and other dairy products, which improve the health condition of the gastrointestinal tract. Many researches confirm the health benefits of probiotics for maintaining gastrointestinal health, avoiding infections through competitive suppression of the development of pathogenic strains, strengthening the immune system, prevention against colorectal cancer, reduction of serum cholesterol, relieving intolerance toward lactose, etc.

Probiotics have healthy effect if taken in specific quantities. According to the Japanese scientists, N. Ishibashi and S. Shimamura, the recommended quantity of live microorganisms in a probiotic product must be at least 107 live microorganisms per gram or per milliliter. According to other scientists, Gomez and Vinderola, the minimum required concentration of live cells in each gram probiotic product at the moment of consumption must be from 10^6 to 10^9 to have any favorable effect.

Today, the market offers a wide range of probiotic products and most of them are in dry forms. A number of factors have influence on the expiry periods of dried probiotic products and their subsequent effect when consumed. The creation of probiotic formulas with lasting durability of the strains and longer expiry periods still continues to be a challenge. Manufacturers of probiotic products constantly apply innovations, which aim to preserve the vitality of probiotic strains during the drying process (lyophilization), rehydration, when passing through the gastrointestinal tract and the strongly alternating pH in the stomach and biliary salts, and during their storage in the sales points. There are numerous researches of the molecular characteristics of probiotic strains and their health effects.

Companies apply different approaches to create new probiotic formulas with preserved vitality of the strains and useful effects. Some Korean and Japanese companies divide probiotic products into four generations:

- First generation – probiotic microorganisms without coating
- Second generation – probiotic microorganisms with single synthetic coating, which protects them when passing through the gastrointestinal tract

http://dx.doi.org/10.5772/61337

- Third generation – microcapsuled probiotic microorganisms with synthetic capsule
- Fourth generation – probiotic microorganisms with two synthetic coatings, protein and mucopolysaccharides, which protect them when passing through the gastrointestinal tract and against high pressure and temperature

Some scientists apply genetic manipulation of known strains to increase their durability. American companies test possible probiotic effects of known spore-carrying microorganisms from the Bacillus family.

Bulgarian manufacturers of probiotics coat the strains of lactic acid microorganisms with natural coating, which consist of ingredients of the food media aiming to raise their durability with the alternating pH and temperature. The Bulgarian scientist, Nikola Alexandrov and his fellow researchers, isolated for the first time in the world 8 completely natural probiotic strains from the Lactobacillus family from pure spring water in Bulgaria [62,63] [Figure 4].

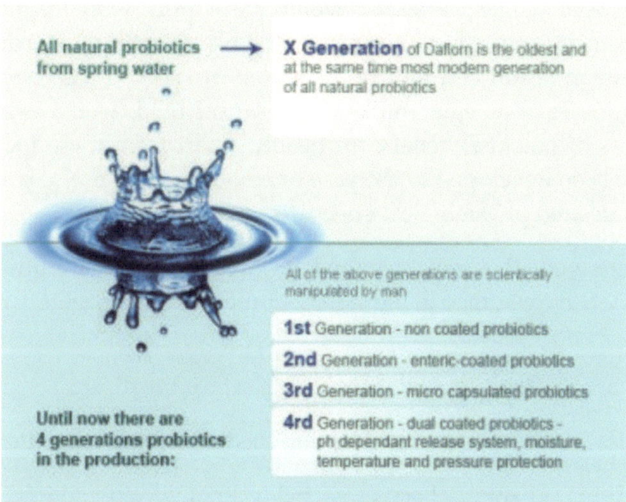

Figure 4. Probiotics from spring water

Research in this field will have major importance for the manufacturers of probiotics, who want to achieve longer term of durability and better health effect of their probiotic products. These researches are also extremely important for the end consumers who demand high-quality functional products to improve the quality of their life.

8. Probiotic functional foods

The oldest concept of functional foods was created by the father of medicine – Hippocrates. He wrote, "Let food be your medicine and medicine – your food."

Food's major role is to provide sufficient nutritive substances, which will satisfy the need for food of the human organism. Today, nutrition science faces new challenges far beyond the concept of food insufficiency.

There are both socioeconomic changes taking place in the world and changes in the demographic structure of population – growing number of elderly people and increase of the expenses for healthcare. Therefore, governments, researchers, health experts, and the foodstuff industry, in general, direct their efforts to identification and creation of functional foods, which may improve the health of the local population, reduce the risk of diseases with social impact, such as cardiovascular diseases, cancer, osteoporosis, and improve the quality of life for the people. In combination with healthy living, the daily use of these functional foods may have positive impact for the health of both working people in active age and their families and for the elderly. This will result in the sharp reduction of the expenses for healthcare and in the optimization of physical and mental health of the population.

Nowadays scientific evidences proved that some foods and food ingredients have favorable physiological and psychological effects beyond the supply with major food substances. Modern researches focus on the identification of the biologically active components in food, which maintain human health and reduce the risk of diseases. It has been found that many traditional foodstuffs, such as eggs, milk, whole-wheat food, fruits, vegetables, soya, etc. contain components of potential benefit for health. Apart from these foods, there are new products that have been developed to increase or combine these useful components because of their benefits or desired physiological effects.

Functional foods are foods that are consumed as part of the normal nutrition process. They have useful effects when consumed in normal quantities within the dietary regime. Functional food could be:

- Food of natural origin – unskimmed milk, whole-wheat bread, etc.
- Food technologically or biotechnologically enriched with some ingredient
- Food from which ingredient has been extracted technologically or biotechnologically
- Food, in which the nature of one or more substances has been modified
- Food, in which bioavailability of one or more substances has been modified
- Food, which is a combination of two or more of the foods described above

Functional food may be addressed to the overall population or separate groups identified in terms of age (e.g., children or adults), genetic and enzyme modifications (intolerance toward gluten, lactose intolerance), functional status (pregnancy, for example), etc. Functional foods must be in conformity with the overall significance of nutrition – potential interrelations with other food substances and ingredients or possible undesired effects, including allergies and intolerance.

The foundations of the modern science of functional foods were laid in Japan during the 1980. The concept of food of specific health use (FOSHU) was established in 1991. Foods defined as

FOSHU are approved by the Minister of Health and Social Cares of Japan after providing detailed and sufficient scientific evidence. Such foods are consumed as part of the standard diet [66]. In USA, the requirements for "reduction of the risk of diseases" for specific foods were made binding by law in 1993. The opinions and conclusions related to health are subject to approval by the Food and Drugs Agency on the base of scientific evidence and their goal is to help consumers by providing information about healthy nutrition, thus avoiding the risk of diseases [67]. In the European Union, the development and the approval of functional foods is regulated by a special organization to the European Commission known as FUFOSE (Functional Food Science in Europe) in cooperation with the European ILSI (International Life Science Institute), which works mainly on issues referring to the harmonization of the legislation in the field of functional foods in the EU Member States. This European Commission has developed two types of health requirements for functional foods: "increased function" and "reduction of the risk of disease" [60]. In Bulgaria, the permit for the production of food with special designation is given by the Bulgarian Food Safety Agency (BFSA) after provision of scientific evidence to the Ministry of Health of the Republic of Bulgaria [63, 67].

The biggest challenge before the scientists in the field of nutrition now and in the future is to research the interrelations between a given food or food ingredient and the improved health and reduced risk of various diseases. The provision of accessible and detailed information for the qualities of the functional foods is of exceptional importance for the consumers' choice of food.

9. Conclusion and future directions

Probiotics are reliable resources for prevention and treatment of immune disorders. There are a lot of encouraging data based on analyses of studies in humans and animal models that probiotics possess clinical efficacy in ulcerative colitis and irritable bowel syndrome as well as other intestinal diseases such as infectious diarrhea, antibiotic-associated diarrhea, necrotizing enterocolitis. The most recent studies suggest the exciting possibility that probiotics can be modified for delivery of vaccines and to potentiate the effects of vaccination [68]. While the paradigm of discovery-based genomics in probiotic LAB has uncovered vital aspects of probiotic mechanisms, it has also revealed the complexity of these interactions with the resident microbiota and the mucosal immune system. Nevertheless, a great opportunity was revealed by this challenge. For example, probiotic bacteria are now being explored as suitable models for vaccine/drug production, due to their close association with host immunity and immunomodulatory action [45, 69]. Latest discoveries show that the role of probiotic bacteria and the resident microbiota extend far beyond gastrointestinal health. It has revealed neuro-chemical importance of intestinal homeostasis. There are studies that show cross talk between gastrointestinal tract and brain (brain–gut axis) [70]. Along with these advancements, it is important that human clinical trials continue with experimental designs that are well-controlled and well-defined, reflecting the great progress that has been made in the field of probiotic and GIT microbiome research [71]. With more than a century passing since Metch-nikoff's observations, keen experimental design using integrated genomics has led to a clearer definition of probiotic bacteria, as well as a model for continued discovery. Bulgaria becomes famous in the world with *Lactobacillus bulgaricus* and the Bulgarian territory is still an important reservoir for isolation of natural strains of lactic acid bacteria, which after an additional selection are used as starter cultures for the production of various fermented foods and probiotic products. The biggest challenge for researchers in the field of nutrition, at present and in the future, is the study of the relationship between a certain food or a nutrient and improved health or reduced risk of various diseases. Provision of accessible and comprehensive information about the properties of functional foods is crucial for food selection by consumers.

Author details

Marieta Georgieva[1*], Kaloyan Georgiev[1] and Peter Dobromirov[2]

*Address all correspondence to: marieta_md@yahoo.com

1 Department of Pharmacology and Toxicology, Faculty of Pharmacy, Medical University, Varna, Bulgaria

2 Medical University, Varna, Bulgaria

References

[1] Frei R, Akdis M, O'Mahony. Prebiotics, probiotics, synbiotics, and the immune system: experimental data and clinical evidence. *Curr Opin Gastroenterol.* 2015;31(2): 153-8. DOI: 10.1097/MOG.0000000000000151.

[2] Johnson BR, Klaenhammer TR. Impact of genomics on the field of probiotic research: historical perspectives to modern paradigms. *Antonie Van Leeuwenhoek.* 2014;106(1): 141-56. DOI: 10.1007/s10482-014-0171-y

[3] Qin J, Li R, Raes J, Arumugam M, Burgdorf KS, Manichanh C, et al. A human gut microbial gene catalogue established by metagenomic sequencing. *Nature.* 2010;464(7285):59-65. DOI: 10.1038/nature08821

[4] Ianiro G, Bibbò S, Gasbarrini A, Cammarota G. Therapeutic modulation of gut microbiota: current clinical applications and future perspectives. *Curr Drug Targets.* 2014;15(8):762-70. DOI: 10.2174/1389450115666140606111402

[5] Masood MI, Qadir MI, Shirazi JH, Khan IU. Beneficial effects of lactic acid bacteria on human beings. *Crit Rev Microbiol.* 2011;37(1):91-8. DOI: 10.3109/1040841X.2010.536522

[6] Foster JA, McVey Neufeld KA. Gut-brain axis: how the microbiome influences anxiety and depression. *Trends Neurosci.* 2013;36(5):305-12. DOI: 10.1016/j.tins.2013.01.005

[7] Vieira AT, Teixeira MM, Martins FS. The role of probiotics and prebiotics in inducing gut immunity. *Front Immunol.* 2013;4:445. DOI: 10.3389/fimmu.2013.00445.

[8] Pfeiler EA, Klaenhammer TR. Role of transporter proteins in bile tolerance of Lactobacillus acidophilus. *Appl Environ Microbiol.* 2009;75(18):6013-6. DOI: 10.1128/AEM.00495-09

[9] Kamada N, Chen GY, Inohara N, Núñez G. Control of pathogens and pathobionts by the gut microbiota. *Nat Immunol.* 2013;14(7):685-90. DOI: 10.1038/ni.2608

[10] Tlaskalova-Hogenova H, Stepankova R, Hudcovic T, Tuckova L, Cukrowska B, Lodinova-Zadnikova R, et al. Commensal bacteria (normal microflora), mucosal immunity and chronic inflammatory and autoimmune diseases. *Immunol Lett.* 2004;93(2-3):97-108.

[11] Borchers AT, Selmi C, Meyers FJ, Keen CL, Gershwin ME. Probiotics and immunity. *J Gastroenterol.* 2009;44(1):26-46. DOI: 10.1007/s00535-008-2296-0

[12] Palmer S. Research Suggests Beneficial Bacteria May Support Immune Health [Internet]. *Today's Dietician.* 2011;13(1):20. Available from: http://www.todaysdietitian.com/newarchives/011211p20.shtml [Accessed: 2015-04-14]

[13] Sommer F, Bäckhed F. The gut microbiota – masters of host development and physiology. *Nat Rev Microbiol.* 2013;11(4):227-38. DOI: 10.1038/nrmicro2974

[14] Artis D. Epithelial-cell recognition of commensal bacteria and maintenance of immune homeostasis in the gut. *Nat Rev Immunol.* 2008;8(6):411-20. DOI: 10.1038/nri2316

[15] Duerr CU, Hornef MW. The mammalian intestinal epithelium as integral player in the establishment and maintenance of host-microbial homeostasis. *Semin Immunol.* 2012;24(1):25-35. DOI: 10.1016/j.smim.2011.11.002

[16] Wells JM, Rossi O, Meijerink M, van Baarlen P. Epithelial crosstalk at the microbiota-mucosal interface. *Proc Natl Acad Sci U S A.* 2011;108(Suppl1):4607-14. DOI: 10.1073/pnas.1000092107

[17] Ouwehand and Salminen. Meeting of the International Scientific Organization for Probiotics and Prebiotics; 2002; 1998.

[18] Lin PW1, Myers LE, Ray L, Song SC, Nasr TR, Berardinelli AJ, et al. Lactobacillus rhamnosus blocks inflammatory signaling in vivo via reactive oxygen species generation. *Free Radic Biol Med.* 2009;47(8):1205-11. DOI: 10.1016/j.freeradbiomed.2009.07.033

[19] Ruiz PA, Hoffmann M, Szcesny S, Blaut M, Haller D. Innate mechanisms for Bifidobacterium lactis to activate transient pro-inflammatory host responses in intestinal

epithelial cells after the colonization of germ-free rats. *Immunology*. 2005;115(4): 441-50. DOI: 10.1111/j.1365-2567.2005.02176.x

[20] Yan F, Cao H, Cover TL, Washington MK, Shi Y, Liu L, et al. Colon-specific delivery of a probiotic-derived soluble protein ameliorates intestinal inflammation in mice through an EGFR-dependent mechanism. *J Clin Invest*. 2011;121(6):2242-53. DOI: 10.1172/JCI44031

[21] Kim SW, Park KY, Kim B, Kim E, Hyun CK. Lactobacillus rhamnosus GG improves insulin sensitivity and reduces adiposity in high-fat diet-fed mice through enhancement of adiponectin production. *Biochem Biophys Res Commun*. 2013;431(2):258-63. DOI: 10.1016/j.bbrc.2012.12.121

[22] Giahi L, Aumueller E, Elmadfa I, Haslberger AG. Regulation of TLR4, p38 MAPkinase, IκB and miRNAs by inactivated strains of lactobacilli in human dendritic cells. *Benef Microbes*. 2012;3(2):91-8. DOI: 10.3920/BM2011.0052

[23] Wang S, Zhu H, Lu C, Kang Z, Luo Y, Feng L, et al. Fermented milk supplemented with probiotics and prebiotics can effectively alter the intestinal microbiota and immunity of host animals. *J Dairy Sci*. 2012;95(9):4813-22. DOI: 10.3168/jds.2012-5426

[24] Granato D, Branco GF, Cruz AG, Faria JA, Shah NP. Probiotic dairy products as functional foods. *Comprehen Rev Food Sci Food Safety*. 2010;9(5):455-470. DOI: 10.1111/j. 1541-4337.2010.00120.x

[25] Cox AJ, Pyne DB, Saunders PU, Fricker PA. Oral administration of the probiotic Lactobacillus fermentum VRI-003 and mucosal immunity in endurance athletes. *Br J Sports Med*. 2010;44(4):222-6. DOI: 10.1136/bjsm.2007.044628

[26] Gleeson M, Bishop NC, Oliveira M, McCauley T, Tauler P, Lawrence C. Effects of a Lactobacillus salivarius probiotic intervention on infection, cold symptom duration and severity, and mucosal immunity in endurance athletes. *Int J Sport Nutr Exerc Metab*. 2012;22(4):235-42.

[27] Ng SC, Hart AL, Kamm MA, Stagg AJ, Knight SC. Mechanisms of action of probiotics: recent advances. *Inflamm Bowel Dis*. 2009;15(2):300-10. DOI: 10.1002/ibd.20602

[28] Henao-Mejia J, Elinav E, Jin C, Hao L, Mehal WZ, Strowig T et al. Inflammasome-mediated dysbiosis regulates progression of NAFLD and obesity. *Nature*. 2012;482(7384):179-85. DOI: 10.1038/nature10809

[29] Vujkovic-Cvijin I, Dunham RM, Iwai S, Maher MC, Albright RG, Broadhurst MJ et al. Dysbiosis of the gut microbiota is associated with HIV disease progression and tryptophan catabolism. *Sci Transl Med*. 2013;5(193):193ra91. DOI: 10.1126/scitranslmed. 3006438

[30] Gordon HA. Morphological and physiological characterization of germfree life. *Ann N Y Acad Sci*. 1959;78:208-20.

[31] Glaister JR. Factors affecting the lymphoid cells in the small intestinal epithelium of the mouse. *Int Arch Allergy Appl Immunol.* 1973;45(5):719-30.

[32] Cebra JJ, Periwal SB, Lee G, Lee F, Shroff KE. Development and maintenance of the gut-associated lymphoid tissue (GALT): the roles of enteric bacteria and viruses. *Dev Immunol.* 1998;6(1-2):13-8.

[33] Moreau MC, Ducluzeau R, Guy-Grand D, Muller MC. Increase in the population of duodenal immunoglobulin A plasmocytes in axenic mice associated with different living or dead bacterial strains of intestinal origin. *Infect Immun.* 1978;21(2):532-9.

[34] Selle K, Klaenhammer TR. Genomic and phenotypic evidence for probiotic influences of Lactobacillus gasseri on human health. *FEMS Microbiol Rev.* 2013;37(6):915-35. DOI: 10.1111/1574-6976.12021

[35] Seksik P, Rigottier-Gois L, Gramet G, Sutren M, Pochart P, Marteau P et al. Alterations of the dominant faecal bacterial groups in patients with Crohn's disease of the colon. *Gut.* 2003;52(2):237-42.

[36] Jeffery IB, O'Toole PW, Ohman L, Claesson MJ, Deane J, Quigley EM, et al. An irritable bowel syndrome subtype defined by species-specific alterations in faecal microbiota. *Gut.* 2012;61(7):997-1006. DOI: 10.1136/gutjnl-2011-301501

[37] Bisgaard H, Li N, Bonnelykke K, Chawes BL, Skov T, Paludan-Muller G, et al. Reduced diversity of the intestinal microbiota during infancy is associated with increased risk of allergic disease at school age. *J Allergy Clin Immunol.* 2011;128(3): 646-52. DOI: 10.1016/j.jaci.2011.04.060

[38] Kalliomäki M, Isolauri E. Pandemic of atopic diseases – a lack of microbial exposure in early infancy? *Curr Drug Targets Infect Disord.* 2002;2(3):193-9.

[39] Rautava S, Kalliomäki M, Isolauri E. Probiotics during pregnancy and breast-feeding might confer immunomodulatory protection against atopic disease in the infant. *J Allergy Clin Immunol.* 2002;109(1):119-21.

[40] Kukkonen K, Savilahti E, Haahtela T, Juntunen-Backman K, Korpela R, Poussa T, et al. Probiotics and prebiotic galacto-oligosaccharides in the prevention of allergic diseases: a randomized, double-blind, placebo-controlled trial. *J Allergy Clin Immunol.* 2007;119(1):192-8.

[41] Barker DJ. The origins of the developmental origins theory. *J Intern Med.* 2007;261(5): 412-7.

[42] Boyle RJ, Mah LJ, Chen A, Kivivuori S, Robins-Browne RM, Tang ML. Effects of Lactobacillus GG treatment during pregnancy on the development of fetal antigen-specific immune responses. *Clin Exp Allergy.* 2008;38(12):1882-90. DOI: 10.1111/j.1365-2222.2008.03100.x

[43] Laitinen K, Poussa T, Isolauri E. Nutrition, allergy, mucosal immunology and intestinal microbiota group. Probiotics and dietary counselling contribute to glucose regu-

lation during and after pregnancy: a randomised controlled trial. *Br J Nutr.* 2009;101(11):1679-87. DOI: 10.1017/S0007114508111461

[44] Petersen ER, Claesson MH, Schmidt EG, Jensen SS, Ravn P, Olsen J, et al. Consumption of probiotics increases the effect of regulatory T cells in transfer colitis. *Inflamm Bowel Dis.* 2012;18(1):131-42. DOI: 10.1002/ibd.21709

[45] Blottière HM, de Vos WM, Ehrlich SD, Doré J. Human intestinal metagenomics: state of the art and future. *Curr Opin Microbiol.* 2013;16(3):232-9. DOI: 10.1016/j.mib.2013.06.006

[46] Le Chatelier E, Nielsen T, Qin J, Prifti E, Hildebrand F, Falony G, et al. Richness of human gut microbiome correlates with metabolic markers. *Nature.* 2013;500(7464):541-6. DOI: 10.1038/nature12506

[47] Lebeer S, Vanderleyden J, De Keersmaecker SC. Host interactions of probiotic bacterial surface molecules: comparison with commensals and pathogens. *Nat Rev Microbiol.* 2010;8(3):171-84. DOI: 10.1038/nrmicro2297

[48] Bron PA, van Baarlen P, Kleerebezem M. Emerging molecular insights into the interaction between probiotics and the host intestinal mucosa. *Nat Rev Microbiol.* 2011;10(1):66-78. DOI: 10.1038/nrmicro2690

[49] Klaenhammer TR, Kleerebezem M, Kopp MV, Rescigno M. The impact of probiotics and prebiotics on the immune system. *Nat Rev Immunol.* 2012;12(10):728-34. DOI: 10.1038/nri3312

[50] Yan F, Polk DB. Probiotics and immune health. *Curr Opin Gastroenterol.* 2011;27(6):496-501. DOI: 10.1097/MOG.0b013e32834baa4d

[51] Mohamadzadeh M, Pfeiler EA, Brown JB, Zadeh M, Gramarossa M, Managlia E, et al. Regulation of induced colonic inflammation by Lactobacillus acidophilus deficient in lipoteichoic acid. *Proc Natl Acad Sci U S A.* 2011;108(Suppl 1):4623-30. DOI: 10.1073/pnas.1005066107

[52] Kamada N, Seo SU, Chen GY, Núñez G. Role of the gut microbiota in immunity and inflammatory disease. *Nat Rev Immunol.* 2013;13(5):321-35. DOI: 10.1038/nri3430

[53] Rakoff-Nahoum S, Paglino J, Eslami-Varzaneh F, Edberg S, Medzhitov R. Recognition of commensal microflora by toll-like receptors is required for intestinal homeostasis. *Cell.* 2004 ;118(2):229-41.

[54] Kwon HK, Lee CG, So JS, Chae CS, Hwang JS, Sahoo A, et al. Generation of regulatory dendritic cells and CD4+Foxp3+ T cells by probiotics administration suppresses immune disorders. *Proc Natl Acad Sci U S A.* 2010;107(5):2159-64. DOI: 10.1073/pnas.0904055107

[55] Cain AM, Karpa KD. Clinical utility of probiotics in inflammatory bowel disease. *Altern Ther Health Med.* 2011;17(1):72-9.

[56] Chomakov H. Bulgarian Yoghurt – unique probiotic, International Symposium on original Bulgarian yoghurt. In: Sofia:2005. p. 21 – 35.

[57] Chomakov H. Probiotics – past, present, future. Esprint, Sofia, 2007.

[58] Chomakov H, Tch Kondareva. Studies on the microflora of chicken digestive system. *Bulg J Agricult Sci.* 1995;1:56-62.

[59] Hosono A. Nutritive and physiological properties of lactic acid bacteria. In: Nagano: Japanese International Cooperation Agency (JICA); 1996. p. 30 – 32.

[60] Commission Regulation (EU) No. 432/2012 [Internet]. May 16, 2012. Available from: https://www.fsai.ie/uploadedfiles/consol_reg432_2012.pdf [Accessed: 2015-04-14]

[61] Alexandrov N. Prophylactic and treatment of multiple organ failure in poisoning with halogenated hydrocarbons. Symp of the Army Medical Services of Member States of Warsaw treaty, published by National Defense Ministry. 1988:17.

[62] Application for Patent No. 13557597/25.07.2012 in the U.S. Patent Office.

[63] Application No. 111161/07.03.2012 in Bulgarian Patent Office, Probiotics for dietary diary product.

[64] Alexandrov N, et al. The probiotics – base of functional nutrition and nutritive treatment in XXI century. In: International Symposium on Original Bulgarian Yoghurt; 2005; Sofia:p. 125-126.

[65] FAO/WHO, London, Canada. Guidelines for the Evaluation of Probiotics in Food [Internet]. 2002. Available from: http://www.fda.gov/ohrms/dockets/dockets/95s0316/95s-0316-rpt0282-tab-03-ref-19-joint-faowho-vol219.pdf [Accessed: 2015-04-14]

[66] Ministry of Health, Labour and Welfare. Available from: http://www.mhlw.go.jp/english/topics/foodsafety/fhc/02.html [Accessed: 2015-04-14]

[67] U.S. Department of Health and Human Services. U.S. Food and Drug Administration [Internet]. [Updated: 04/13/2015]. Available from: http://www.fda.gov/ [Accessed: 04-15-2015]

[68] Moeini H, Rahim RA, Omar AR, Shafee N, Yusoff K. Lactobacillus acidophilus as a live vehicle for oral immunization against chicken anemia virus. *Appl Microbiol Biotechnol.* 2011;90(1):77-88. DOI: 10.1007/s00253-010-3050-0

[69] Kajikawa A, Zhang L, Long J, Nordone S, Stoeker L, LaVoy A, et al. Construction and immunological evaluation of dual cell surface display of HIV-1 gag and Salmonella enterica serovar Typhimurium FliC in Lactobacillus acidophilus for vaccine delivery. *Clin Vaccine Immunol.* 2012;19(9):1374-81. DOI: 10.1128/CVI.00049-12

[70] Bercik P, Collins SM, Verdu EF. Microbes and the gut-brain axis. *Neurogastroenterol Motil.* 2012;24(5):405-13. DOI: 10.1111/j.1365-2982.2012.01906.x

[71] Sartor RB, Sherman PM, Mayer EA. An update on the use and investigation of probiotics in health and disease. Gut. 2913;62(5):787-96. DOI: 10.1136/gutjnl-2012-302504

Chapter 10

Bruton's Disease

Yıldız Camcıoğlu

Additional information is available at the end of the chapter

http://dx.doi.org/10.5772/61173

Abstract

Bruton's disease, in other terms X-linked agammaglobulinemia (XLA), is the first reported primary immunodeficiency in 1952, caused by a single genetic defect. The development of B cell is under control of signals transmitted by the B-cell antigen receptor (BCR) complex. Lyn, Syk, and Bruton's tyrosine kinase (BTK) are cytoplasmic protein tyrosine kinases. XLA is caused by mutations in the Btk gene, and Btk mutations are responsible for 85% of all antibody deficiencies. Btk mutation interrupts the B-cell development at the pre-B-cell stage, resulting in the absence of B lymphocytes and plasma cells in peripheral blood and peripheral lymphoid tissues. Up till now, 380 unique mutations have been identified. Autosomal recessive forms of agammaglobulinemia also result in B-cell defects, but more severe bacterial infections are seen in XLA patients due to absolute block in early B-cell development. All serum immunoglobulin isotypes are decreased, and antibody production especially against vaccine antigens is impaired.

Most of the XLA patients have clinical signs and symptoms after 6 to 9 months of age due to diminished protective maternal antibodies transmitted through placenta. The most frequent symptoms are recurrent upper and lower respiratory tract infections, some of them may suffer from neutropenia.

These patients are susceptible to enteroviral infection, which causes chronic meningoencephalitis and dermatomyositis-like syndrome. Recurrent respiratory tract infections lead to chronic lung disease and bronchiectasis. These infections may disable the patient and result in death. B-cell dysfunction may also cause autoimmunity and B-cell malignancies.

Patients with recurrent infections have to be evaluated for the primary immunodeficiency. X-linked agammaglobulinemia has to be considered with low serum IgG, IgA, and IgM levels and severely decreased B-cell number in the peripheral blood by lymphocyte subset analysis. A definitive diagnosis can be made by genetic studies. The majority of patients are diagnosed at the age of 5 years.

Immunoglobulin replacement therapy and antibiotic for infections are current choice of treatment to prevent life-threatening infections and organ damage. Hematopoietic stem cell (HSC)-based gene therapy can be curative.

Neonatal screening assays (KRECs) have been developed to determine the absence of B cells, seen in XLA.

Keywords: Absence of B cells, Bruton's disease, X-linked agammaglobulinemia, agammaglobulinemia, *Btk* gene mutation, Bruton's tyrosine kinase defect

---

1. Introduction

Bruton's disease is an X-linked agammaglobulinemia (XLA OMIM No. 300300) that was first described as primary immunodeficiency in 1952 by Dr. Bruton. It is the best-known antibody deficiency [1–5]. More than half of the patients with Bruton's diseases characterized by recurrent bacterial infections such as otitis, sinusitis, and sinopulmonary infections are developing after 7 to 9 months of age when transplacental maternal immunoglobulin G (IgG) levels decrease below protective levels in infants. In this disorder, genetic abnormalities lead to blockage in the maturation of B cells in the bone marrow and only confined to the B-cell lineage. *Streptococcus pneumoniae* and *Haemophilus influenzae* are the most common responsible encapsulated pathogens for recurrence of otitis and sinusitis. Pneumonia, empyema, meningitis, septicemia, and septic arthritis are severe infections, which may be the first warning signs of disease for physician to suspect immunodeficiency. The distinctive clinical features of the disease are early onset bacterial infections, absent mature B cells or remarkably reduced circulating B cells, severe reduction in the basal serum immunoglobulins, inability to produce antibodies against antigens, and occurrence of autoimmune diseases paradoxically. Based on these principal findings, approximately 90% of male patients presumed with XLA are likely to have mutation in *Btk* [6–9].

2. History

In 1952, an American pediatrician, Dr. Ogden Carr Bruton, described the clinical case of an 8-year-old boy who had recurrent episodes of pneumococcal sepsis [1, 2]. Dr. Bruton vaccinated the patient to prevent infections, but the boy did not produce antibodies to *Pneumococcus*. Electophoretic analysis revealed a lack of gammaglobulins in the patient's serum. Dr. Bruton treated this patient with monthly injections of exogenous gamma globulin. The patient remained free of sepsis episodes for 14 months during which he received injections. The disorder was observed only in male patients. Based on the observation of five additional male patients similar to Bruton's disease by Janeway and colleagues, the disorder later became known as X-linked agammaglobulinemia [9, 10, 11]. This disease was named Bruton's X-linked agammaglobulinemia after having discovered the first immunodeficient patient [12].

3. Prevalence

The frequency of Bruton's disease has been estimated as 1 per 200,000 live births. Prevalence is approximately 1 per 10,000. The prevalence of XLA varies in different countries obtained from published reports. Based on national registries, the prevalence was ranging between 0.09 and 11.25 per 100,000 population [13–17]. The minimum prevalence has been reported as 0.09 (minimum) from Germany [14], while it has been reported as 11.25 (maximum) in the USA [16]. The prevalence of XLA in Eastern and Central European (ECE) countries (total population, 145,530,870) was found to be 1 per 1,399,000 individuals.

4. *Btk* genes and function

X-linked agammaglobulinemia is caused by mutations in the gene encoding a cytoplasmic protein tyrosine kinase, called Bruton's tyrosine kinase (Btk), in honor of the discoverer of the disorder, Colonel Ogden Bruton, MD. Btk is signal transduction molecule downstream of pre-B-cell receptor (PreBCR) and the B-cell receptor (BCR). It is a key regulator for B-lymphocyte precursors to differentiate into B cells in bone marrow. Mutation in Btk results in the defective production and function of the enzyme. In a healthy person, the enzyme is activated by the pre-B-cell receptor, and it delivers biochemical signals that prompt the B cells to divide or mature and survive. Therefore, patients with defective Btk have almost complete absence of B cells and plasma cells due to arrest in maturation beyond pre-B cell [5–9].

The gene for this enzyme was identified in 1993 by two independent groups [18, 19]. It is located on the Xq21.3-Xq22, the long arm of the X chromosome [18–24]. Btk belongs to a distinct family of protein kinases. Tec, Itk, Bmx, and Txk are other members of this family. The protein contains five regions, PH, TH, SH3, SH2, and kinase domains, and any of these domains may be affected by mutations causing XLA [23, 24]

Since 1993, the number of genetic studies has increased. XLA is a variable disease in certain patients [25, 26]. The types of mutations causing XLA include missense, nonsense, point, frameshift, slice site, deletion, insertion, and premature stop codon mutations [27]. In general, missense mutations account for 40% of all mutations, whereas nonsense mutations account for 17%, deletions account for 20%, insertions account for 7%, and slice site accounts for 16%. This distribution is similar to those listed in Immunodeficiency mutation database [28].

In a study conducted on 56 patients, mutations affecting the *Btk* gene were demonstrated in 51 patients. It was shown that 22 mutations were missense [29]. In another study, the number of missense mutations was found to be higher [30]. In the study by Chan et al., 12 patients were evaluated, and 3 deletion mutations, 8 nucleotide substitution mutations, and 1 insertion–deletion mutation were detected [31]. In the study carried out in Central European patients with agammaglobulinemia, the point mutations were observed to be more frequent [32]. The first study in 16 Turkish XLA patients was done by Wang et al. [33], seven novel mutations were identified: 2 missense and 4 deletions resulting in frameshift and premature stop codon, novel mutations were determined in 7 cases; 2 missense, 1 nonsense, and 4 deletion mutations were detected. In the last update, lists of the online BTKbase, 1155 entries have been compiled from 974 unrelated families with 602 unique molecular events [32]. The genetic profile of XLA has been studied in 122 patients from 109 families in Eastern and Central European (ECE) countries in 2009 [17]. BTK sequence analysis revealed 98 different mutations, in which 46 of them were reported for the first time. The mutations included single nucleotide changes in the coding exons (35 missense and 17 nonsense), 23 splicing defects, 13 small deletions, 7 large deletions, and 3 insertions.

We conducted a study in Istanbul University, Cerrahpaşa Medical School, Children's Hospital, to determine the BTK mutation in a total of 19 Turkish boy from 18 unrelated families with recurrent infections, almost no CD19(+) B cells and agammaglobulinemia (Table 1) [34].

Patient no.	Age at diagnosis	IgG (mg/dL)	IgA (mg/dL)	IgM (mg/dL)	$CD19^{+}$ B cells	Family history	Consanguinity
P 1	4	<166	0	<128	3	(–)	(–)
P 2	1.5	29	0	<29	0	(–)	(+)
P 3	3	0	0	32	-	(–)	(+)
P 4	3.5	250	0	31	0	(–)	(–)
P 5a	3.5	-	-	-	0	(+)	(–)
P 5b	3 months	21	3	<18	0	(+)	(–)
P 6	1.5	611	179	55	2	(–)	(+)
P 7	1.5	157	<25	<18	0	(–)	(–)
P 8	8	307	28	121	0	(–)	(+)
P 9	6	<145	0	28	0	(–)	(–)
P 10	5	83	4	12	0	(–)	(–)
P 11	4	447	6	4	0	(–)	(+)
P 12	2	<140	<6	<16	0	(–)	(–)
P 13	9	<153	0	<2	0	(–)	(+)
P 14	5	<143	<23	70	0	(+)	(–)
P 15	7	681	188	25	2	(+)	(–)
P 16	3	180	<28	<29	0	(–)	(–)
P 17	8	302	152	8	0	(–)	(–)
P 18	1	315	60	33	2	(–)	(–)

Table 1. Clinical data of 18 male patients with agammaglobulinemia

BTK gene mutations were determined within 10 patients. The types of the mutations were 3 missense, 4 frameshift and premature stop codon; 2 splice site; and 1 point. Missense mutations were determined in the three patients (patients 2, 4, and 17). In one patient (patient 17), a novel amino acid substitution was determined within the TH domain in exon 6 (c. 491G > A) (p.G164D), which was not included previously in the ESID database. A novel point mutation within the PH domain in exon 2 (c. 49A > T) (p.K17X) was detected in Patient 7. This mutation as well has not been defined previously in the ESID database. The frameshift and premature stop codon mutations were observed to be frequent, followed by missense mutations (Table 2). Although four of the patients have features relevant with a clinical and immunological diagnosis of XLA, a BTK gene mutation could not be determined. In such cases, other autosomal recessive gene defects (μ heavy chain, surrogate light chain λ5, Igα and Igβ signaling molecules, and B-cell linker adaptor protein (BLNK)) should be investigated [35–40]. These genes map proteins involved in maturation of pro-B cells into pre-B cells. These defects have also been shown to result in agammaglobulinemia and an absence of circulating B cells, which cannot be clinically distinguished from XLA.

Patient no.	Localization	Nucleotide aberration	Amino acid aberration	Protein domain
P 2	Exon 18	c.1762T>G	p.W588G	TK
P 4	Exon 2	c.40T>C	p.S14P	PH
P 5a	Exon 13	c.1157_1161delCCACT	p.S386fsX10	TK
P 5b	Exon 13	c.1157_1161delCCACT	p.S386fsX10	TK
P 7	Exon 2	c.49A>T	p.K17X	PH
P 10	Exon 9	c.839+4_+7delAGTA		
P 12	Exon 15	c.1461_1465delGA	p.E488fsX19	TK
P 14	Exon 8	c.713delG	p.G238fsX39	SH3
P 16	Exon 12	c.1102+1G>A		
P 17	Exon 6	c.491G>A	p.G164D	TH

Table 2. *Btk* mutations identified in 10 XLA patients

In the light of these studies, gene defect has to be defined for the accurate diagnosis of XLA, carrier detection, and prenatal diagnosis.

5. Genetic counseling

XLA is inherited in sex-linked diseases (x-linked). As the defects are connected with the X-chromosome and the inheritance is recessive, only male infants are affected. If a boy inherits a defective gene, since he does not have a healthy gene from his father, the boy may have the disease. Women who carry a mutant allele of the *Btk* gene on one of their chromosomes are carrier of the disease. Therefore, mothers, sisters, and maternal aunts should be investigated for carrier status because they are obligate carriers. Brothers, uncles, or nephews of the mother must be questioned for this disorder. The family history of XLA is nonexistent in approximately 50% of patients. Some of these patients (15–20%) with XLA may have a de novo mutation in *Btk* gene, and their mothers are not carriers. If the mutant *Btk* allele is known previously in the family, carrier testing for at-risk female relatives or prenatal diagnosis is possible [41–43].

6. Immunology of XLA

B cells arise from hematopoietic stem cells in the bone marrow. B cells begin to generate and express B-cell receptors (BCRs) (Fig. 1). The entire developmental process of B cells occurs within the bone marrow. A common lymphoid progenitor (CLP) gives rise to pro-B lymphocytes, which next develop into pre-B lymphocytes and then to B lymphocytes. Stimulated B cells may further differentiate into plasma cells that synthesize and secrete immunoglobulins. Mutation in Bruton tyrosine kinase causes arrest in the development of B lymphocyte at the early stage of large pre-B-cell ($CD19^+$ cytoplasmic μ^+) stage in the bone marrow (Fig. 2). This defect is leaky, resulting in a few immature B cell. B-cell developmental defects in bone marrow lead to a marked decrease or absence of fully mature B lymphocytes in peripheral blood, absent or few follicles, and germinal centers in lymphoid organs. Plasmocytes are absent, and reticuloendothelial tissue and lymphoid organs (tonsils, spleen, Peyer plaques, and lymph nodes) are poorly developed. Therefore, secondary lymphoid organs such as lymph nodes and tonsils are reduced in size. The consequence of decreased immunoglobulin-producing B cell is diminished in all serum immunoglobulin isotypes, resulting in inability to produce antibodies against protein and polysaccharide antigens. The percentage of T cell is increased, and T cell functions are intact. These patients have the ability to control viral and fungal infections because of intact cell-mediated immunity. The thymus is in normal size and architecture.

Antibodies are produced by plasma cells that are terminally differentiated B cells. When B lymphocytes identify and interact with a specific antigen in the body, it is triggered to mature into a plasma cell that is able to produce specific antibodies. Plasmocytes produce nine antibody isotypes: immunoglobulins G (IgG1, IgG2, IgG3, and IgG4), immunoglobulins M (IgM), immunoglobulins A (IgA1 and IgA2), immunoglobulins D (IGD), and immunoglobulins E (IgE). Antibodies are soluble molecules that bind to antigens to render them harmless by agglutination and neutralization or "tag" the antigens to facilitate destruction and removal by phagocytes and via activating complement components. Antibodies are an important component of humoral immune responses and integral part of body's defense mechanism against bacteria. During the first 6–9 months of life, infants with XLA are protected from infections by transferred maternal IgG antibodies. Reduced maternal antibodies by 6–9 months of age and failures in humoral immunity leave the affected XLA patient with a reduced ability to resist infections and increased susceptibili-

http://dx.doi.org/10.5772/61173

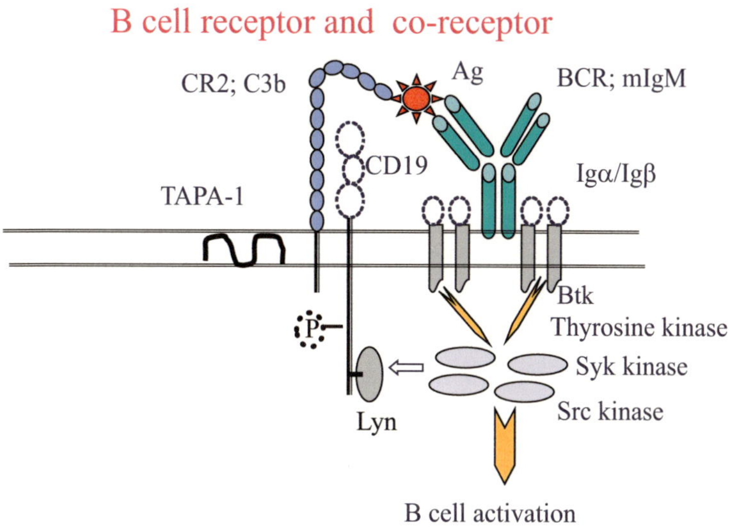

Figure 1. Btk, delivering signals for maturation of B cell.

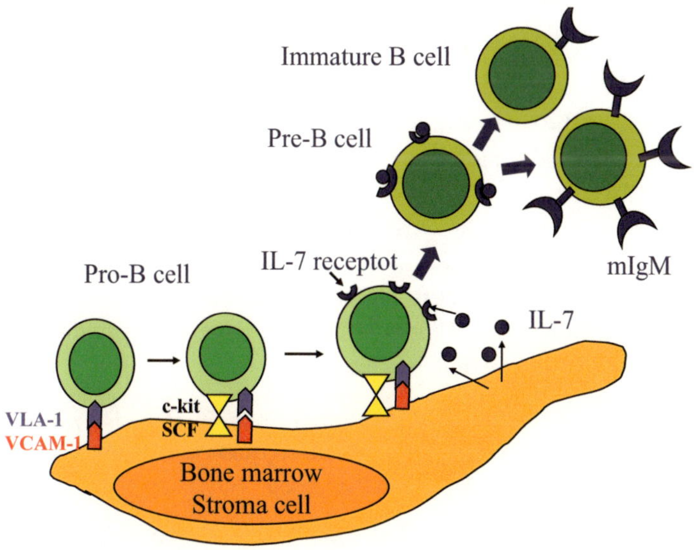

Figure 2. Development of B cells in bone marrow.

ty to encapsulated bacteria and enteroviruses as well. As a consequence, there is a virtual absence of humoral response to recall antigens [9, 12, 44–47].

7. Clinical presentation

Symptoms of patients with XLA most often begin at about 6 to 9 months of age, when the transferred maternal immunoglobulin has been catabolized and the infant becomes dependent on his own immune system. Widespread use of antibiotics may often mask the presentation of disease and despite recurrent sinopulmonary infections diagnosis of XLA may delay until 3–5 years of age or adolescence in some cases [8]. In a small subpopulation of cases with XLA, about 10% to 15%, who are not recognized to have immunodeficiency until 5 years of age, serum immunoglobulin levels may be high [46]. Patients with XLA are clinically characterized by an onset of recurrent bacterial infections due to remarkable decrease in immunoglobulin levels [5–9, 47–50].

The clinical findings leading to the diagnosis of XLA were determined in 82 patients with proven mutations in Bruton's tyrosine kinase. The authors reported that the majority of patients with XLA had a history of recurrent otitis at the time of diagnosis. The physical findings of decreased or absent tonsils and cervical lymph nodes could have alerted physicians to the diagnosis of XLA [51].

Clinical presentations of X-linked agammaglobulinemia have been defined by a multicenter retrospective survey of 96 patients. The onset of infections was in the first 4 months of life (25% of cases), 8 months of life (50% of cases), 12 months of life (75% of cases), and 18 months of life (90% of cases). The most frequent infections involved the upper respiratory tract (75%), the lower respiratory tract (65%), the gastrointestinal tract (35%), the skin (28%), and the central nervous system (16%) [52].

Infection usually develops at the surface of mucous membranes, namely, middle ear, sinuses, and lungs. Pneumonia, otitis media, sinusitis, conjunctivitis, and diarrhea are the hallmark of XLA patients. In some cases, infection can spread through the bloodstream, and septicemia, meningitis, septic arthritis, cellulitis, and osteomyelitis may occur. *S. pneumoniae* and *H. influenzae* are the most common responsible encapsulated pathogens of infections. These microorganisms also affect all patients with antibody deficiency, such as common variable immunodeficiency (CVID); however, patients with XLA have susceptibility to enteroviral infection in contrast to other antibody deficiencies.

There are many published data about the clinical presentation of XLA. They are reflecting the results of different population of XLA patients. The frequency of clinical presentations is variable due to different cohorts of XLA patients assessed.

Infection was the most common initial clinical presentation (85%), followed by a positive family history (41%) and neutropenia (11%) in 201 XLA patients included in the United States Registry. The average age of diagnosis was significantly younger in patients with a positive family history (2.59 years) than in patients with a negative family history (5.37 years) ($p < 0.001$). Seventy percent of patients had at least 1 episode of otitis, 62% at least 1 episode of pneumonia, 60% at least 1 episode of sinusitis, 23% at least 1 episode of chronic/recurrent diarrhea, 21% at least 1 episode of conjunctivitis, 18% at least 1 episode of pyoderma and/or cellulitis, 11% at least 1 episode of meningitis/encephalitis, 10% at least 1 episode of sepsis, 8% at least 1 episode of septic arthritis, 6% at least 1 episode of hepatitis, and 3% at least 1 episode of osteomyelitis. Of 201 patients, 14 (6.9%) were dead at the time they were entered in the registry. Causes of death were disseminated enterovirus infection (n = 6), pulmonary insufficiency (n = 5), adenovirus infection (n = 1), sepsis (n = 1), acquired immunodeficiency disease syndrome (AIDS) (n = 1), myocarditis (n = 1), hepatitis (n = 2), and stem cell transplantation (n = 1) [53].

The median age at the onset of the disease was 8 months, and the median age of diagnosis was 48 months based on the records of 33 Iranian XLA patients. The most frequent infections were seen in the respiratory tract (93.9%), gastrointestinal tract (75.8%), central nervous system (33.3%), and musculoskeletal system (21.2%). Chronic otitis media, chronic sinusitis, chronic diarrhea, and bronchiectasis were developed complications in 75.8% of cases [54].

The mean age of onset was 2.5 years, and the mean age at diagnosis was 7.3 years in six patients with XLA from northern Thailand. Patients had a history of otitis media, pneumonia, arthritis, and sinusitis (5/6); pericarditis (1/6), meningitis (1/6), and pyoderma (1/6) were other experienced infections. *Pseudomonas aeruginosa* and *Staphylococcus aureus* were isolated on multiple occasions in five patients. Five cases had developed bronchiectasis and three patients septicemia [55].

Recurrent pulmonary infections and an unusual course of common pulmonary infection should alert physician for underlying immunodeficiency. Lung infections were evaluated in 39 Iranian patients with XLA. The authors reported that 82% (32/39) of patients with XLA experienced at least one episode of pneumonia, and 84% (27/32) of those patients had more than one episode. An average rate of pneumonia episode per patient per year was 1.67 for XLA patients [56].

A patient with XLA presenting with respiratory distress, was reported to have *Pneumocystis jirovecii* pneumonia. This patient is a reminder that the potential consequences of BTK deficiency in cells other than B-cells should be considered [57].

Mycoplasma infections may involve the respiratory tract, the urogenital tract, and joints, leading to prolonged than severe course or asymptomatic in some cases [58, 59].

Skin infections such as impetigo, abscesses, and furuncles due to group A streptococcus or staphylococcus had been also reported.

Although patients with XLA experience childhood viral infections uneventful, they have susceptibility to certain viruses. Enteroviral infections (echovirus, coxsackievirus, and polio virus) frequently run a severe course and often resist therapy in affected patients. Enterovirus may cause severe and, eventually, fatal progressive encephalitis [5–9, 52, 60, 61].

Clinical manifestations of enteroviral meningoencephalitis demonstrate great variation changing from severe infection to chronic enteroviral infection. Illness may be overt as acute infection with fever, headache, and seizures or tend to progress slowly throughout the years with loss of cognitive skills, ataxia, paresthesia, neurosensory hearing loss, and lethargy [60, 61]. The laboratory assessment of cerebrospinal fluid (CSF) may reveal clear fluid, pleocytosis ($<1000/mm^3$), elevated protein level (0.5–5 g/dL), and in a few cases hypoglycorrhachia or normal CSF results. Polymerase chain reaction (PCR) techniques may detect virus in CSF.

Initial magnetic resonance imaging (MRI) or computed tomography (CT) scan reveal no abnormality; however, cortical or subcortical atrophy, ventricular dilatation, periventricular changes, and hydrocephaly may be observed later in life. There are no typical histopathology findings at brain biopsy. Illness is progressive and mortality is very high. As a result of disseminated enteroviral infection, dermatomyositis-like syndrome may develop with erythematous rash and peripheral edema. Hepatitis with increased alanine aminotransferase (ALT) may accompany [60–63].

Gastrointestinal disorders are common problems of XLA patients. Patients may have infections, autoimmunity, or rarely malignancy. *Campylobacter jejuni* is the most frequent pathogen causing gastrointestinal tract infection. Typically, affected patients suffer from fever, skin rash, and persistent diarrhea [64–66]. Parasitic infection especially *Giardia lamblia* infection may cause abdominal pain, diarrhea, poor growth, or loss of serum proteins. *Giardia* can be isolated from stool samples of patients and too hard to eradicate.

Inflammatory disorders in XLA patients unexpectedly occur. A web-based patient survey was conducted in patients with XLA. Based on 128 patient responses, the majority of respondents (69%) reported having at least one inflammatory symptom. Just 28% of them had been diagnosed with an inflammatory condition. Arthritis had been diagnosed only in 7% XLA patients, despite 20% reported painful joints and 11% reported swelling of the joints. Similarly, 21% reported symptoms of chronic diarrhea and 17% reported abdominal pain. However, only 4% had been diagnosed with Crohn's disease. Data from the United States Immune Deficiency Network (USIDNET) Registry on 149 patients with XLA revealed that 12% had pain, swelling, or arthralgia, while 18% had been diagnosed with arthritis [67]. Kawasaki disease is also reported in an XLA patient, providing opportunity to understand the relationship between autoimmunity and XLA [68].

Noninfectious or infectious arthritis may occur in patients with X-linked agammaglobulinemia. Juvenile rheumatoid is relatively common in patients with XLA. The mechanisms are not clear of noninfectious arthritis. *H. influenzae, S. pneumoniae,* and mycoplasma are pathogens causing septic arthritis. Pain and swelling of joints are presenting symptoms. Erythrocyte sedimentation rate increase, rheumatoid factor (RF), and antinuclear antibody (ANA) tests are negative. Arthritis may be the first presenting symptom of X-linked agammaglobulinemia. That is the reason why physicians must be aware of immunodeficiencies [69, 70].

Growth hormone deficiency associated with XLA patient has been reported [71].

Although the relationship between the Bruton kinase mutation and the development of malignant tumors is unknown, XLA patients seem to be at risk for colorectal cancer and lymphoid malignancies. B-cell precursor acute lymphoblastic leukemia (BCP-ALL) has been reported in a case with XLA. It has been reported that somatic mutation found in MLL2 suggests that the alterations of BTK and MLL2 synergistically function as leukemogenesis [72, 73].

Cases with vaccine-associated paralytic poliovirus infection as a consequence of attenuated oral polio (Sabin) have been reported in XLA patients [74]. The incubation period of the infection is more than 30 days, and chronic encephalomyelitis develops eventually [75].

http://dx.doi.org/10.5772/61173

8. Physical Examination

Remarkable physical findings of XLA patients are the absence or hypoplasia of tonsils and lymph nodes. Chronic otitis, sinusitis, mastoiditis, or bronchiectasis are consequences of recurrent infections.

9. Diagnosis

Significant progress in the field has been achieved in the light of collaborative studies. Guidelines for screening primary immunodeficiencies have been published by experts, non-immunologists and immunologists [51, 76–78]. The classification of primary immunodeficiency diseases had been updated by the *ad hoc* Expert Committee of the International Union of Immunological Societies [79]. The hallmark of clinical features and laboratory evidences were provided for each immunodeficiency, which help physicians to recognize and diagnose patients with immunodeficiency timely.

9.1. Clinical clues

X-linked agammaglobulinemia (XLA) should always be considered in children with recurrent, persistent, unusual sinopulmonary infections or a life-threatening severe bacterial infection below 5 years of age. Small tonsils and lymph nodes on physical examination are warning signs of disorder. Patients with strong family history of immunodeficiency relevant with X-linked inheritance should be investigated further.

9.2. Laboratory approach

Based on studies, detailed family and medical history combined with careful physical examination further guide specific blood tests of the immune system, which will be performed step by step to confirm the diagnosis of XLA. Severe defects of immune systems should be ruled out at the first steps of diagnostic protocol for suspected immunodeficiency. Infection with human immunodeficiency virus (HIV) has to be excluded rapidly. Tests have to be performed and interpreted by a specialist immunologist. The use of age-matched reference values for lymphocyte subsets and immunoglobulin levels are highly recommended to avoid misinterpretation.

Baseline blood tests give useful information. The complete blood test (CBC) is a crucial test to reveal anemia, neutropenia, lymphopenia, thrombocytopenia, or eosinophilia, which may give a clue to which type of PID is present. Neutropenia is associated with a small subpopulation of patients with XLA (11%), which can be misdiagnosis as congenital neutropenia [8, 80, 81]. Severe neutropenia is usually in association with pseudomonas or staphylococcal sepsis. A CBC and a manual leukocyte differential can aid in the identification of striking lymphopenia, which is a very important clue for severe combined immunodeficiencies (SCID) accepted as medical emergency.

Screening tests for antibody deficiencies as recommended by experts are presented as follows [8, 50, 76–78, 82]:

- Serum total protein level
- Serum immunoglobulin assay: IgG, IgA, IgM
- Isohemagglutinins (IgM antibodies to A and B blood group antigens)
- Specific antibody responses
- Tetanus, diphtheria (IgG1)
- Pneumococcal and meningococcal polysaccharides (IgG2)
- Viral respiratory pathogens (IgG1 and IgG3)
- Other vaccines: hepatitis B, influenza, MMR, and polio (killed vaccine)
- Lymphocyte subpopulation by flow cytometry (B-cell quantitation)
- Lymphocyte proliferation tests
- B-cell maturation analysis in bone marrow
- Genetic determinations of defect

Serum immunoglobulin concentration should be measured by quantitative techniques, and IgG, IgA, and IgM are routinely measured in serum. Values of determined immunoglobulin levels have to be compared with normal-for-age values. The majority of patients with XLA have less than 200 mg/dL serum IgG level. However, serum IgG concentration is more than 200 mg/dL in 10% of children with XLA. Serum IgM and IgA are classically less than 20 mg/dL. Low serum IgG concentration may also be determined in patients who have protein-losing enteropathy and nephrosis. The concomitant serum protein levels of these patients are low; hence, they produce antibodies normally. Under certain conditions, the determination of IgE and IgD levels may be required.

Isohemagglutinins are natural IgM-class antibodies against A and B blood group antigens. Therefore, they are not found in patients who have type AB blood group. In addition, the measurement of isohemagglutinin titers in the serum is not reliable below 6 months of age. Normal values for anti-A titer is 1:16 or higher and anti-B titer is 1:8 or higher. Isohemagglutinins titer is low in XLA patients due to poor IgM synthesis.

Individuals with XLA fail to make antibodies against vaccine antigens or pathogens such as tetanus, *H. influenzae*, or *S. pneumoniae*. Since children are vaccinated with diphtheria–tetanus —acellular pertussis (DTaP), conjugated *H. influenzae* type b, and conjugated pneumococcal vaccine (PVC), the measurement of antibodies against these antigens is informative. The measurement of specific antibodies against diphtheria and tetanus before and 2 weeks after DTaP or booster DT immunization reveals a patient's ability to produce IgG antibodies against protein antigens. Pneumococcal polysaccharide vaccine or conjugated pneumococcal vaccine (PVC) is used to evaluate a patient's ability to respond to polysaccharide antigen (IIb C). The

http://dx.doi.org/10.5772/61173

measurement of pneumococcal antibody titers before and 4 to 8 weeks after vaccination should be done in patients more than 2 years of age (Ib A). The normal response to each pneumococcal serotype is defined as a titer equal to or greater than 1.3 mg/mL antibody (IIb C) [83]. The ability of antibody production against antigens and the response to vaccination are severely impaired in XLA patients.

Patients who have agammaglobulinema need lymphocyte phenotyping. The number of B lymphocytes in the peripheral blood can be enumerated by flow cytometry using dye-conjugated monoclonal antibodies (CD 19 and CD 20), which are specific B-cell markers. B cells constitute 4–10% of the peripheral lymphocyte. The reduced number of $CD19^+$ B cells in the peripheral blood would be indicative of defective B-cell differentiation and would suggest XLA if not combined with depleted T-cell numbers. B cell is markedly reduced below <1% in patients with XLA [76–79, 83].

Mutations in *BTK* gene can be scanned by sequence analysis, which can detect approximately 90% of mutations in *BTK*.

10. BTK protein testing

BTK mutations occur in the absence of the BTK protein in monocytes. The detection of BTK protein in monocytes by immunofluorescence or western blot [84, 85] can confirm the diagnosis of XLA.

Female carriers may be determined by mutation analysis or Btk protein expression on blood cells by flow cytometry. They have normal immune functions, but they have a 50% chance of transmitting the disease to each of her sons.

The following diagnostic criteria for X-linked agammaglobulinemia were published by Conley et al. in 1999 [86]:

Definitive diagnosis—males with less than 2% $CD19^+$ B cells and at least one of the following:

- Mutation in *BTK*
- Absent Btk mRNA on northern blot analysis of neutrophils or monocytes
- Absent Btk protein in monocytes or platelets
- Maternal cousins, uncles, or nephews with less than 2% $CD19^+$ B cells

Probable diagnosis—males with less than 2% $CD19^+$ B cells and the following:

- Onset of recurrent bacterial infections in the first 5 years of life
- Serum IgG, IgM, and IgA more than 2 SD below normal for age
- Absent isohemagglutinins and/or poor response to vaccines
- Exclusion of other causes of hypogammaglobulinemia

Possible diagnosis—males with less than 2% CD19⁺ B cells in whom other causes of hypogammaglobulinemia have been excluded and who has at least one of the following:

- Onset of recurrent bacterial infections in the first 5 years of life
- Serum IgG, IgM, and IgA more than 2 SD below normal for age
- Absent isohemagglutinins

Chest X-ray or CT scan of patients with XLA reveals bronchiectasis most commonly distributed in the middle or lower lobes, atelectasis, and bronchial wall thickening. CT scan of sinuses may suggest the presence of chronic sinusitis.

Prenatal diagnosis—this may be achieved by using mutation analysis in amniotic fluid cells and Btk protein expression on cord blood cells by flow cytometry.

11. Newborn screening

Kappa-deleting recombination excision circles (KRECs) are chosen as markers for B lymphopenia at birth, indicative of X-linked agammaglobulinemia. The measurement of KRECs in newborn would help the early diagnosis of XLA patients [87].

12. Differential diagnosis

Differential diagnosis should be done by other disorder with hypogammaglobulinemia such as CVID, X-linked hyper IgM syndrome, and X-linked lymphoproliferative disease.

It had been known for several years that there were girls who had an immunodeficiency that looked just like XLA, and immunologists had suggested that there were forms of agammaglobulinemia with autosomal recessive inheritance (ARA). Since 1996, several genes (μ heavy chain deficiency, λ5 deficiency, Igα deficiency, Igβ deficiency, BLNK deficiency, PI3 kinase deficiency, and E47 transcription deficiency) that can cause ARA have been identified. All of these genes code for proteins that work with BTK to support the maturation of pro-B cells into pre-B cells. Patients with mutations in any of these genes have clinical and laboratory findings that are very similar to those seen in patients with mutations in Btk (Table 3) [35–39].

Disease	Genetic defect	Inheritance	Serum Ig	Associated features
Btk deficiency	Mutation in Btk, a cytoplasmic tyrosine kinase activated by cross-linking the BCR	XL	All isotypes decreased	Severe bacterial infections: normal numbers of pro-B cells

Disease	Genetic defect	Inheritance	Serum Ig	Associated features
μ heavy chain deficiency	Mutation in μ heavy chain: essential component of the pre-BCR	AR	All isotypes decreased	Severe bacterial infections: normal numbers of pro-B cells
λ5 deficiency	Mutation in 15: part of the surrogate light chain in the pre-BCR	AR	All isotypes decreased	Severe bacterial infections: normal numbers of pro-B cells
Igα deficiency	Mutation in Igα (CD79α) : part of pre-BCR and BCR	AR	All isotypes decreased	Severe bacterial infections: normal numbers of pro-B cells
Igβ deficiency	Mutation in Igβ (CD79β) : part of pre-BCR and BCR	AR	All isotypes decreased	Severe bacterial infections: normal numbers of pro-B cells
BLNK deficiency	Mutation in BLNK: a scaffold protein that binds to Btk	AR	All isotypes decreased	Severe bacterial infections: normal numbers of pro-B cells
PI3 kinase deficiency	Mutation in PIK3R1; a kinase involved in signal transduction in multiple cell types	AR	All isotypes decreased	Severe bacterial infections: decreased or absent pro-B cells
E47 transcription deficiency	Mutation in TCF3:a transcription factor required for control of B-cell development	AD	All isotypes decreased	Recurrent bacterial infections
Myelodysplasia with hypogammaglobulinemia	May have monosomy 7, trisomy 8,or dyskeratosis congenita	Variable	One or more isotypes may be decreased	Infections: decreased numbers of pro-B cells
Thymoma with immune deficiency	Unknown	None	One or more isotypes may be decreased	Bacterial and opportunistic infections: autoimmunity: decreased numbers of pro-B cells

Table 3. Diseases with absent or decreased B cells and markedly reduced in serum immunoglobulin isotypes (Al-Herz et al., *Front Immunol*, 2014)

13. Treatment

There is no curative treatment for XLA. Therapeutic measures consist of intravenous immunoglobulins (400–600 mg/kg monthly in order to maintain the IgG levels at 500–800 mg/dL), specific treatment of bacterial infections with antibiotics, and bronchodilators. The mainstay of treatment consists of immunoglobulin replacement therapy and prolonged antibiotic treatment of suspected bacterial infections. Immunoglobulin replacement therapy is essential for the XLA patients who are unable to produce sufficient antibodies against antigens. IgG is purified from thousand of human plasma and contains a wide range of antibodies against so many infections. Thus, it is life saving for XLA patients, and they have to continue to receive to survive. The aim of immunoglobulin treatment given by intravenous (IVIG) or subcutaneous (SCIG) infusions is to avoid acute infections, to decrease the number of bacterial infections, to improve quality of life, and to increase life expectancy of patients [8, 9, 47, 88–92].

IVIG infusions have to be done at hospital or home by professionally educated staff if possible. The common recommended dose of IVIG treatment for antibody replacement is between 0.3 and 0.6 g/kg, administered every 2 to 4 weeks via the intravenous route. The first IVIG infusion must be given slowly starting with a rate of 0.5 to 1.0 mg/kg per minute. Patient should be monitored closely for any adverse reactions during infusion. If the patient tolerates well, the infusion rate may be increased to 1.5 to 2.5 mg/kg per minute after 15 to 30 minutes. The maximal infusion rate is 4 mg/kg per minute, and infusion of an IVIG product should last 2 to 4 hours. The aim of IVIG therapy in patients with PID is to maintain serum IgG levels between 350 and 500 mg/ dL. Since there is a large variation in individual IgG elimination rates, the periodic measurement of serum IgG concentration is critical to monitor the adequacy of replacement during therapy. Retrospective studies in patients with XLA revealed that the severity and the number of infections especially pulmonary diseases are decreased depending on IVIG dose [88]. Serious bacterial illnesses and enteroviral meningoencephalitis were prevented when maintained IgG levels were above 800 mg/dL [89–95].

A 5-year multicenter prospective study on 201 patients with CVID and 101 patients with XLA was conducted to identify the effects of long-term immunoglobulin treatment and the IgG trough level to be maintained over time required to minimize infection risk. Overall, 24% of patients with XLA remained infection free during the study. In addition, in XLA, the comorbidity risk factor identified for pneumonia was the presence of bronchiectasis [96].

Infusion-related adverse effects and transmission of blood-borne viruses are adverse effects of immunoglobulin replacement therapy [97]. Reduced adverse reactions are reported with improved and new IVIG products. The subcutaneous IG (SCIG) therapy was reported to be effective, safe, and well tolerated in children and adults. High treatment satisfaction (TS) scores and health-related quality of life (HRQOL) were advantages of SCIG. Subcutaneous infusions are recommended to patients who are small children, reactive to IVIG, or have problem with vascular access. SCIG is given as a parent-managed or a self-managed treatment. Norway, Sweden, United Kingdom, and Belgium are the countries in which SCIG is often applied to children [98, 89]. Clinical records of 1151 XLA patients identified from ESID were included in ESID registry. According to ESID registry, 305 XLA patients were treated with IVIG (73%) and 114 patients were treated with SCIG (27%) [98, 99].

Bacterial infections treated with a high dose of selected antibiotics or antibiotics sensitive to yielded pathogens for prolonged periods.

Six young patients with XLA treated with cord blood or bone marrow transplants were reported. No one benefited from transplantation, and expected increase in serum IgM or blood B-cell number was not observed [100].

http://dx.doi.org/10.5772/61173

14. Vaccination

Live viral vaccines, such as oral polio, rotavirus, yellow fever, live attenuated influenza, and live bacterial (e.g., typhoid [*Salmonella typhi*, Ty21a]) vaccines should not be applied to patients with X-linked agammaglobulinemia. Therefore, inactivated polio vaccine (Salk) should be given to patients with XLA and their family contacts. These patients may develop vaccine-acquired diseases such as central nervous system infection due to oral poliovirus vaccine.

The effectiveness of the measles and varicella vaccines are uncertain because most patients receive IVIG and do not have capacity to produce antibody responses [101, 102].

However, bacille Calmette–Guérin (BCG) vaccine applied to 50 patients with X-linked agammaglobulinemia did not reveal any systemic infection [102].

15. Complications

The most common secondary complications of XLA are chronic sinusitis, chronic lung disease, malabsorption, and enteroviral infection. The delay in diagnosis of XLA remains a significant problem, as a consequence of recurrent pneumonias, bronchiectasis, pulmonary hypertension, and finally cor pulmonale may develop. Many patients have been diagnosed after chronic sequel had already been existed. The aggressive use of antibiotics can decrease the incidence of chronic sinusitis and lung disease. Hearing loss is a consequence of chronic otitis media. Early diagnosis and treatment of bowel infections may decrease the risk of inflammatory bowel disease. Renal AA amyloidosis had been reported in 38-year-old patient with Bruton's disease [103].

16. Mortality

Chronic lung diseases and infections, especially disseminated viral infections, and meningoencephalitis due to enterovirus are major causes of mortality. Treatment with newly developed and improved immunoglobulin products and antibiotics and improvement of care of immunodeficient patients would reduce the mortality rates and increase the survival of XLA patients. Registered 41 XLA patients were followed up 20 years until 2010. Among 41 patients, 26.8% died during the follow-up period. All of the complications existed before the initiation of treatment was reduced after immunoglobulin replacement therapy, except sinusitis and conjunctivitis. The associations between some immunological and clinical characteristics such as lymphocyte subsets, consanguinity marriage, and mortality were documented [104].

17. Prognosis

In the case of the early diagnosis of XLA and an appropriate therapy before the appearance of sequel, prognosis is well. They are encouraged a full active lifestyle and children can attend to all regular school. Attention should be paid to pulmonary infections and complications in the long-term follow-up of patients. XLA is a chronic disease; patients need immunoglobulin replacement therapy to avoid infections and care of a multidisciplinary team of specialists for the rest of their lives [98, 99].

Author details

Yıldız Camcıoğlu*

Address all correspondence to: camciy@yahoo.com

Division of Infectious Diseases, Clinical Immunology and Allergy, Department of Pediatrics, Cerrahpasa Medical School, Istanbul University, Cerrahpasa, Turkey

Disclosure: The author has no conflict of interest.

References

[1] Bruton OC Agammaglobulinemia. Pediatrics. 1952:9:722–728.

[2] Bruton OC, APT L, Gitlin D, Janeway CA. Absence of serum gammaglobulins. AMA Am J Dis Child. 1952:84(5):632–636.

[3] Conley ME. X-linked immunodeficiencies. Curr Opin Genet Dev. 1994 Jun;4(3):401–406

[4] Sideras P, Smith CI. Molecular and cellular aspects of X-linked agammaglobulinemia. Adv Immunol. 1995:59:135–223

[5] Ochs HD, Smith CIE. X-linked agammaglobulinemia. A clinical and molecular analysis. Medicine1996;75:287–299

[6] Conley ME, Parolini O, Rohrer J, Campana D. X-linked agammaglobulinemia: new approaches to old questions based on the identification of the defective gene. Immunol Rev. 1994 Apr;138:5–21

[7] Ballow M. Approach to the patient with recurrent infections. Clin Rev Allergy Immunol. 2008 Apr;34(2):129–140.

[8] Driessen G, van der Burg M. Educational paper: primary antibody deficiencies. Eur J Pediatr. 2011 Jun;170(6):693–702.

[9] van der Burg M, van Zelm MC, Driessen GJ, van Dongen JJ. New frontiers of primary antibody deficiencies. Cell Mol Life Sci. 2012 Jan;69(1):59–73.

[10] Janeway CA Apt L, Gitlin D. Agammaglobulinemia. Trans Assoc Am Physicians. 1953;66:200–202

[11] Conley ME. Hypogammaglobulinemia: fifty years later. Clin Immunol. 2002 Sep; 104(3):201–203

[12] Khan WN. Colonel Bruton's kinase defined the molecular basis of X-linked agammaglobulinemia, the first primary immunodeficiency. J Immunol. 2012 Apr 1;188(7): 2933–2935.

[13] Stonebraker JS, Farrugia A, Gathmann B. ESID Registry Working Party, Orange JS. Modeling primary immunodeficiency disease epidemiology and its treatment to estimate latent therapeutic demand for immunoglobulin. J Clin Immunol. 2014 Feb;34(2): 233–244.

[14] Gathmann B, Goldacker S, Klima M, Belohradsky BH, Notheis G, Ehl S, Ritterbusch H, Baumann U, Meyer-Bahlburg A, Witte T, Schmidt R, Borte M, Borte S, Linde R, Schubert R, Bienemann K, Laws HJ, Dueckers G, Roesler J, Rothoeft T, Krüger R, Scharbatke EC, Masjosthusmann K, Wasmuth JC, Moser O, Kaiser P, Groß-Wieltsch U, Classen CF, Horneff G, Reiser V, Binder N, El-Helou SM, Klein C, Grimbacher B, Kindle G. The German national registry for primary immunodeficiencies (PID). Clin Exp Immunol. 2013 Aug;173(2):372–380.

[15] Hashimoto S, Tsukada S, Matsushita M, Miyawaki T, Niida Y, Yachie A, Kobayashi S, Iwata T, Hayakawa H, Matsuoka H, Tsuge I, Yamadori T, Kunikata T, Arai S, Yoshizaki K, Taniguchi N, Kishimoto T. Identification of Bruton's tyrosine kinase (Btk) gene mutations and characterization of the derived proteins in 35 X-linked agammaglobulinemia families: a nationwide study of Btk deficiency in Japan. Blood. 1996 Jul 15;88(2):561–573.

[16] Boyle JM, Buckley RH. Population prevalence of diagnosed primary immunodeficiency diseases in the United States. J Clin Immunol. 2007 Sep;27(5):497–502.

[17] Tóth B, Volokha A, Mihas A, Pac M, Bernatowska E, Kondratenko I, Polyakov A, Erdos M, Pasic S, Bataneant M, Szaflarska A, Mironska K, Richter D, Stavrik K, Avcin T, Márton G, Nagy K, Dérfalvi B, Szolnoky M, Kalmár A, Belevtsev M, Guseva M, Rugina A, Kriván G, Timár L, Nyul Z, Mosdósi B, Kareva L, Peova S, Chernyshova L, Gherghina I, Serban M, Conley ME, Notarangelo LD, Smith CI, van Dongen J, van der Burg M, Maródi L. Genetic and demographic features of X-linked agammaglobulinemia in Eastern and Central Europe: a cohort study. Mol Immunol. 2009 Jun; 46(10):2140–2146.

[18] Vetrie D, Vorechovský I, Sideras P, Holland J, Davies A, Flinter F. The gene involved in X-linked agammaglobulinaemia is a member of the src family of protein-tyrosine kinases. Nature. 1993:361:226–233

[19] Tsukada S, Saffran DC, Rawlings DJ, Parolini O, Allen RC, Klisak I. Deficient expression of a B cell cytoplasmic tyrosine kinase in human X-linked agammaglobulinemia. Cell. 1993:72:279–290

[20] Rohrer J, Parolini O, Belmont JW, Conley ME. The genomic structure of human BTK, the defective gene in X-linked agammaglobulinemia. Immunogenetics. 1994:40:319–324.

[21] Mattsson PT, Vihinen M, Smith CI. X-linked agammaglobulinemia (XLA): a genetic tyrosine kinase (Btk) disease. Bioessays. 1996 Oct;18(10):825–834.

[22] Conley, ME, Broides, A, Hernandez-Trujillo, V, Howard, V, Kanegane, H, Miyawaki, T. Genetic analysis of patients with defects in early B-cell development. Immunol Rev. 2005:203:216–234

[23] Smith CI, Islam TC, Mattsson PT, Mohamed AJ, Nore BF, Vihinen M. The Tec family of cytoplasmic tyrosine kinases: mammalian Btk, Bmx, Itk, Tec, Txk and homologs in other species. BioEssays News Rev Mol Cell Dev Biol. 2001:23:436–446.

[24] Ohta Y, Haire, RN, Litman RT Fu, SM Nelson, RP Kratz, J. Genomic organization and structure of Bruton agammaglobulinemia tyrosine kinase: localization of mutations associated with varied clinical presentations and course in X chromosome-linked agammaglobulinemia. Proc Natl Acad Sci U S A. 1994:91:9062–9066.

[25] Piirilä H, Väliaho J, Vihien M. Immunodeficiency mutation databases. Hum Mutat. 2006;27:1200–1208.

[26] Broides A, Yang W, Conley ME. Genotype/phenotype correlations in XLA. Clin Immunol. 2006;118:195–200

[27] Rohrer J, Minegishi Y, Richter D, Eguiguren J, Conley ME. Unusual mutations in Btk: an insertion, a duplication, an inversion, and four large deletions. Clin Immunol. 1999 Jan;90(1):28–37

[28] Väliaho, J, Smith, CI, Vihinen, M. BTKbase: the mutation database for X-linked agammaglobulinemia. Hum Mutat. 2006:27:1209–1217.

[29] Holinski-Feder, E, Weiss, M, Brandau, O, Jedele, KB, Nore B, Bäckesjö, CM. Mutation screening of the BTK gene in 56 families with X-linked agammaglobulinemia (XLA): 47 unique mutations without correlation to clinical course. Pediatrics. 1998:101:276–284.

[30] Granodos EL, de Diego RP, et al. A genotype/phenotype correlation study in a group of 54 patients with X-linked agammaglobulinemia. J Allergy Clin Immunol. 2005;116

[31] Chan KW, Chen T, Jiang L, et al. Identification of Bruton tyrosine kinase mutations in 12 Chinese patients with X-linked agammaglobulinemia by long PCR-direct sequencing. Int J Immunogenet. 2006;33:205–209.

[32] Kristutek D, Aspalter RM, et al. Characterization of novel Bruton's tyrosine kinase gene mutations in Central European patients with agammaglobulinemia. Mol Immunol. 2007;44:1639–1643.

[33] Wang Y, Kanegane H, Sanal Ö, Ersoy F, Tezcan T, Futatani T, Tsukada S, Miyawaki T. Bruton tyrosine kinase gene mutations in Turkish patients with presumed X-linked agammaglobulinemia. Hum Mutat. 2001Oct;18 (4):356.

[34] Aydogmus C, Camcloglu Y, van der Burg M, Cokugras H, Akçakaya N, vanDongen JJ. Bruton's tyrosine kinase gene mutations in Turkish patients with X-linked agammaglobulinemia from a single center: novel mutations in BTK gene. Turkiye Klinikleri J Med Sci. 2013;33(4):1042–1046

[35] Yel L, Minegishi Y, Coustan-Smith E, Buckley RH, Trübel H, Pachman LM, Kitchingman GR, Campana D, Rohrer J, ConleyME. Mutations in the mu heavy-chain gene in patients with agammaglobulinemia. N Engl J Med. 1996 Nov;14;335(20):1486–1493.

[36] Minegishi Y, Smith EC, Wang YH, Cooper MD, Campana D, Conley ME. Mutations in the human λ5/14.1 gene result in B cell deficiency and agammaglobulinemia. J Exp Med. 1998;187:71–77.

[37] Minegishi Y, Coustan-Smith E, Rapalus L, Ersoy F, Campana D, Conley ME. Mutations in Igα (CD79a) result in a complete block in B-cell development. J Clin Invest. 1999a;104:1115–1121.

[38] Minegishi Y, Rohrer J, Smith EC, Lederman HM, Pappu R, Campana D, Chan AC, Conley ME. An essential role for BLNK in human B cell development. Science. 1999b; 286:1954–1957.

[39] Dobbs AK, Yang T, Farmer D, Kager L, Parolini O, Conley ME. A hypomorphic mutation in Igbeta (CD79b) in a patient with immunodeficiency and a leaky defect in B cell development. J. Immunol. 2007;179:2055–2059.

[40] Conley ME, Dobbs AK, Quintana AM, Bosompem A, Wang YD, Coustan-Smith E, Smith AM, Perez EE, Murray PJ. Agammaglobulinemia and absent B lineage cells in a patient lacking the p85α subunit of PI3K. J Exp Med. 2012 Mar 12;209(3):463–470. doi:10.1084/jem.20112533. Epub 2012 Feb 20

[41] Wengler GS, Parolini O, Fiorini M, Mella P, Smith H, Ugazio AG, Notarangelo LD. A PCR-based non-radioactive X-chromosome inactivation assay for genetic counseling in X-linked primary immunodeficiencies. Life Sci. 1997;61(14):1405–1411.

[42] Allen RC, Nachtman RG, Rosenblatt HM, Belmont JW. Application of carrier testing to genetic counseling for X-linked agammaglobulinemia. Am J Hum Genet. 1994 Jan; 54(1):25–35.

[43] Lau YL, Levinsky RJ, Malcolm S, Goodship J, Winter R, Pembrey M. Genetic prediction in X-linked agammaglobulinaemia. Am J Med Genet. 1988 Oct;31(2):437–448.

[44] Conley ME. B cells in patients with X-linked agammaglobulinemia. J Immunol. 1985:134:3070–3074

[45] Conley ME. Early defects in B cell development. Curr Opin Allergy Clin Immunol. 2002 Dec;2(6):517–522.

[46] Pieper K, Grimbacher B, Eibel H. B-cell biology and development. J Allergy Clin Immunol. 2013 Apr;131(4):959–971.

[47] Conley ME, Howard VC. In: Pagon RA, Adam MP, Ardinger HH, Wallace SE, Amemiya A, Bean LJH, Bird TD, Dolan CR, Fong CT, Smith RJH, Stephens K, editors. GeneReviews® [Internet]. Seattle (WA): University of Washington, Seattle; 1993–2015. 2001 Apr 05 [updated 2011 Nov 17].

[48] Slatter MA, Gennery AR Clinical immunology review series: an approach to the patient with recurrent infections in childhood. Clin Exp Immunol. 2008 Jun;152(3):389–396.

[49] Casanova JL, Abel L. Primary immunodeficiencies: a field in its infancy. Science. 2007 Aug 3;317(5838):617–619.

[50] deVries E, Driessen G. Educational paper: primary immunodeficiencies in children: a diagnostic challenge. Eur J Pediatr. 2011 Feb;170(2):169–177.

[51] Conley ME, Howard V. Clinical findings leading to the diagnosis of X-linked agammaglobulinemia. J Pediatr. 2002 Oct;141(4):566–571.

[52] Lederman, HM, Winkelstein, JA (1985) X-linked agammaglobulinemia: an analysis of 96 patients. Medicine (Baltimore) 1985;64:145–156.

[53] Winkelstein, JA, Marino, MC, Lederman, HM, Jones, SM, Sullivan, K, Burks, AW. X-linked agammaglobulinemia: report on a United States registry of 201 patients. Medicine (Baltimore). 2006;85:193–202.

[54] Moin M, Aghamohammadi A, Farhoudi A, Pourpak Z, Rezaei N, Movahedi M, Gharagozlou M, Ghazi BM, Zahed A, Abolmaali K, Mahmoudi M, Emami L, Bashashati M. X-linked agammaglobulinemia: a survey of 33 Iranian patients. Immunol Invest. 2004 Feb;33(1):81–93.

[55] Trakultivakorn M, Ochs HD. X-linked agammaglobulinemia in northern Thailand. Asian Pac J Allergy Immunol. 2006 Mar;24(1):57–63.

[56] Aghamohammadi A, Allahverdi A, Abolhassani H, Moazzami K, Alizadeh H, Gharagozlou M, Kalantari N, Sajedi V, Shafiei A, Parvaneh N, Mohammadpour M, Karimi N, Sadaghiani MS, RezaeiN. Comparison of pulmonary diseases in common variable immunodeficiency and X-linked agammaglobulinaemia. Respirology. 2010 Feb;15(2): 289–295.

[57] Dittrich AM, Schulze I, et al. X-linked agammaglobulinemia and *Pneumocystis carinii pneumonia*—an unusal co-incidence? Eur J Pediatr. 2003;162(6):432–433.

[58] Roifman CM, Rao CP, Lederman HM, Lavi S, Quinn P, Gelfand EW. Increased susceptibility to Mycoplasma infection in patients with hypogammaglobulinemia. Am J Med. 1986;80(4):590–594.

[59] Webster D, Windsor H, Ling C, Windsor D, Pitcher D. Chronic bronchitis in immunocompromised patients: association with a novel Mycoplasma species. Eur J Clin Microbiol Infect Dis. 2003;22(9):530–534.

[60] McKinney RE Jr, Katz SL, Wilfert CM. Chronic enteroviral meningoencephalitis in agammaglobulinemic patients. Rev Infect Dis. 1987;9:334–356.

[61] Quartier P, Foray S, Casanova JL, et al. Enteroviral meningoencephalitis in XLA: intensive immunoglobulin therapy and sequential viral detection in cerebrospinal fluid by polymerase chain reaction. Pediatr Infect Dis J. 2000;19(11):1106–1108.

[62] Misbah SA, Spickett GP, Ryba PC, Hockaday JM, Kroll JS, Sherwood C, Kurtz JB, Moxon ER, Chapel HM. Chronic enteroviral meningoencephalitis in agammaglobulinemia: case report and literature review. J Clin Immunol. 1992 Jul;12(4):266–270.

[63] Agarwal S, Mayer L. Diagnosis and treatment of gastrointestinal disorders in patients with primary immunodeficiency. Clin Gastroenterol Hepatol. 2013 Sep;11(9): 1050–1063.

[64] Staines Boone AT, Torres Martínez MG, López Herrera G, de LeijaPortilla JO, Espinosa Padilla SE, Espinosa Rosales FJ, Lugo Reyes SO. Gastric adenocarcinoma in the context of X-linked agammaglobulinemia: case report and review of the literature. J Clin Immunol. 2014 Feb;34(2):134–137.

[65] Maarschalk-Ellerbroek LJ, Oldenburg B, Mombers IM, Hoepelman AI, Brosens LA, Offerhaus GJ, Ellerbroek PM. Outcome of screening endoscopy in common variable immunodeficiency disorder and X-linked agammaglobulinemia. Endoscopy. 2013;45(4):320–323.

[66] Washington K, Stenzel TT, Buckley RH, Gottfried MR. Gastrointestinal pathology in patients with common variable immunodeficiency and X-linked agammaglobulinemia. Am J Surg Pathol. 1996 Oct;20(10):1240–1252

[67] Hernandez-Trujillo VP, Scalchunes C, Cunningham-Rundles C, Ochs HD, Bonilla FA, Paris K, Yel L, Sullivan KE. Autoimmunity and inflammation in X-linked agammaglobulinemia. J Clin Immunol. 2014 Aug;34(6):627–632.

[68] Behniafard N, Aghamohammadi A, Abolhassani H, Pourjabbar S, Sabouni F, Rezaei N. Autoimmunity in X-linked agammaglobulinemia: Kawasaki disease and review of the literature. Expert Rev Clin Immunol. 2012 Feb;8(2):155–159.

[69] Machado P, Santos A, Faria E, Silva J, Malcata A, Chieira C. Arthritis and X-linked agammaglobulinemia. Acta Reumatol Port. 2008 Oct–Dec;33(4):464–467.

[70] Verbruggen G, De Backer S, Deforce D, Dewetter P, Cuvelier C, Veys E, Elewaut D. X-linked agammaglobulinaemia and rheumatoid arthritis. Ann Rheum Dis. 2005;64:1075–1078.

[71] Stewart DM, Notarangelo LD, Kurman CC, Staudt LM, Nelson DL. Molecular genetic analysis of X-linked hypogammaglobulinemia and isolated growth hormone deficiency. J Immunol. 1995 Sep 1;155(5):2770–2774.

[72] Hoshino A, Okuno Y, Migita M, Ban H, Yang X, Kiyokawa N, Adachi Y, Kojima S, Ohara O, Kanegane H. X-linked agammaglobulinemia associated with B-precursor acute lymphoblastic leukemia. J Clin Immunol. 2015 Feb;35(2):108–111. doi:10.1007/s10875-015-0127-7. PMID :25591849.

[73] Conley ME. Are patients with X-linked agammaglobulinemia at increased risk of developing acute lymphoblastic leukemia? J Clin Immunol. 2015 Feb;35(2):98–99.

[74] Hidalgo S, Garcia Erro M, Cisterna D, Freire MC. Paralytic poliomyelitis caused by a vaccine-derived polio virus in an antibody deficient Argentinean child. Pediatr Infect Dis J. 2003;22(6):570–572.

[75] Fiore L, Plebani A, et al. Search for poliovirus long-term excretors among patients affected by agammaglobulinemia. Clin Immunol. 2004;111:98–102.

[76] deVries E, Noordzij JG, Kuijpers TW, van Dongen JJ. Flow cytometric immunophenotyping in the diagnosis and follow-up of immunodeficient children. Eur J Pediatr. 2001 Oct;160(10):583–591.

[77] Bousfiha AA, Jeddane L, Ailal F, Al Herz W, Conley ME, Cunningham-Rundles C, Etzioni A, Fischer A, Franco JL, Geha RS, Hammarström L, Nonoyama S, Ochs HD, Roifman CM, Seger R, Tang ML, Puck JM, Chapel H, Notarangelo LD, Casanova JL. A phenotypic approach for IUIS PID classification and diagnosis: guidelines for clinicians at the bedside. J Clin Immunol. 2013 Aug;33(6):1078–1087

[78] deVries E. Patient-centred screening for primary immunodeficiency, a multi-stage diagnostic protocol designed for non-immunologists: 2011update. European Society for Immunodeficiencies (ESID) members. Clin Exp Immunol. 2012 Jan;167(1):108–119.

[79] Al-Herz W, Bousfiha A, Casanova JL, Chatila T, Conley ME, Cunningham-Rundles C, Etzioni A, Franco JL, Gaspar HB, Holland SM, Klein C, Nonoyama S, Ochs HD, Oksenhendler E, Picard C, Puck JM, Sullivan K, Tang ML. Primary immunodeficiency diseases: an update on the classification from the international union of immunological societies expert committee for primary immunodeficiency. Front Immunol. 2014 Apr 22;5:162.

[80] RodrÃquez PF, Garcia Rodriguez MC, et al. Neutropenia as early manifestation of XLA: Report on 4 patients. An Esp Pediatr. 1999;51(3):235–240.

[81] Rezaei N, Farhoudi A, Pourpak Z, etal. Neutropenia in patients with primary antibody deficiency disorders. Iran J Allergy Asthma Immunol. 2004;3(2):77–81.

[82] Folds JD, Schmitz JL. Clinical and laboratory assessment of immunity. J Allergy Clin Immunol. 2003 Feb;111(2 Suppl):S702–S711.

[83] Orange JS, Ballow M, Stiehm ER, Ballas ZK, Chinen J, De La Morena M, Kumararatne D, Harville TO, Hesterberg P, Koleilat M, McGhee S, Perez EE, Raasch J, Scherzer R, Schroeder H, Seroogy C, Huissoon A, Sorensen RU, Katial R. Use and interpretation of diagnostic vaccination in primary immunodeficiency: a working group report of the Basic and Clinical Immunology Interest Section of the American Academy of Allergy, Asthma & Immunology. J Allergy Clin Immunol. 2012 Sep; 130(3 Suppl):S1–S24.

[84] Gaspar HB, Lester T, Levinsky RJ, Kinnon C. Bruton's tyrosine kinase expression and activity in X-linked agammaglobulinemia (XLA): the use of protein analysis as a diagnostic indicator of XLA. Clin Exp Immunol. 1998;111:334–338.

[85] Futatani T, Miyawaki T, Tsukada S, et al. Deficient expression of Bruton's tyrosine kinase in monocytes from X-linked agammaglobulinemia as evaluated by a flow cytometric analysis and its clinical application to carrier detection. Blood. 1998;91:595–602.

[86] Conley ME, Notarangelo LD, EtzioniA. Diagnostic criteria for primary immunodeficiencies. Representing PAGID (Pan-American Group for Immunodeficiency) and ESID (European Society for Immunodeficiencies). Clin Immunol. 1999 Dec;93(3):190–197.

[87] Borte S, von Döbeln U, Hammarström L. Guidelines for newborn screening of primary immunodeficiency diseases. Curr Opin Hematol. 2013 Jan;20(1):48–54.

[88] Sweinberg SK[1], Wodell RA, Grodofsky MP, Greene JM, Conley ME. Retrospective analysis of the incidence of pulmonary disease in hypogammaglobulinemia. J Allergy Clin Immunol. 1991 Jul;88(1):96–104.

[89] Camcioglu Y. Immunoglobulin treatment of immunodeficient patients. In: Metodiev K, editor. Immunodeficiency, Croatia, InTech; 2012:89–112.

[90] Shapiro RS, Borte M. 7th International Immunoglobulin Conference: Immunoglobulin in clinical practice. Clin Exp Immunol. 2014 Dec;178Suppl 1:65–66.

[91] Cunningham-Rundles C. Key aspects for successful immunoglobulin therapy of primary immunodeficiencies. Clin Exp Immunol. 2011 Jun;164Suppl 2:16–19.

[92] Ballow M. Optimizing immunoglobulin treatment for patients with primary immunodeficiency disease to prevent pneumonia and infection incidence: review of the current data. Ann Allergy Asthma Immunol. 2013 Dec;111(6 Suppl):S2–S5.

[93] Hoernes M, Seger R, Reichenbach J. Modern management of primary B-cell immunodeficiencies. Pediatr Allergy Immunol. 2011 Dec;22(8):758–769

[94] Quinti I, Pierdominici M, et al. European surveillance of immunoglobulin safety—results of initial survey of 1243 patients with primary immunodeficiencies in 16 countries. Clin Immunol. 2002;104:231–236.

[95] Plebani A, Soresina A, Rondelli R, Amato GM, Azzari C, Cardinale F, Cazzola G, Consolini R, De Mattia D, Dell'Erba G, Duse M, Fiorini M, Martino S, Martire B, Masi M, Monafo V, Moschese V, Notarangelo LD, Orlandi P, Panei P, Pession A, Pietrogrande MC, Pignata C, Quinti I, Ragno V, Rossi P, Sciotto A, Stabile A; Italian Pediatric Group for XLA-AIEOP. Clinical, immunological, and molecular analysis in a large cohort of patients with X-linked agammaglobulinemia: an Italian multicenter study. Clin Immunol. 2002 Sep;104(3):221–230.

[96] Quinti I, Soresina A, Guerra A, Rondelli R, Spadaro G, Agostini C, Milito C, Trombetta AC, Visentini M, Martini H, Plebani A, Fiorilli M; IPINet Investigators. Effectiveness of immunoglobulin replacement therapy on clinical outcome in patients with primary antibody deficiencies: results from a multicenter prospective cohort study. J Clin Immunol. 2011 Jun;31(3):315–322.

[97] Palabrica FR, Kwong SL, Padua FR. Adverse events of intravenous immunoglobulin infusions: a ten-year retrospective study. Asia Pac Allergy. 2013 Oct;3(4):249–256.

[98] Howard V, Greene JM, Pahwa S, Winkelstein JA, Boyle JM, Kocak M, Conley ME. The health status and quality of life of adults with X-linked agammaglobulinemia. Clin Immunol. 2006 Feb–Mar;118(2–3):201–208.

[99] Šedivá A, Chapel H, Gardulf A; Europe immunoglobulin map. European Immunoglobulin Map Group (35 European countries) for European Society for Immunodeficiencies (ESID) Primary Immunodeficiencies Care in Development Working Party. Clin Exp Immunol. 2014 Dec;178:Suppl 1:141–143. PMID12763478.

[100] Howard V, Myers LA, Williams DA, Wheeler G, Turner EV, Cunningham JM, Conley ME. Stem cell transplants for patients with X-linked agammaglobulinemia. Clin Immunol. 2003 May;107(2):98–102

[101] Medical Advisory Committee of the Immune Deficiency Foundation, Shearer WT, Fleisher TA, Buckley RH, Ballas Z, Ballow M, Blaese RM, Bonilla FA, Conley ME, Cunningham-Rundles C, Filipovich AH, Fuleihan R, Gelfand EW, Hernandez-Trujillo V, Holland SM, Hong R, Lederman HM, Malech HL, Miles S, Notarangelo LD, Ochs HD, Orange JS, Puck JM, Routes JM, Stiehm ER, Sullivan K, Torgerson T, Winkelstein J. Recommendations for live viral and bacterial vaccines in immunodeficient patients and their close contacts. J Allergy Clin Immunol. 2014 Apr;133(4):961–966.

[102] Principi N, Esposito S. Vaccine use in primary immunodeficiency disorders. Vaccine. 2014 Jun 24;32(30):3725–3731.

[103] Gonzalo-Garijo MA, Sánchez-Vega S, Pérez-Calderón R, Pérez-Rangel I, Corrales-Vargas S, Fernández de Mera JJ, Robles R. Renal amyloidosis in a patient with X-

linked agammaglobulinemia (Bruton's disease) and bronchiectasis. J Clin Immunol. 2014 Jan;34(1):119–122.

[104] Abolhassani H, Hirbod-Mobarakeh A, Shahinpour S, Panahi M, Mohammadinejad P, Mirminachi B, Shakari MS, Samavat B, Aghamohammadi A· Mortality and morbidity in patients with X-linked agammaglobulinaemia. Allergol Immunopathol (Madr). 2015 Jan–Feb;43(1):62–66.

Section 3

Research Data

Chapter 11

Multicentric Castleman's Disease

Moosa Patel, Vinitha Philip, Atul Lakha, Sugeshnee Pather, Muhammed Faadil Waja, Lucille Singh and Mohamed Arbee

Additional information is available at the end of the chapter

http://dx.doi.org/10.5772/61709

Abstract

Castleman's disease (CD) is a lymphoproliferative disorder, manifesting clinically as unicentric or multicentric disease and pathologically as hyaline vascular, plasma cell or mixed variants.

Multicentric Castleman's disease (MCD) is the most common form of CD encountered at Chris Hani Baragwanath Academic Hospital (CHBAH). From being a rare disease, MCD has increased in the last five years, primarily as a result of the association of human immunodeficiency virus (HIV), being highly prevalent in our patient population. The dominant clinical manifestations of the disease include constitutional symptoms, fever, anaemia, lymphadenopathy and hepatosplenomegaly.

We present a series of 35 adult patients with MCD, who were seen over a 25-year period at CHBAH, and highlight the similarities and differences compared with other published series.

Based on our local experience, we observed that the prognosis of HIV-associated MCD has improved with optimization and control of HIV replication (use of combination antiretroviral therapy), prophylaxis and treatment of opportunistic infections, as well as etoposide and rituximab based chemotherapy.

In the setting of HIV, MCD should no longer be regarded as a rare disease with a fatal outcome.

Keywords: Multicentric Castleman's disease, Human immunodeficiency virus infection, Human herpes virus-8, South Africa, immunosuppression

1. Introduction

Castleman's disease (CD), also known as angiofollicular or giant lymph node hyperplasia, is a rare B-cell lymphoproliferative disorder, first described by Benjamin Castleman in a series of patients in 1956 [1]. It is a heterogeneous disorder, manifesting clinically as a unicentric (solitary; localised) or multicentric disease and pathologically as hyaline vascular, plasma cell or mixed variants [2–6].

The multicentric variety is aetiologically linked to human herpes virus-8 (HHV-8) [7]. It is strongly associated with immunosuppression and is now being encountered with increasing frequency in patients with HIV (human immunodeficiency virus) infection [8].

This review will focus on CD, with particular reference to Multicentric Castleman's disease (MCD), and it will include a description of the disease as seen at Chris Hani Baragwanath Academic Hospital (CHBAH), Johannesburg, South Africa over a 25-year period (1990 to 2014). The renewed interest in MCD stems from its association with HIV, particularly in areas such as sub-Saharan Africa where HIV has reached pandemic proportions, with South Africa being home to approximately 6.4 million people living with HIV/AIDS (acquired immunodeficiency syndrome) [9].

2. Epidemiology

Castleman's disease (CD), from being rare, is now more commonly encountered. In the last three decades since the discovery of HIV, the incidence of MCD has progressively increased over time. The median age at presentation of MCD is 40 (21–67) years, with a male predominance of 90%, based on a systematic review of published cases in the literature up to 2007 [10]. A younger age at presentation is noted in HIV-seropositive individuals with MCD compared to HIV-seronegative MCD [11,12].

3. Pathology

Two distinct variants have been described in CD: the hyaline vascular and plasma cell variant. Where features of both these varieties occur, it is referred to as the mixed type or variant [2,5].

The hyaline vascular variant is characterised by follicles which show prominent vascular proliferation and hyalinization of the central portion. There is concentric layering of the lymphocytes at the periphery of the follicles (mantle zone) – referred to as 'target follicles' and imparting a classical 'onion-skin' appearance (see Figure 1). Another feature of this variety is the presence of prominent sclerotic blood vessels which penetrate radially into the germinal centres and transfix it, resulting in a 'lollypop' follicle appearance (see Figure 2). The interfollicular stroma is also prominent, with numerous hyperplastic vessels, plasma cells, eosinophils, and immunoblasts. The hyaline vascular variety is most commonly associated with UCD [2,6].

The plasma cell variant is characterised by a diffuse interfollicular plasma cell proliferation. Intermingled with the plasma cells are immunoblasts, lymphocytes, and histiocytes. Features of the hyaline vascular variant are typically inconspicuous or absent. This variety is most commonly associated with MCD [2,5,6]. The histopathological characteristic of MCD is the presence of large, abnormal plasmablasts located within the mantle zones of involved lymph nodes [13,14].

The mixed variant or type of CD shares morphological features between the hyaline vascular variant and plasma cell variant. It is classically encountered in MCD and is typically seen in HIV-associated MCD [4,5].

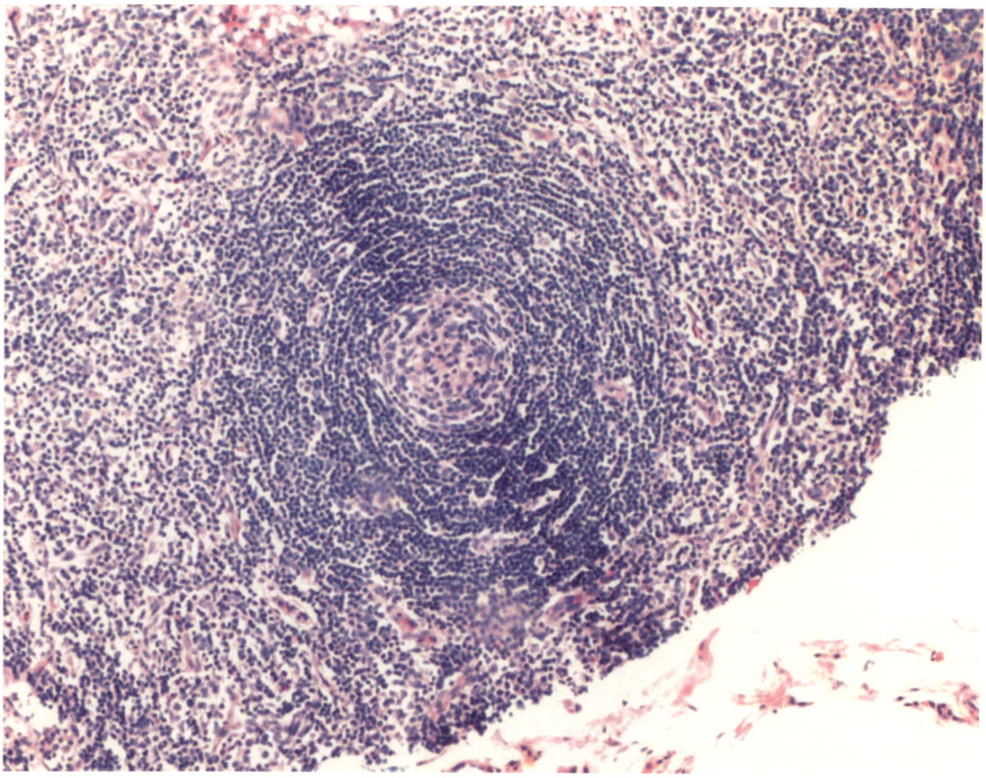

Figure 1. Haematoxylin and Eosin stained section of lymph node (100× magnification) showing the concentric layering of lymphocytes in the mantle zone of the lymphoid follicle – 'onion-ring' appearance

The pathogenesis of CD involves an interplay between viruses, namely HHV-8 and HIV, cytokines such as IL-6 (interleukin-6) and IL-10, and growth factors such as VEGF (vascular endothelial growth factor) [15,16].

Multicentric Castleman's disease (MCD) is aetiologically linked to HHV-8 [7]. Human Herpesvirus 8 is a gamma herpes virus and the causative organism in KS [17]. Soulier et al, 1995 [7], showed that HHV-8 sequences were detected in lymph nodes in 14/14 (100%) cases of HIV-associated MCD, compared to 7/17 (41%) cases with HIV-negative MCD. Other studies have demonstrated an almost universal association of HHV-8 with HIV-associated MCD [11,18].

Interleukin-6 levels are increased in CD. A raised CRP, a surrogate marker for IL-6, anaemia, hypergammaglobulinemia, plasmacytosis, splenomegaly, and lymphadenopathy are all

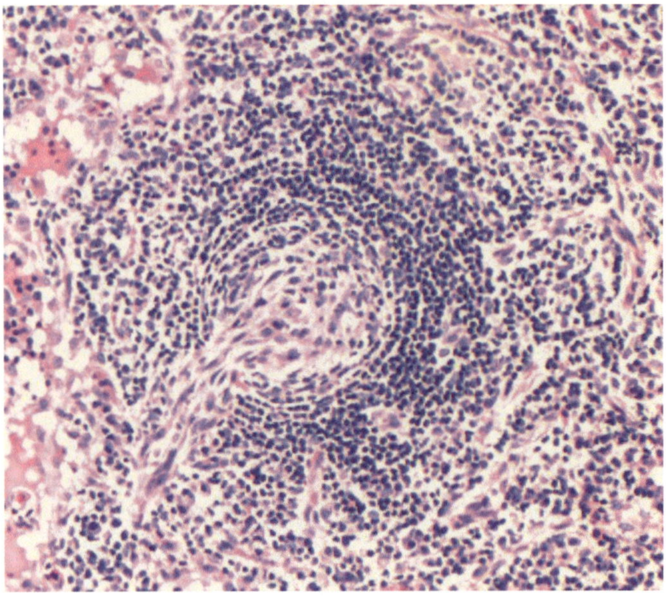

Figure 2. Haematoxylin and Eosin stained section of lymph node (200× magnification) showing the radially penetrating blood vessels transfixing the germinal centre – 'lollipop' appearance

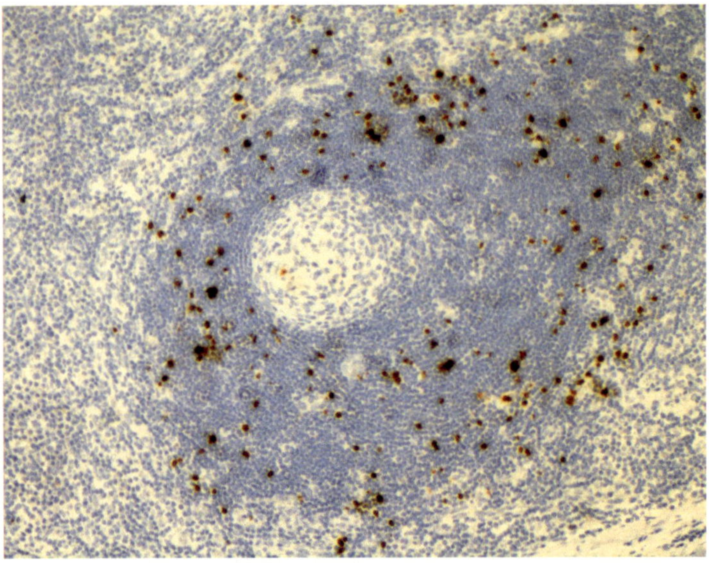

Figure 3. Human Herpesvirus-8 immunohistochemical stain showing mantle zone concentricity and distinct HHV-8 positive nuclear staining of lymphoid cells in the mantle zone (100× magnification)

associated with elevated levels of IL-6 [15,16]. Increased VEGF expression is also noted in CD and is likely to be responsible for the increased angiogenesis component of the disease [19].

The diagnosis of CD is based on a combination of compatible clinical features together with distinct histopathological features characteristic of the disease. Importantly, other benign and malignant disorders with overlapping clinical and histological features should be excluded. Recently, diagnostic criteria have been proposed for patients with MCD, particularly in association with HIV [20,21]. These include the French ANRS (Agence Nationale de Recherchesurle SIDA) criteria and the National Cancer Institute (NCI) criteria [20,21]. The diagnostic criteria devised by these two groups complement the histopathological findings and are particularly useful in those with idiopathic MCD. However, in HIV and HHV-8 associated MCD, the histopathological diagnosis has been made much easier due to the presence of DNA tests to detect HHV-8 in the blood and HHV-8 immunostaining of the tissue. Thus, Bower et al, 2014 [22], suggest that in these individuals a triad of 'B' symptoms, elevated plasma HHV-8 levels and histopathological findings should suffice in making the diagnosis of MCD.

4. Clinical features and management

Two distinct clinical variants of Castleman's disease are recognised: MCD and UCD. Unicentric Castleman's disease (UCD) refers to localized disease, presenting at a single site, such as the chest (most commonly the mediastinum), neck, abdomen, or other sites. Typically patients are asymptomatic and come to clinical attention when an enlarged lymph node is noted on physical examination or at imaging studies [1,2, 23].

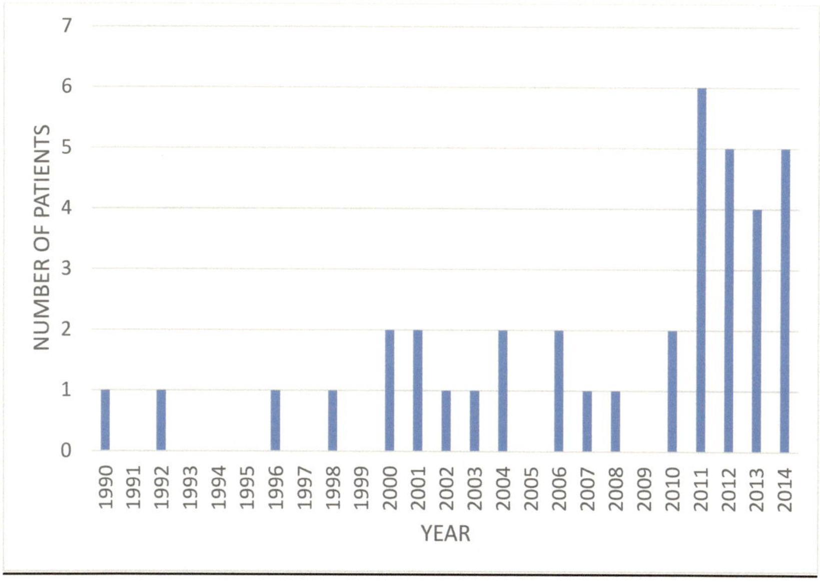

Figure 4. Bar graph which depicts the number of patients seen with Castleman's disease at Chris Hani Baragwanath Academic Hospital from 1990 to 2014

Multicentric Castleman's disease (MCD) refers to a systemic disease with constitutional symptoms (fever, night sweats, weight loss), generalized lymphadenopathy and hepatosplenomegaly. It is usually associated pathologically with the plasma cell or mixed variant. Unlike UCD, MCD is strongly associated with HIV, immunosuppression and HHV-8 [11,23,24]. Laboratory studies usually reveal the presence of anaemia, a raised ESR, elevated CRP, thrombocytopenia, hypoalbuminemia and polyclonal hypergammaglobulinemia [3, 4,11,15].

At Chris Hani Baragwanath Academic Hospital (CHBAH), Soweto, Johannesburg, a total of 38 patients were seen with CD over a 25-year period. Three of the patients (7.9%) were diagnosed with UCD and 35 (92.1%) with MCD. Of all the patients with CD, 22/38 (57.9%) were seen in the last 5 years compared to 42.1% in the first 20 years. The increase in the number of patients with CD in the last 5 years is primarily as the result of the ongoing HIV pandemic in South Africa and the contribution from HIV. Ninety five percent (21/22) of the patients seen in the last five years and 100% of those with MCD were HIV seropositive.

	Age	Gender	Site of lymphadenopathy	Localised or systemic disease	Anaemia (A) or thrombocytopenia (T)	Treatment	HIV	Response	Outcome
1	18	M	Mediastinum	Localised	No A or T	Surgical resection	Negative	Complete response	Alive
2	64	F	Inguino-femoral	Localised	No A or T	Surgical resection	Negative	Complete response	Alive
3	59	F	Axilla	Localised	No A or T	Surgical resection	Negative	Complete response	Alive

Table 1. Clinical characteristics of Unicentric Castleman's disease

With regard to UCD, there were 2 females and 1 male, with a female to male ratio of 2:1. The mean age at presentation was 47 years. All the patients were diagnosed post biopsy/resection of localised nodal disease. None of the patients were HIV seropositive. No further treatment was required in these patients after the initial surgical resection. All the patients are alive and are well on observation (see Table 1).

A summary of the clinical characteristics of the patients with MCD is depicted in Table 2.

Characteristic	Result/Finding
Number of patients	35
Median age; Mean age; Range	Median = 36 years; Mean = 37years; Range = 18–64 years
Gender; ratio	Males = 19, Females = 16; M:F ratio – 1.2:1
Multicentric disease	35/35 = 100%

http://dx.doi.org/10.5772/61709

Characteristic	Result/Finding
Fever	16/35 = 46%
'B' symptoms	23/35 = 66%
Lymphadenopathy	35/35 = 100%
Hepatomegaly	18/35 = 51%
Splenomegaly	20/35 = 57%
Anaemia (Hb<12 g/dl)	32/35 = 91%; Mean Hb = 7.8g/dl; Range = 2.8 – 13.5 g/dl
Thrombocytopenia (Platelets <100 × 10^9/l)	9/35 = 26%; Mean platelet count = 211 x 10^9/l; Range = 22 – 602 × 10^9/l
HIV status (positive or negative)	30/35 = 86% positive; 5/35 = 14% negative
CD4 count × 10^6/l – mean and range; <350 × 10^6/l; <200 x 10^6/l	Mean CD4 count = 257 × 10^6/l; Range = 12 – 829 × 10^6/l; <350 × 10^6/l = 79%; <200 × 10^6/l = 46%
Morphology: i) Hyaline vascular (HV); ii) Plasma cell (PC); Mixed (M)	HV only = 1/35 (3%); PC only = 1/35 (3%); Mixed = 34/35 (94%)
HHV-8 immunostain on biopsy	Early part of the current series – not done. In the patients from 2010–2014, performed in 19/21 patients with MCD. The result was positive in 19/19 patients = 100%
Associations	Tuberculosis 15/35 = 43%; Kaposi's sarcoma 8/35 = 23%; Autoimmune haemolytic anaemia 6/35 = 17%; Pure red cell aplasia 2/35 = 6% and 1/35 = 3% with each of the following – primary effusion lymphoma, microlymphoma, adenocarcinoma, bullous pemphigoid, immune thrombocytopenia, hepatitis B, hepatitis C, hypoglycaemia and nephrotic syndrome
Response to treatment (evaluable patients – CR = complete response; PR = partial response)	17/35 evaluable patients; CR 9/17 = 53%; PR = 47%
Outcome: Alive; Died (mean survival, range); Lost to follow up (LTFU)	Alive 14/35 = 40%; Died = 34% (mean survival = 13 months, range 0.25 – 64 months); LTFU = 26%

Table 2. Summary of the clinical characteristics of Multicentric Castleman's disease

5. Associations

Castleman's disease may be seen in association with other diseases including POEMS syndrome (polyneuropathy, organomegaly, endocrinopathy, monoclonal protein/gammopathy, and skin changes/sclerotic bone lesions), paraneoplastic pemphigus, Kaposi's sarcoma, Hodgkin lymphoma, Non Hodgkin lymphoma (in particular, primary effusion lymphoma (PEL), and diffuse large B-cell lymphoma -DLBCL) [2,11, 22, 25,26,27].

6. Management

Treatment modalities for CD include supportive care and specific modalities of treatment.

In the unicentric form of the disease, surgical resection of the localised site of the disease is usually curative. However, follow up is recommended as patients may rarely relapse or develop complications (such as an increased risk of lymphoma development) [23,26,28].

For MCD, a variety of specific treatment options are available, in addition to supportive care (such as analgesia, allopurinol, transfusion of blood and blood products where indicated). Specific treatment modalities include antiviral (anti-herpesvirus) and antiretroviral drugs where a viral association is documented, corticosteroids, monoclonal antibodies, immunomodulatory agents (such as thalidomide), splenectomy, and radiotherapy [29].

Chemotherapy has evolved from single-agent (e.g. chlorambucil) to combination chemotherapy (cyclophosphamide, doxorubicin, vincristine, prednisone – CHOP), to the addition of rituximab and etoposide [3,11,20,29,30,31]. Bower, 2010 [29], in his excellent review on 'How I treat HIV-associated multicentric Castleman disease', uses a combination of weekly IVI rituximab (375 mg/m^2) with IVI etoposide (100 mg/m^2) for 4 weeks for aggressive HIV-associated MCD, with an overall 2 year survival of 85% and rituximab monotherapy (375 mg/m^2 weekly for 4 weeks) for low-risk HIV-associated MCD, with an overall 2 year survival of 100% [29].

For HIV-negative, HHV-8 negative MCD, other therapeutic options have been explored. This includes monoclonal antibodies directed against IL-6 (siltuximab) or the IL-6 receptor (tocilizumab) [27].

Multicentric Castleman's disease (MCD) is increasingly being recognised as a relapsing and remitting disease and in the HIV-seropositive setting is not necessarily suppressed or diminished by combination antiretroviral therapy [29]. As such, the role of both rituximab and antiherpesvirus agents such as valganciclovir have been explored as maintenance therapies [20,29,32,33]. However, the role of maintenance therapy in this disease remains controversial and requires further evaluation.

7. Discussion

Human immunodeficiency virus infection (HIV) is endemic in South Africa and is associated with an increased risk of infection and malignancy, primarily as a consequence of immunodeficiency [9]. The major impact of HIV on the haematological malignancies in South Africa has been in regards to an increased prevalence of Non-Hodgkin lymphoma and, more recently, Hodgkin lymphoma [34,35].

In South Africa, CD is rare. However, there has been a noticeable increase in MCD in the last five years, with more than doubling of the number of patients in the last five years, compared to the previous twenty years (see Figure 4). This is attributable to the ongoing burden of HIV, as the majority of patients in this series with MCD are HIV seropositive (86%).

There were 35 adult patients diagnosed with MCD over a 25-year period at CHBAH, a large, tertiary, public sector, University of the Witwatersrand linked hospital, located in Soweto, Johannesburg. The median age at presentation was 36 years (18–64 years), with a male to female ratio of 1.2:1. The age is similar to that described in the literature. However, in our series, there is no marked male predominance, as the major risk factor in our patients for acquisition of HIV is heterosexual contact as compared to intravenous drug use or homosexuality.

The clinical presentation of MCD is similar to that described in the literature (see Table 2). Fever, 'B' symptoms, lymphadenopathy, hepatosplenomegaly, and anaemia are commonly encountered. Pathologically, the mixed variant is seen in 94% of the patients. The mean CD4 count in the HIV seropositive patients (86%) was $257 \times 10^6/l$, with 46% of the patients having a CD4 count of $< 200 \times 10^6/l$. Fifty three percent of the patients had newly diagnosed HIV (at the time of the diagnosis of MCD) and 47% were known to be seropositive (86% of the positive patients were on combination antiretroviral therapy). Concomitant Kaposi's sarcoma was diagnosed in 23% of patients. The HHV-8 immunostain performed on 19/21 patients with MCD in the last five years was positive in 100% of the patients (see Figure 3). Other associations are detailed in Table 2, most of these are related to coexistent HIV or HHV-8. Of note is the high prevalence of concomitant tuberculosis (43%).

A variety of treatments were used over the past twenty years, ranging from symptomatic/ supportive treatment to corticosteroids, single agent chemotherapy, combination chemotherapy (such as CHOP and more recently the addition of etoposide to CHOP → CHOEP), rituximab together with CHOP or CHOEP, radiotherapy, and splenectomy. Of the evaluable patients, 53% achieved a complete response to treatment and 47% manifested a partial response to treatment. As our patients have more aggressive and advanced disease, the etoposide and rituximab combinations are now being favoured. All the HIV seropositive patients receive concomitant combination antiretroviral therapy.

Long term follow up is necessary to exclude relapse and complications of the disease, such as the development of large cell lymphoma, which has a 15-fold increased incidence in patients with HIV-associated MCD [36].

8. Conclusion

Multicentric Castleman's disease is the most common form of CD encountered in our patients at CHBAH. From being a rare disease, MCD has increased over the past few years, primarily as a result of the association of HIV, being highly seroprevalent in our patient population. The dominant clinical manifestation of MCD is lymphadenopathy. Therefore, the cause of significant lymphadenopathy should always be defined, particularly in the setting of HIV. Most of the patients were initially suspected of having a lymphoma, while others with HIV and Kaposi's sarcoma or autoimmune haemolytic anaemia had a lymph node biopsy to define the possible cause of the lymphadenopathy in association with the KS or AIHA. The prognosis of HIV-associated MCD has improved with optimization and control of HIV replication (use of combination antiretroviral therapy), prophylaxis, and treatment of opportunistic infections, as well as etoposide and rituximab based chemotherapy. In the setting of HIV, MCD should no longer be regarded as a rare disease with a fatal outcome.

Acknowledgements

We thank all the medical, nursing and allied healthcare professionals who were involved in the diagnosis, management and follow up of the patients with Castleman's disease. In particular, we would like to thank all the staff of the Clinical Haematology unit, Infectious Disease unit, Department of Medicine and National Health Laboratory Service, CHBAH, and, most importantly, the patients whose data have been used in this study.

Author details

Moosa Patel[1*], Vinitha Philip[1], Atul Lakha[1], Sugeshnee Pather[2], Muhammed Faadil Waja[1], Lucille Singh[1] and Mohamed Arbee[1]

*Address all correspondence to: moosa.patel@wits.ac.za

1 Clinical Haematology Division, Department of Medicine, Chris Hani Baragwanath Academic Hospital and Faculty of Health Sciences, University of the Witwatersrand, Johannesburg, South Africa

2 Department of Anatomical Pathology, National Health Laboratory Service, Chris Hani Baragwanath Academic Hospital and Faculty of Health Sciences, University of the Witwatersrand, Johannesburg, South Africa

References

[1] Castleman B, Iverson L, Menendez V. Localized mediastinal lymph node hyperplasia resembling thymoma. *Cancer* 1956;9(4):822–30, 1956.

[2] Keller AR, Hochholzer L, Castleman B. Hyaline-vascular and plasma-cell types of giant lymph node hyperplasia of the mediastinum and other locations. Cancer 1972;29:670–683.

[3] Oksenhendler E, Duarte M, Soulier J, et al. Multicentric Castleman's disease in HIV infection: a clinical and pathological study of 20 patients. AIDS 1996;10(1):61–7.e.

[4] Weisenburger DD, Nathwani BN, Winberg CD, et al. Multicentric angiofollicular lymph node hyperplasia: A clinicopathological study of 16 cases. Human Path 1985;16:62.

[5] Gaba AR, Stein RS, Sweet DL, et al. Multicentric giant lymph node hyperplasia. Am J Clin Path 1978;69:86.

[6] Flendrig JA. Benign giant lymphoma: clinicopathologic correlation study. In: Clark RL, Cumley RW eds. The year book of cancer. Chigaco: Year Book Medical, 296–299, 1970.

[7] Soulier J, Grollet L, Oksenhendler E, et al. Kaposi's sarcoma-associated herpesvirus-like DNA sequences in multicentric Castleman's disease. Blood 1995;86(4):1276–80.

[8] Stebbing J, Pantanowitz L, Dayyani F, et al. HIV-associated multicentric Castleman's disease. Am J Hematol 2008;83(6):498–503.

[9] Shisana O, Rehle T, Simbayi LC, et al. South African national HIV prevalence, HIV incidence, behaviour and communication survey. HSRC Press, Cape Town, 2014

[10] Mylona EE, Baraboutis IG, Lekakis LJ, et al. Multicentric Castleman's disease in HIV infection: a systematic review of the literature. AIDS Rev 2008;10(1):25–35.

[11] Bower M, Newsom-Davis T, Naresh K et al. Clinical Features and Outcome in HIV-Associated Multicentric Castleman's disease. J Clin Oncol 2011;29:2481–2486.

[12] Dossier A, Meignin V, Fieschi C, et al. Human Herpesvirus 8-Related Castleman Disease in the absence of HIV infection. Clinical Infectious diseases 2013;56:833–842.

[13] Menke DM, Tierman M, Camoriano JK, et al. Diagnosis of Castleman's disease by identification of an immunophenotypically aberrant population of mantle zone B lymphocytes in paraffin-embedded lymph node biopsies. Am J Clin Pathol 1996;105:268–276.

[14] Dupin N, Diss TL, Kellam P, et al. HHV-8 is associated with a plasmablastic variant of Castleman disease that is linked to HHV-8 positive plasmablastic lymphoma. Blood 2000;95:1406–1412.

[15] Oksenhendler E, Carcelain G, Aoki Y, et al. High levels of HHV-8 viral load, human interleukin-6, interleukin-10, and C reactive protein correlate with exacerbation of multicentric Castleman disease in HIV-infected patients. Blood 2000;96:2069–2073.

[16] Polizzotto MN, Uldrick TS, Wang V, et al. Human and viral interleukin-6 and other cytokines in Kaposi sarcoma herpesvirus-associated multicentric Castleman disease. Blood 2013;122(26):4189–4198.

[17] Chang Y, Cesarman E, Pessin MS, et al. Identification of herpesvirus-like DNA sequences in AIDS-associated Kaposi's sarcoma. Science 1994;266:1865–1869.

[18] Suda T, Katano H, Delsol, et al. HHV-8 infection status of AIDS-unrelated and AIDS-associated multicentric Castleman's disease. Pathol Int 2001;51(9):671–679.

[19] Nishi J, Arimura K, Utsunomiya A, et al. Expression of vascular endothelial growth factor in the sera and lymph nodes of the plasma cell type of Castleman's disease. Br J Haematol 2013;104:482.

[20] Gérard L, Bérezné A, Galicier L, et al. Prospective study of rituximab in chemotherapy-dependent human immunodeficiency virus associated multicentric Castleman's disease: ANRS 117 CastlemaB Trial. J Clin Oncol 2007;25:3350–3356.

[21] Uldrick TS, Polizzotto MN, Yarchoan R. Recent advances in Kaposi sarcoma herpesvirus-associated multicentric Castleman disease. Curr Opin Oncol 2012;24:495–505.

[22] Bower M, Pria AD, Coyle C, et al. Diagnostic criteria schemes for multicentric Castleman disease in 75 cases. J Acquir Immune Defic Syndr 2014;65(2):e80–82.

[23] Talat N, Belgaumkar AP, Schulte KM. Surgery in Castleman's disease: a systematic review of 404 published cases. Ann Surg 2012;255(4):677–84.

[24] Powles T, Stebbing J, Bazeos A, et al. The role of immune suppression and HHV-8 in the increasing incidence of HIV-associated multicentric Castleman's disease. Ann Oncol 2009;20(4):775–9.

[25] Munoz G, Geijo P, Moldenhauer F, et al. Plasmacellular Castleman disease and POEMS syndrome. Histopathology 1990;17:172.

[26] Herrada J, Cabanillas F, Rice L, et al. The clinical behaviour of localized and multicentric Castleman's disease. Ann Int Med 1998;128:657.

[27] Kawabata H, Kadowaki N, Nishikori M, et al. Clinical features and treatment of Multicentric Castleman's disease: A retrospective study of 21 Japanese patients at a single institute. J Clin Exp Hematop 2013;53(1):69–77.

[28] Larroche C, Cacoub P, Soulier J, et al. Castleman's disease and lymphoma: report of eight cases in HIV-negative patients and literature review. Am J Hematol 2002;69:119.

[29] Bower M. How I treat HIV-associated multicentric Castleman disease. Blood 2010;116(22):4415–4421.

[30] Scott D, Cabra L, Harrington WJ Jr. Treatment of HIV-associated multicentric Castleman's disease with oral etoposide. Am J Hematol 2001;66(2):148–150.

[31] Bestawros A, Michel R, Seguin C, et al. Multicentric Castleman's disease treated with combination chemotherapy and rituximab in four HIV-positive men: a case series. Am J Hematol 2008;83(6):508–511.

[32] Oksenhendler E. HIV-associated multicentric Castleman disease. Curr Opin HIV AIDS 2009;4(1):16–21.

[33] Casper C, Krantz EM, Corey L, et al. Valganciclovir for suppression of human herpesvirus-8 replication: a randomized, double-blind, placebo-controlled, cross-over trial. J Infect Dis 2008;198(1):23–30.

[34] Patel M, Philip V, Omar T, et al. The impact of Human Immunodeficiency Virus Infection (HIV) on Lymphoma in South Africa. Journal of Cancer Therapy 2015;6:527–535.

[35] Patel M, Philip V, Fazel F. Human Immunodeficiency Virus Infection and Hodgkin's Lymphoma in South Africa – An emerging problem. Advances in Hematology http://dx.doi.org/10.1155/2011/578163, 2011.

[36] Oksenhendler E, Boulanger E, Galicier L, et al. High incidence of Kaposi's sarcoma-associated herpes virus-related non-Hodgkin's lymphoma in patients with HIV infection and multicentric Castleman's disease. Blood 2002;99(7):2331–2336.

Chapter 12

Pharmacological Properties of Monoclonal Antibodies Directed Against Interleukins

Kaloyan Georgiev and Marieta Georgieva

Additional information is available at the end of the chapter

http://dx.doi.org/10.5772/61774

Abstract

The road to individualized therapy goes through detecting specific targets (e.g., antigens), suitable for influence, and their selective targeting by using specially designed molecules (e.g., antibodies). A significant advance in this area is the development of therapeutic monoclonal antibodies. This approach enables maximizing the therapeutic effect on one hand, and reducing systemic toxicity on the other hand. In recent years, significant progress was made in improving their pharmacological performance – pharmacokinetics (longer half-life) and pharmacodynamics properties (better efficacy because of stronger affinity to human receptor), and safety profile (less antigenic and immunogenic reactions). Interleukins are a diverse, multifunctional group of proteins that carry out communication between various immune cells and control their gene expression. They manage the intensity and magnitude of an inflammatory response, and control differentiation, proliferation, and secretion of antibodies. Therefore, interleukin network represents an interesting pharmacological target, modulation of which using either biological or small chemical agents could contribute to suppression of excessive activated immune system and successfully treat the diseases that they are involved in.

Keywords: Monoclonal antibodies, pharmacological properties, pharmacokinetics, pharmacodynamics, cytokines, interleukins

1. Introduction

An effective immune response is possible only through the interaction of several cell types. To coordinate this process, there are a number of mechanisms for communication between immune cells, including a plurality of immunomodulating signaling molecules, such as cytokines. An officially recognized definition of the cytokines does not exist. Cytokines are a group of regulatory molecules with protein or glycoprotein structure (relatively small molecular mass ~10-35 kDa) that carry intercellular signals between immune system cells. The name "cytokine" was coined to describe both – a cell, cyto, and a movement, kinos. Due to the immense structural and functional differences between cytokines their classification is very difficult. In natural immunity, the effector cytokines are mostly produced by mononuclear phagocytes and therefore often called monokines. Although monokines can be elicited directly by microbes, they can be also secreted by mononuclear phagocytes in response to antigen-stimulated T-cells, i.e., as part of specific immunity. Most cytokines in specific immunity are made by activated T-lymphocytes, and these molecules are often called lymphokines. T-cells produce several cytokines that function primarily to regulate the growth and differentiation of various lymphocytes and play important roles in the activation phase of immune response. The major group among cytokines is the group of interleukins, which are produced by a plurality of nuclear cells in response to various stimuli. The main functions of the interleukins are:

- Mediating the inflammatory response.
- Involved in the Th1- and Th2-immune response.
- Lymphocyte growth and differentiation.
- Chemoattractants for lymphocytes and polymorph nuclear leukocytes.
- Play role in hematopoiesis.
- Some of them could inhibit inflammatory process (e.g., IL-10, IL-13).

Therefore, the interleukins represent a huge interest for researchers. Their role in plenty of diseases with excessive activity of the immune system contributes to this as well. Antagonists of the interleukins or their receptors act immunosuppressive and are successfully applied in such disorders. The name "interleukins" was proposed by scientists in 1979 during the Second International Lymphokine Workshop in Switzerland and comes from the prefix inter, which means between (carrying out communication) and leukins, which determines their origin and their action (production from and influence on leukocytes). [1] By 1978, with the introduction of modern methods of purification of proteins, it became clear that interleukin (IL) can be separated into two proteins – IL-1 and IL-2 – depending on cell targets and functions. By that time, it was known that Interleukin-1, which is produced by monocytes/macrophages, was a lymphocyte-activating factor and Interleukin-2 was a T-cell growth factor, thymocyte-stimulating factor, and costimulator. Today it is clear that IL-2 supports the growth of natural-killer (NK) T-cells and especially the subpopulation of NK cells known as lymphokine activated killer (LAK) cells, which are involved in killing tumor cells. This discovery contributed to the approval of IL-2 as a cancer therapeutic drug that is able to stimulate the recruitment and expansion of natural killer cells in order to attack tumor cells.

Nowadays 37 different interleukins are known, the numbering of which is in order of increase in numbers from 1 to 37. [2] Approved monoclonal antibodies affect certain members of the family of interleukins, such as IL-1, IL-2, IL-6, IL12/23, or IL-17, the function of which is considerably studied and proven (Tables 1 and 2).

Interleukins	Origin	Biological function	References
IL-1	Macrophage, Monocytes, Fibroblast, and Dendritic cells	Inflammation, fever, activation of T- and B-cells	[2, 3, 4]
IL-2	Th type 1-cells	T-cell proliferation and expansion	[7, 8]
IL-6	Macrophage, Monocytes, Th type 2-cells, B-cells	Inflammation, fever, activation of B-cells	[14, 15]
IL-12	Macrophage, B and T-cells, Dendritic cells	Synergistic with IL-2, INF-γ, and TNF-α production in T-cells	[20, 21, 22, 23]
IL-17	Th type 17-cells	Inflammation, angiogenesis	[27]
IL-23	Antigen-presenting cells (APC)	INF-γ production, reduce CD8+ T-cell proliferation, angiogenesis	[20, 21, 22, 23]

Table 1. Some interleukins, their origin, and biological function.

MAb	Molecular type	Interleukin target(s)	Indication(s)
Canakinumab	Human	IL-1β	Cryopyrin-associated periodic syndromes (CAPS), active systemic juvenile idiopathic arthritis (SJIA)
Basiliximab	Chimeric	IL-2 (CD25)	Prevention of acute organ rejection
Daclizumab	Humanized	IL-2 (CD25)	Prevention of acute organ rejection
Tocilizumab	Humanized	IL-6	Rheumatoid arthritis (RA)
Ustekinumab	Human	IL-12/23	Plaque psoriasis, psoriatic arthritis
Secukinumab	Human	IL-17A	Plaque psoriasis

Table 2. Approved monoclonal antibodies directed against interleukins.

1.1. Therapeutic monoclonal antibodies

Therapeutic monoclonal antibodies have gained large attention over recent decades because of their desirable features, such as high potency and safety profile. Nowadays, they are used in almost all clinical fields, ranging from toxin and pathogen neutralization or clearance to influence endogenous cytokine, treating cancer, and in modulation of many other diseases. [3] The first monoclonal antibodies were generated in mice in 1975 using a hybridoma technique, first described by Kohler and Milstein [4]. They were rewarded ten years later, in 1984, with the Nobel Prize in Medicine for their discovery. The key feature of a monoclonal antibody is its unique specificity. Monoclonal antibodies are monovalent antibodies that bind to the same epitope and are produced from a single B-lymphocyte clone. This homogeneity will give rise to the same immunological effector functions. In principle, monoclonal antibodies can be produced in unlimited quantities, because the hybridoma cell itself survives after cryopreservation at least for decades. Monoclonal antibodies are classified according to an international terminology (Table 3).

Prefix	Target infix	Origin infix	Suffix
Variable	-o(s)-: Bone	-u-: Human	-mab
	-vi(r)-: Virus	-o-: Mouse	
	-ba(c)-: Bacteria	-a-: Rat	
	-li(m)-: Immune system	-e-: Hamster	
	-ci(r)-: Cardiovascular System	-xi-: Chimeric (e.g., mouse-human or hamster-human)	
	-tu(m)-: Tumor (general)	-zu-: Humanized	
	-neu(r)-: Nervous system	-axo-: Hybrid (rat-mouse	
	-ki(n)-: Interleukin		
	-mu(l)-: Musculosceletal System		
	-tox(a)-: Toxine		

Table 3. Classification of monoclonal antibodies according to an international terminology.

Single syllables of the name suggest the origin and therapeutic area in which they are used. Examples: Cana-kin-u-mab – human monoclonal antibody directed against interleukins; Basi-li-xi-mab – chimeric immunotropic monoclonal antibody, etc.

The first licensed monoclonal antibody was Orthoclone OKT3 (muromonab-CD3), which was approved in 1986 for use in preventing kidney transplant rejection. [5] It is a monoclonal mouse IgG2a antibody whose cognate antigen is CD3. It works by binding to ε (epsilon) – chain of the CD3-proteins expressed on T-lymphocytes, inhibits CD3-associate effects and interrupts T-cell receptor mediated signal transduction. However, due to significant reported side effects, its use was limited to acute cases. [6] One of the most important adverse effects is a cascade of systemic cytokine release that has been termed cytokine release syndrome (CRS) or cytokine storm. CRS is associated with increased serum levels of cytokines (e.g., TNFα, IL-2, IL-6, INF-γ) that peak between 1 and 4 h after dose, duration 12–16 h, and severity could be mild to life-threatening. Signs and symptoms include fever, chilling, dyspnea, wheezing, chest pain and tightness, nausea, vomiting, and diarrhea. Hypervolemic pulmonary edema, nephrotoxicity, meningitis, and encephalopathy are possible [7].

1.2. Targeting IL-1

Although the family of interleukin-1 incorporates many members, two of them are studied best – IL1α and IL-1β, encoded by two related but distinct IL-1 genes – IL1A and IL1B, respectively. The both interleukins are strongly proinflammatory molecules that modulate the peripheral immune response during infection and inflammation [8]. These cytokines increase the expression and activity of adhesion molecules (e.g., VCAM-1, ICAM-1, L-selectine) that promote attraction of immunocompetent cells to the site of infection. The more potent inflammatory cytokine is IL-1β, which has been demonstrated in numerous in vitro and in vivo animal models [9]. Two types of IL-1 receptor are cloned with different physiological and

http://dx.doi.org/10.5772/61774

pharmacological characteristics: IL-1R1 and IL-1R2, respectively [10]. There is also a natural glycoprotein inhibitor of the receptors for IL-1, IL-1Ra (IL-1 receptor antagonist), which modulates the effects of both cytokines by competing with them for binding sites of the receptor, and a number of other molecules that directly regulate IL-1 activity, such as the IL-1 receptor type I (IL-1RI), the decoy receptor IL-1 receptor type II (IL-1RII), its coreceptor IL-1 receptor accessory protein (IL-1RAcP), and soluble receptor forms.

In humans, IL-1 plays a major role in bone resorption and cartilage destruction by inducing prostaglandin E2 and proteolytic enzymes, such as matrix metalloproteinase. [11] This led to the development of interleukin-1 inhibitors, as a possible therapeutic strategy in rheumatoid arthritis and other chronic inflammatory diseases.

IL-1β plays a crucial role in the pathogenesis of multiple myeloma (MM) [12]. This is based on the fact that IL-1β is the main cytokine in the bone marrow, which increases production of the paracrine IL-6, the primary growth factor, responsible for survival and expansion of the myeloma cells. Reducing IL-1β activity could be a possible way for slowing disease progression and induction of the chronic disease state in patients with smoldering or indolent multiple myeloma, as shown the results from phase II clinical trial with IL-1RA [13]. Since the receptor antagonist – anakinra – has a short plasma half-life and the need for frequent administration, the monoclonal antibodies would be superior options due to their longer plasma half-lives and less frequent administration.

The role of IL-1β was established in both types of diabetes. In very low concentrations (picomolar), IL-1β is able to destroy insulin-producing pancreatic β-cells [14]. High glucose concentrations stimulate IL-1β production from the β-cell itself [15], thus implicating a self-destructive role for IL-1β autoinflammation by the β-cell and the recruitment of immune cells via IL-1β-driven chemokines [16]. The IL-1β derives either from the β-cell itself or from the infiltrated blood monocytes in the islet. Caspase-1 dependent IL-1β production has been observed in macrophages available in human adipose tissues, which demonstrate the connection between obesity and type 2 diabetes [17, 18]. Improved insulin sensitivity and decreased insulin resistance have been shown in diabetic mice, administered with caspase-1 inhibitor [17].

IL-1 takes part in cardiovascular events, such as stroke, myocardial infarction, kidney failure, liver failure, acute lung injury, each one of them with rapid loss of function. The ischemic event in the myocardial infarction and thrombotic stroke starts with a sudden blockage of a blood vessel by a clot formatted after atherosclerotic plaque rupture. The result of the blockage is hypoxia (decreased oxygen supply) and death of the cells [19].

Pharmacological approaches affecting the function of IL-1 include:

- Using recombinant nonglycosylated molecule of human IL-1 receptor antagonist (IL-1RA) produced in E.coli – Anakinra, marketed as Kiniret® (Amgen). It was introduced to the practice in 1993 and it blocks the activity of both IL-1α and IL-1β. Anakinra currently dominates the field of IL-1 therapeutics and is the drug of choice in cryopyrin-associated periodic syndromes (CAPS), and it is also prescribed to treat rheumatoid arthritis in patients in whom one or more disease-modifying anti-rheumatic drugs (DMARDs) have failed.

- Using fusion protein, consisting of the ligand-binding domains of the extracellular portions of the human interleukin-1 receptor component (IL-1R1) and IL-1 receptor accessory protein (IL-1RAcP) linked to the Fc region of human IgG1 – Rilonacept (Arcalyst®), currently in use to treat CAPS.
- Using human monoclonal antibody against IL-1β – Canakinumab or Gevokizumab.
- Orally active small-molecule inhibitors of IL-1 production, such as caspase 1 inhibitors, which are under investigation.

1.3. Pharmacological properties of canakinumab

Canakinumab (ACZ885) is a high-affinity human monoclonal anti-interleukin-1β antibody, with molecular size ~150 kDa, designed to bind and neutralize the activity of human IL-1β. It is registered under trade name Ilaris® (Novartis) and is approved for treatment of cryopyrin-associated periodic syndromes (CAPS) and active systemic juvenile idiopathic arthritis (SJIA). The CAPS cover various progressive, hereditary inflammatory diseases caused by a mutation of the NALP3 gene. The NALP3 protein (cryopyrin) is a component of a protein complex, named inflammasome. The active inflammasome complex activates the enzyme caspase-1, which cleaves pro-IL-1β to the biologically active IL-1β. NALP3 regulates IL-1β levels. If there is a mutation, even a relatively weak stress agent such as cold is enough to stimulate the synthesis of IL-1β [20]. After administration, canakinumab bind with high affinity to IL-1β and form a complex – canakinumab-IL-1β. This complex is eliminated very slowly, due to its larger size, and this leads to increasing plasma concentrations of both unbound and bound IL-1β. Total IL-1β concentrations can therefore be used as a surrogate pharmacodynamic marker of "drug activity" (i.e., binding of IL-1β by the antibody), as it is easily detected following canakinumab administration [21]. From the following mechanism of action can be expected typical pharmacokinetic properties of human IgG-type immunoglobulins like slow serum clearance (0.174 L/day), low total volume of distribution at steady state (Vss ~ 6.0 L), and a long elimination half-life of 26 days. Bioavailability after subcutaneous administration is 70%. Canakinumab shows dose-dependent (linear) pharmacokinetics both given as an intravenous infusion and as a single subcutaneous administration [21]. In clinical trials, canakinumab achieved a complete and sustained remission in patients with CAPS and a mutation in the NALP3 gene, regardless of phenotype and severity. The effect occurs rapidly. After a single subcutaneous administration 97% of IL-1β-mediated symptoms (such as fever, joint and muscle pain, skin rashes, tissue damage and inflammation) had disappeared after eight weeks. A 90% remained symptom-free for up to one year if they received canakinumab injection in eight-week intervals [22]. In general, the adverse effects of canakinumab are mild to moderate. The most common adverse effects (>10% of treated patients) are reactions at the injection site, inflammation of the upper respiratory tract or sinuses, and headache [23].

1.4. Pharmacological properties of gevokizumab

Gevokizumab (XOMA 052, XOMA Corporation, Berkeley, CA, USA) is a recombinant, humanized IgG2 monoclonal antibody that binds to IL-1RI allosterically, reducing the formation of the IL-1RI:IL1RAcP signaling complex [24], which distinguishes it from other monoclonal antibodies. The clinical significance of these differences is not known.

Gevokizumab is produced in Chinese hamster ovary cells and has shown activity on animal models against RA, gout, and Type 2 diabetes. Additionally, in mouse models of myocardial infarction and atherosclerosis, gevokizumab maintained left ventricular function [25] and decreased markers of atherosclerosis [26], respectively. Gevokizumab was investigated in a randomized, placebo-controlled, dose-escalation first-in-human study conducted in the United States (NCT00513214) and Switzerland (NCT00541983) on patients with Type 2 diabetes. For the purposes of the study, single and multiple doses of gevokizumab were given i.v. or s.c. to 98 patients with poor-controll diabetes, which are treated with standard anti-diabetes therapy [27]. In this study, gevokizumab was well-tolerated. The most serious adverse reactions were carcinomatous appendix and occlusion of carotid artery, which were not considered to be drug-related. One insulin-dependent patient experienced episodic symptoms of hypoglycemia, which was not considered to be related to treatment. The changes of pharmacokinetic parameters of gevokizumab were dose-related. The mean half-life was 22–23 days, which allows subcutaneous application once a month. After this study, XOMA started a IIb phase study of gevokizumab in 421 Type 2 diabetic patients at multiple sites in the United States during 2010 with metformin therapy on background (NCT01066715). The initial endpoint of the study (change in HbA1c levels from baseline compared to placebo) was not reached, but the development in cardiovascular diseases is ongoing. Another two studies are exploring the effects of gevokizumab on beta islet cell function in patients with Type 1 diabetes.

Gevokizumab is in phase III clinical trial in treatment of both acute and controlled noninfectious uveitis (NIU) and Behcet uveitis – EYEGUARD™ – A, B, C [28]. Previous results were quite encouraging. Seven patients received a single infusion of 0.3 mg kg^{-1} gevokizumab. Rapid and long-lasting clinical response was established in all patients after the treatment with gevokizumab. Intraocular inflammation was resolved completely in 4–21 days (median 14 days), with a median duration of response of 49 days (range 21–97 days). One of the patients during the study was exacerbation-free. No one needed rescue therapy during the study period [29].

There are recent reports of a novel fully human anti-IL-1β IgG1 – P2D7KK, with greater affinity for IL-1β than canakinumab, which potently neutralizes human, mouse, and monkey (rhesus macaque) IL-1β, and significantly reduces pathological signs of various models of animal diseases [30]. Authors of that publication argue that in animal model of MM the new monoclonal antibody showed significant protection from myeloma-induced lethality, as 70% of P2D7KK-treated mice survived compared with 20% in the isotype group, and are hopeful that it has potential as an anticancer therapeutic.

1.5. Targeting IL-2

Interleukin (IL)-2 is a small (15-kDa), α-helical cytokine produced primarily by recently activated T-cells. It binds to a receptor (IL-2R) that is composed of three subunits, an α-chain that functions only for IL-2 binding (IL-2Rα, CD 25) and the β (IL-2Rβ, CD 122) and γ (IL-2Rγ, CD 132) subunits (Figure 1), which function to augment ligand binding and induce cellular signaling.

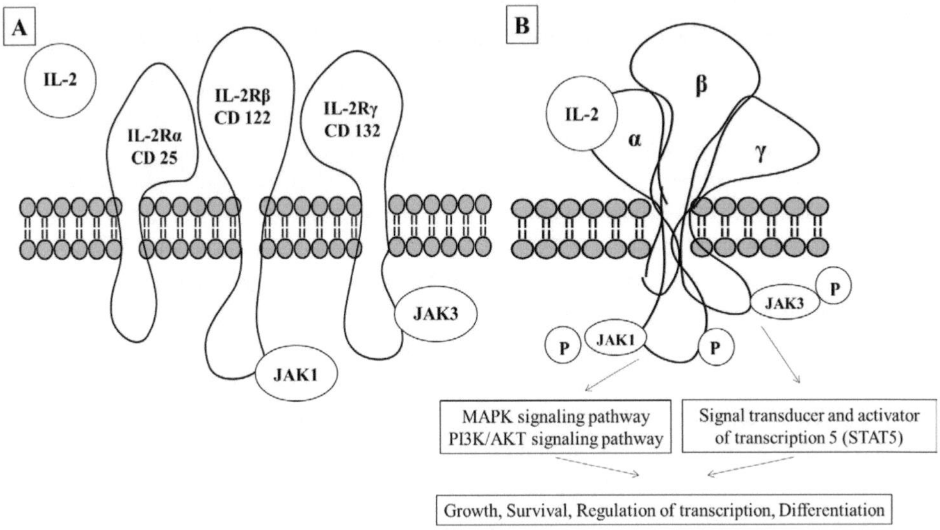

Figure 1. Structure of IL-2 receptor. **A.** In the absence of binding of IL-2 **B.** After binding to IL-2 and forming a stable heterotrimer, which then leads to the initiation of signal transduction.

IL-2 is an essential cytokine produced mainly by CD4+ T lymphocytes for promoting the clonal expansion of recently antigen-activated T cells [31]. Beside acting as T-lymphocyte growth factor, it has been found that IL-2 takes part in the activation of apoptosis and the development of regulatory T-cells and cytotoxic T lymphocytes [32]. This cytokine is of a great interest in pharmacology because, on one hand, the activation of interleukin-2 receptor results in stimulation of the immune system and can be used for inducing cytotoxicity on NK-resistant tumor cells; on the other hand, its inhibition could lead to suppression of unwanted immune responses, especially those that occur in autoimmune diseases or transplant rejection reactions. Recombinant human interleukin-2 (rhIL-2, Aldesleukin, Proleukine®, Chiron Corporation, Emeryville, CA) is used in clinical practice. It differs from the native IL-2 that lacks the first amino acid (alanine) and the cysteine at position 125 is replaced by serine. In contrast to the natural IL-2, aldesleukin is not glycosylated [33]. Aldesleukin stimulates the growth of activated T- and B-cells as well as NK (natural killer) cells by the IL-2 receptor. It can activate lymphokine-activated killer (LAK) cells and tumor-infiltrating lymphocytes (TIL) cells. It was approved in 1993 for treatment of metastatic renal cell cancer and later for metastatic melanoma. Aldesleukin displays biphasic pharmacokinetics, with an alpha (distribution) half-life of 13 min and a beta (terminal) half-life of 85 min. In cancer patients, the mean clearance rate of aldesleukin is 268 ml/min. The dose of aldesleukin in metastatic renal cell carcinoma and melanoma is 600,000 int. units/kg every 8 h for a maximum of 14 doses. Repeat after 9 days for a total of 28 doses per course. If needed, retreatment is made 7 weeks after previous course. The other product with IL-2 is denileukin diftitox (Ontac®, Seragen, Inc., Hopkinton, MA) consisting of diphtheria toxin fragments A and B fused to interleukin-2. In the recurrent or refractory cutaneous T-cell lymphoma, (CTCL), a rare slow-growing form of non-Hodgkin's lymphoma, in patients whose malignant cells express the CD25 component of the interleukin-2

http://dx.doi.org/10.5772/61774

receptor is indicated. It interacts with high-affinity interleukin-2 receptor on the surface of malignant cells and, via receptor-mediated endocytosis enters intracellular. Then enzymatically active fragment A portion of diphtheria toxin inhibits protein synthesis and leads to cell death. The pharmacokinetic parameters of Denileukin diftitox include terminal half-life of 70–80 min, Vd ~0.06 to 0.08 L/kg, and CL_{tot} ~1–2 ml/min/kg. Clearance could be significantly affected by the development of antibodies to denileukin diftitox, reducing mean systemic exposure by approximately 75%. In patients with CTCL, intravenous dose of denileukin diftitox is 9 or 18 mcg/kg/day; days 1 through 5 days every 21 days for 8 cycles.

1.6. Pharmacological properties of basiliximab and daclizumab

The chimeric monoclonal antibody basiliximab (Simulect®, Novartis, New York, NY, USA) and humanized monoclonal antibody daclizumab (Zenapax®, Roche Pharmaceuticals, Nutley, NJ, USA) have identical mechanisms of action, specifically bind the alpha subunit of the interleukin-2 (CD25) receptor on activated T-lymphocytes, thereby reducing IL-2-mediated T-cell proliferation. Daclizumab was approved by the FDA in 1997 as the first humanized therapeutic mAb, composed of 90% human and 10% murine antibody sequences with a binding affinity of 3 nM to IL-2Ra, about one-third that of its murine parental antibody. The both antibodies are indicated for prevention of acute organ rejection in adult and pediatric renal and liver transplant recipients in combination with other immunosuppressive agents [34], with no increase in opportunistic infections or adverse effects, proven to be a class of effective and specific immunosuppressive agents. Basiliximab requires only two doses. The first dose 20 mg should be given within 2 h prior to transplantation surgery. The recommended second dose 20 mg should be given 4 days after transplantation. Pharmacokinetic parameters of basiliximab are: total body clearance (Cltot ~0.075 L/h), volume of distribution at steady state (Vss ~8 L), and an elimination half-life of approximately 7,4 days [35]. Basiliximab was found to be safe and effective when used in a maintenance regimen consisting of cyclosporine, mycophenolate mofetil, and prednisone. [36] Although, daclizumab has a longer half-life (20 days), it is applied more frequently than basiliximab. The standard course of treatment with daclizumab requires administration of five doses. The first dose (1 mg/kg given intravenously over 15 min in 50–100 mL of normal saline) should be given no more than 24 h before transplantation. The four remaining doses should be given at intervals of 14 days [37]. Both drugs are well-tolerated, but anaphylactic reactions can occur. The risk of incidents of lymphoproliferative disorders and opportunistic infections is low [38]. There are many other diseases, with pathological immune response, which are a subject to the therapy with anti-IL-2 receptor antibodies, like multiple sclerosis, psoriasis, uveitis, etc. However, clinical trials are still ongoing.

1.7. Targeting IL-6

Interleukin-6 (IL-6) is a cytokine of approximately 26 kDa, which is synthesized by mononuclear phagocytes, vascular endothelial cells, fibroblasts, and other cells in response to IL-1 and, to a lesser extent, TNF. It exerts pleiotropic effects on many cells and plays a central role in diverse host defense mechanisms such as the immune response, hematopoiesis, and acute-phase reactions [39]. IL-6 is capable of stimulating the proliferation and activation of synoviocyte and osteoclasts, which leads to formation of synovial pannus. In combination with IL-1, they increase production of matrix metalloproteinases, which induces joint and cartilage destruction [40]. IL-6 induces the synthesis of the major mediators of the acute phase response, such as serum C-reactive protein (CRP) and amyloid A. IL-6 high levels correlate with disease activity and clinical manifestations of rheumatoid arthritis, systemic-onset juvenile idiopathic arthritis (sJIA), Castleman's disease, and systemic lupus erythematosus (SLE) [41, 42].

IL-6 transmits its signals in two pathways: binding to a membrane receptor (mIL6R or CD126) or to its soluble form (sIL6R) (Figure 2).

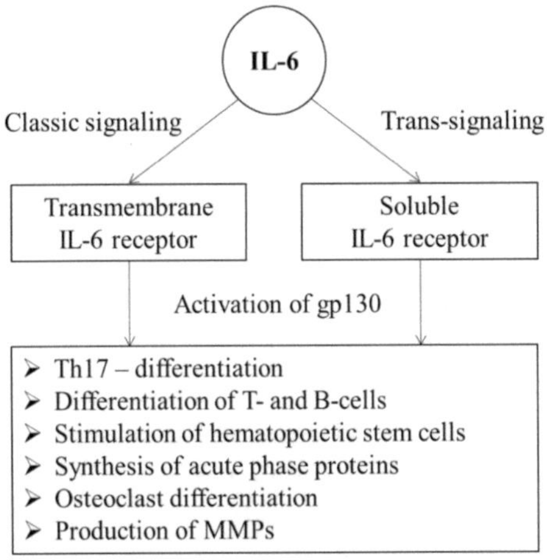

Figure 2. Pleiotropic effects of IL-6.

For both pathways, IL-6 stimulation activates Janus family tyrosine kinases (JAKs), which are associated with gp130 IL6 transducer (CD130), leading to the induction of two major signal transduction pathways, signal transducer and activator of transcription (STAT-3) pathway and mitogen-activated protein kinases (MAPKs) pathway [42]. Targeting and inhibiting IL-6R is a new promising pharmacological approach leading to a significant improvement of signs and symptoms in dysimmune diseases, such as rheumatoid arthritis (RA) or Castleman's disease, which was demonstrated in many clinical trials with a marked reduction in disease activity and the acute-phase response. Lately, modulating the function of IL-6 is used in treatment of cancers.

1.8. Pharmacological properties of tocilizumab and other newly developed monoclonal antibodies against IL-6

Tocilizumab (TCZ, Actemra®, Chugai Pharmaceutical Co Ltd, Tokyo, Japan; now a member of the Roche Group) is a humanized anti-IL-6 receptor antibody, licensed for the treatment of rheumatoid arthritis (RA), polyarticular and systemic juvenile idiopathic arthritis by intravenous administration of 8 mg/kg (and no less than 4.8 mg) in combination with methotrexate (MTX) or monotherapy [43]. The subcutaneous formulation (162 mg weekly) is now entering phase III trials and the preliminary data have shown comparable efficacy and safety profiles to the established intravenous formulation [44]. Tocilizumab can simultaneously bind to both receptors – mIL6R and sIL6R – thereby interrupting the IL-6 signal pathway but does not affect signaling of other IL-6 family cytokines [45], and without increasing the IL-6 half-life [46]. Pharmacokinetic parameters of tocilizumab include – Vdss – 2.54–4.08 L (children) and 6.4 L (adults), the half-life is 6.3 days, but in steady state could be increased to 16–23 days (children) and 11–13 days (adults) [47]. Adverse events associated with the usage of tocilizumab include increased serum cholesterol and liver enzymes (ALT, AST), infusion-related reaction and infections (especially respiratory infection, and skin and soft tissue infections). Total cholesterol, low-density lipoproteins, triglycerides, and high-density lipoproteins are increased in 20–30% of patients treated with tocilizumab. The possible explanation of this effect is that IL-6 modulates lipoprotein receptor expression and lowers blood lipid levels via upregulation of the very-low-density lipoprotein (VLDL) receptor. If tocilizumab reduces the levels of IL-6, it will increase the levels of plasma proteins [48]. According to recent studies, this elevation of lipids does not show apparent increase in cardiac events in a follow-up of 5 years [49]. The most common adverse events of treatment with tocilizumab were infections (such as upper respiratory tract infection, nasopharyngitis, skin infections, pneumonia, gastroenteritis, and urinary tract infection, both viral and bacterial), nonsignificantly higher than the placebo group [50, 51]. Resolution of infections such as pneumonia, herpes zoster, limb abscess, osteomyelitis, sepsis, staphylococcal cellulitis, acute pyelonephritis, and staphylococcal polyarthritis have improved with appropriate treatment [52].

Siltuximab (CNTO 328, Sylvant®, Janssen Biotech) is a chimeric monoclonal antibody, an interleukin-6 (IL-6) antagonist, which is indicated for the treatment of patients with multicentric Castleman's disease (MCD) who are human immunodeficiency virus (HIV) negative and human herpesvirus-8 (HHV-8) negative. It is tested in clinical trials for multiple myeloma (MM), metastatic renal cell carcinoma (MRCC), and prostate cancer [53]. The clearance of siltuximab in patients is 0.23 L/day, according to population pharmacokinetic analysis and body weight is the only significant determinant for siltuximab clearance. The mean serum terminal half-life (t ½) for siltuximab in patients after the first i.v. infusion of 11 mg/kg is 21 days (range: 14–30 days). The CYP450 enzyme activity may reach its normal levels (previously downregulated by IL6), due to binding of bioactive IL6 by siltuximab. This may result in increased metabolism of CYP450 substrates compared with metabolism before treatment with siltuximab. If siltuximab is coadministered with CYP450 substrate drugs with a narrow therapeutic range, the dose of the concomitant medication may need to be adjusted. On the basis of the population pharmacokinetic analysis, no initial dosage adjustment is necessary for patients with baseline mild-to-severe renal impairment (CLCr ≥ 15 mL/minute) or for patients with baseline mild-to-moderate hepatic impairment (Child-Pugh Class A and B). Patients with baseline severe hepatic impairment (Child-Pugh Class C) were not included in clinical trials. Within the serum siltuximab exposure range observed following administration of 11 mg/kg i.v. every 3 weeks, no exposure–response relationships between serum CRP and siltuximab exposure or between durable tumor and symptomatic response rate and siltuximab exposure were identified. Following siltuximab dosing, 0.2% (1/411) of patients tested positive for anti-siltuximab antibodies. Further immunogenicity analyses of the single positive sample revealed a low titer of anti-siltuximab antibodies with nonneutralizing capabilities [54].

Sarilumab (SAR153191/REGN88) is a fully human anti-IL-6Rα monoclonal antibody that binds membrane-bound and soluble human IL-6Rα with high affinity. It blocks cis and trans IL-6-mediated inflammatory signaling cascade. There was no reported evidence of complement-dependent or antibody-dependent cell-mediated cytotoxicity [55]. Sarilumab inhibits IL-6 signaling in a dose-dependent manner [56, 57]. Subcutaneous application in phase I studies in patients with RA has shown that sarilumab is generally well-tolerated, [58, 59] and reduces the acute-phase reactants such as C reactive protein (CRP) [60]. Sarilumab improves clinical signs and symptoms in RA patients with moderate-to-severe disease with tolerability similar to other IL-6 inhibitors. After completing the phase II clinical trial, the most favorable efficacy, safety, and dosing convenience were obtained by using 150 mg and 200 mg sarilumab q2w. Those doses will be further evaluated in phase III clinical trials [61].

Sirukumab (CNTO 136) is another human monoclonal antibody that targets only soluble IL-6 and is designed for the treatment of rheumatoid arthritis. It is currently in clinical phase III.

1.9. Modulating IL-11

Interleukin-11 is an ~20 kDa cytokine produced by bone marrow stromal cells. It stimulates megakaryopoiesis and may prove to be of therapeutic benefit in patients with platelet deficiencies. It also enhances the development of macrophages and perhaps other cells from marrow precursors. Neumega (oprelvekin) is a recombinant IL-11 protein product (MW ~19 kDa) approved for prevention of severe thrombocytopenia and reducing the need for platelet transfusions following myelosuppressive chemotherapy. The recommended dose for adults 50 mcg/kg/day once daily for ~10–21 days (until postnadir platelet count ≥50,000 cells/mcL) is administering subcutaneously. The most serious adverse effects reported are allergic or hypersensitivity reactions, including anaphylaxis. They may occur with the first or with subsequent doses. Patients who developed allergic reactions need to permanently discontinue the administration.

1.10. Targeting IL-12/23

Psoriasis is a chronic inflammatory disease of the skin, affecting 2–3% of the general population [62]. Plaque psoriasis, the most frequent form, has skin lesions in the form of scaly, red plaques. In psoriasis, destruction of normal immune-mediated signaling is caused by the overproduction and immature migration of keratinocytes to the surface of the skin [63]. Initially perceived as a skin disease, psoriasis can influence physical and mental condition of the body and lead to the development of joint disorders (psoriatic arthritis) and depression, thus significantly affecting the quality of life. Interleukins 12 and 23 play an important role in the formation of plaques of psoriasis. IL-12 stimulates production of IFN-gamma and tumour necrosis factor alpha (TNFα) and it is involved in differentiating naive T-cells into T-helper (Th)-1 cells, while IL-23 activates IL-17-producing T-cells (Th17) (Figure 3) [64, 65].

http://dx.doi.org/10.5772/61774

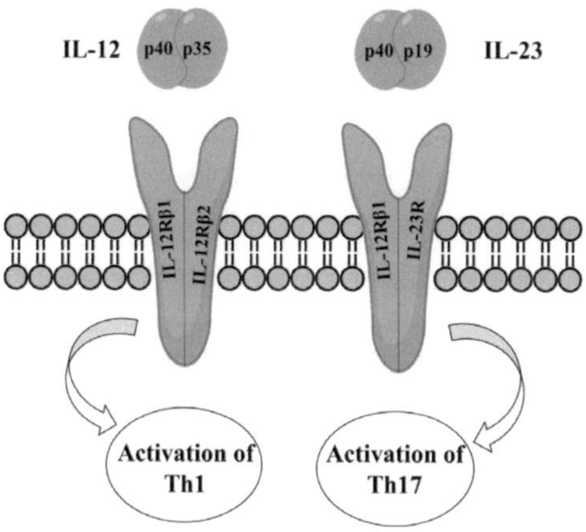

Figure 3. IL-12 family members.

1.11. Pharmacological properties of ustekimumab

Ustekinumab (UST, Stelara®) is an IgG1/kappa human monoclonal antibody composed of 1326 amino acid residues, with a molecular weight of approximately 148.6 kDa, directed against the shared p40 subunit of IL-12 and IL-23, thereby preventing IL-12 and IL-23 from binding to the receptor chain IL-12Rb1 to trigger downstream signaling pathways. It is currently approved for treatment of plaque psoriasis and psoriatic arthritis. The pharmacokinetic properties of ustekinumab in human population do not show any serious differences in patients with psoriatic arthritis and those with plaque psoriasis [66]. Absolute bioavailability after subcutaneous administration is approximately 57% and biological half-life is ~10–126 days. In clinical trials, ustekinumab has improved rapidly and sustainedly the symptoms of psoriasis. Even after one injection there was a significant improvement that persisted over the 1.5-year study period. It achieved the primary endpoint of 75% reduction in the Psoriasis Area and Severity Index (PASI) score in a large proportion of patients in the phase III PHOENIX trials (defined as 75% clinical improvement of affected skin areas determined by the size, severity of erythema, plaque thickness, and scaling) compared to 3% for placebo [67]. The effect lasted for 76 weeks after treatment with ustekinumab at more than 80% of the responders. In a randomized, multicenter study ustekinumab was compared with etanercept in the treatment of more than 900 patients with moderate-to-severe plaque psoriasis. After 12 weeks, 55% of patients receiving ustekinumab reached (45 mg at weeks 0 and 4) PASI-75; under etanercept (50 mg twice a week) it was 39% [68].

1.12. Targeting IL-17

Interleukin 17 (IL-17), similarly as interferon gamma, increases the production of chemokines in the various tissues that stimulate recruitment of monocytes and neutrophils to the site of inflammation. It was classified as a proinflammatory cytokine stimulating the production of IL-6 and IL-8, and the surface expression of the intracellular adhesion molecule-1 (ICAM-1) in human fibroblasts [69]. IL-17 is produced by the recently identified T-cell subset Th17 and is under the influence of IL-23, a cytokine belonging to the IL-12 family [70]. IL-23 is proinflammatory mediator, which induces chronic inflammation through the activation of Th17 cells and the secretion of Th17 by non-T-cells, as mentioned earlier. This pathway is essential for production of many other mediators that are involved in chronic inflammatory responses in autoimmune diseases. Large amounts of Th17 cells are found in blood and skin lesions of people with psoriasis. Although many signaling pathways including that of Th17 are investigated in psoriasis, IL-17A inhibitors are able to relieve psoriatic symptoms in forms resistant to anti-TNF agents and have higher specificity than inhibitors of IL-12 and IL-23. The combination of IL-17A and TNF-α induces a proinflammatory signaling cascade; patients who are refractory to anti-TNF agents may respond to therapies that target IL-17A [71]. As opposed to the agents that target IL-12 and IL-23 (ustekinumab), inhibitors of IL-17A may induce a more specific response.

1.13. Pharmacological properties of secukinumab, izekizumab, and brodalumab

Secukinumab (AIN-457, Cosentyx®, Novartis Pharma AG) is a fully human IgG1κ monoclonal antibody that selectively binds and neutralizes the effects of IL-17A. It is indicated for the treatment of adult patients with moderate-to-severe plaque psoriasis who are candidates for phototherapy or systemic therapy. In the pivotal studies, 70% of the subjects achieved a clear or almost clear skin. For the subjects, the antibody was injected once a week for 16 weeks. The effect was greater than the treatment with the TNF-α inhibitor etanercept (Enbrel®) and it was held in the majority of patients on continued therapy at one year. First improvements of the skin image appeared after two weeks only. On average, the skin symptoms had reduced after three weeks to half of what was achieved with etanercept after seven weeks. In addition, fewer and milder side effects than the reference were registered. [72]

Ixekizumab is a humanized IgG4 monoclonal antibody (mAb) neutralizing IL-17A. The safety and efficacy of ixekizumab was assessed in a phase II, double-blind, placebo-controlled trial with 142 moderate-to-severe plaque-type psoriasis patients. Patients were randomized into five groups administering subcutaneously 150, 75, 25, 10 mg ixekizumab or placebo, at 0, 2, 4, 8, 12, and 16 weeks [73]. The achievement of 75% reduction of Psoriasis Area and Severity Index (PASI) after 12 weeks of treatment constituted the primary endpoint of the study occurring in 82.1, 82.8, 76.7, 29 and 7.7% of patients treated with 150, 75, 25, 10 mg ixekizumab or placebo, respectively. The amelioration of PASI score was significantly greater in all ixekizumab groups compared with placebo ($p < 0.001$ for each comparison), with the exception of the lowest dose (10 mg) [73]. Furthermore, a statistically significant reduction of PASI score by at least 90% was observed in the 150 mg (71.4%), 75 mg (58.6%), and 25 mg (50.0%) groups versus placebo 0% ($p < 0.001$). Regarding the safety profile, the occurrence of adverse events including nasopharyngitis, upper respiratory infection, injection site reaction, and headache was similar across all study groups, and no serious adverse events were reported. Phase III studies are currently ongoing; among them are a head-to-head trial with etanercept, another head-to-head trial with adalimumab on psoriatic arthritis, and a study evaluating ixekizumab efficacy and safety on psoriatic arthritis patients [74].

Brodalumab is a human mAb, which blocks IL-17RA, the receptor subunit shared by IL-17A, IL-17F, and IL-17A/F heterodimer ligands. The antagonism of IL-17 signaling by brodalumab was primary proven clinical, genomic, and histological in 10 patients with psoriasis after only 1 week in a phase I, proof-of-concept study [75]. Its efficacy is confirmed in recent phase II, randomized, double-blind, placebo-controlled, dose-ranging study involving 198 patients. They received subcutaneously brodalumab of 280 mg monthly, or 70, 140, 210 mg brodalumab or placebo at weeks 0, 1, 2, 4, 6, 8, and 10 [76]. The monthly administration of 280 mg improved PASI score, with 45%, while other dosages (210, 140, and 70 mg) achieved 85.9%, 86.3%, and 16% of PASI score, respectively, after 12-week study assessment. The greater frequency of adverse effects was observed in patients receiving the high-dose regimen of brodalumab. There were two cases of mild neutropenia (grade III) among the serious adverse events [76]. Presently, phase II trials are being conducted to assess brodalumab as a therapeutic option for psoriatic arthritis, while its ability to treat plaque-type psoriasis has already progressed to phase III studies. Brodalumab is currently being investigated for the treatment of psoriatic arthritis on phase II and III trials for the treatment of plaque-type psoriasis. Of relevance, one trial evaluates clinical to withdrawal-and-retreatment with brodalumab in psoriatic patients, and another study compares efficacy and safety of brodalumab compared with ustekinumab (anti-IL-12/IL-23p40 agent) and placebo [77].

1.14. Potential of pharmacokinetic and pharmacodynamics drug interactions using monoclonal antibodies

Most of the pharmacokinetic drug–drug interactions (DDIs) of small molecules occur at the level of modulation of activity/levels of the enzymes and/or transporters involved in their biodegradation/bioactivation and/or disposition. Because these enzymes and/or transporters are not involved in the elimination processes of mAbs and functional derivatives, it is believed that potential future interactions with concomitant administration of mAbs with small molecules are unlikely. Despite that, monoclonal antibodies are not metabolized by cytochrome enzymes (CYPs) and these are not suspected for drug interactions. However, it is known from in vitro studies [78-82] that the increased activity of certain cytokines is capable of reducing the activity of CYP enzymes:

- CYP1A2 levels by IFN-a, IFN-a-2b, IFN-b, IL-2 and IL-6
- CYP2C8 levels by IL-1
- CYP2C9 levels by IL-2 and IL-10
- CYP2C19 levels by IFN-a-2b, IFN-b, TNF-a, IL-2, and IL-6
- CYP2D6 levels by IFN-a-2b
- CYP2E1 levels by IFN-a-2b and IL2
- CYP3A levels by IL-1, IL-2, IL-6, and IL-10

In contrast to other cytokines, IL-4 was shown to increase the activity of CYP2E1, suggesting that another mechanism of enzyme activity regulation could be involved [78]. The molecular mechanisms underlying downregulation of drug-metabolizing enzyme and transporter levels by cytokines are not fully defined but lower gene and protein expressions have been reported for some nuclear receptors involved in regulation of CYPs and transporters including pregnane X receptor (PXR), constitutive androstane receptor (CAR), and farnesoid X activated receptor (FXR) [83, 84]. Although in vitro systems (e.g., microsomes and hepatocytes) are routinely employed to predict in vivo DDIs of small molecules [85], the use of in vitro systems to predict in vivo interactions between small-molecule drugs and therapeutic proteins is still in development. Most of the problems are caused by poor correlation and extrapolation between in vitro and in vivo results.

Influencing the levels of expression of P-glycoprotein (P-gp), also known as multidrug resistance protein 1 (MDR1), can also contribute to DDIs. Several studies have shown that intestinal P-gp was inversely correlated with the inflammatory disease activity. Cytokine-mediated downregulation of P-gp in inflamed intestine of ulcerative colitis (UC) patients was presumably dependent on disease activity, with a possible contribution from IL-8 [86]. Presence of P-gp in the membranes of blood-brain-barrier (BBB) restricts passage of drug molecules into the brain. Some studies show that activity of P-gp was downregulated after short-term exposure to inflammatory mediators, whereas its activity was upregulated following more prolonged exposure [87, 88].

Modulation of activity of CYP enzymes by monoclonal antibodies, through interactions with ILs, can enter into interactions with drugs, which are metabolized by CYPs. Clinical studies have shown that IL-6 inhibits function of CYP1A2, 2C9, 2C19, and CYP3A4 and the function is normalized by anti-IL-6 receptor antibody – tocilizumab [89]. When patients taking drugs with a narrow therapeutic index that are metabolized by these CYP enzymes, for example, atorvastatin, calcium channel blockers, theophylline, warfarin, phenytoin, cyclosporine, or benzodiazepines, blood levels of these drugs should be monitored and clinicians should be alert for possible interactions. It should be taken into account that monoclonal antibodies have long elimination half-life and the effect on CYP enzymes activity may continue after treatment for several weeks.

Pharmacodynamic (PD) interactions using monoclonal antibodies are also possible. The basic mechanisms that are involved include reduction in target number or target-bearing cell number, thus affecting receptor-mediated clearance [90]. The use of pharmacodynamic interactions to improve the pharmacological effect of monoclonal antibodies is growing [91, 92]. In nonhuman primates, paclitaxel in combination with trastuzumab resulted in a 1.5-fold increase in trastuzumab serum concentration [93]. Similarly, paclitaxel enhances the therapeutic benefit of cetuximab, possibly through inhibition of angiogenesis and the induction of apoptosis [94]. Pharmacodynamic interactions have also been reported in other clinical and preclinical experiments [95-97]. A combination of cetuximab (mAb-targeting epidermal growth factor receptor, EGRF) with either gefitinib or erlotinib (EGRF tyrosine kinase inhibitors) was used to maximize EGRF signaling inhibition [98]. Synergism between these drugs has been reported in vivo in athymic nude mice and in vitro across a variety of human cancer cell models. Synergistic antitumor activity has been reported between a taxane compound (BMS-275183) and cetuximab using athymic nude mice [99].

http://dx.doi.org/10.5772/61774

In addition, a recently published study demonstrated in mice that coadministration of anti-VEGF antibodies reduced the delivery of a second mAb to tumor tissues. This pharmacokinetic–pharmacodynamic interaction was only observable when tumor tissue levels were analyzed as no change in plasma pharmacokinetics was observed [100].

2. Conclusions and future directions

Interleukins represent an attractive target for pharmacological interventions to fine-tune immune cell functions for treatment of human diseases. Discovery and development of therapeutic monoclonal antibodies is an option for achieving these objectives. However, the impact on these intracellular signaling molecules hides many pitfalls, as the border between useful and harmful influence is very thin. Examples of this can be the case with humanized monoclonal antibody directed against CD28 – TGN 1412. During the phase I clinical trial, all six volunteers receiving the drug were hospitalized, at least four of them developed multiple organ dysfunction, despite being administered at a supposed sub-clinical dose of 0.1 mg/kg; approximately 500 times lower than the dose found safe in animals. [101] Another case in this regard is the occurrence of progressive multifocal leukoencephalopathy (PML) in subjects treated with natalizumab. [102] Therefore, it is necessary to extrapolate properly the results obtained from preclinical studies to humans by knowing very well the pharmacological characteristics and evaluation of the risk benefits in order to prevent future tragedies.

Author details

Kaloyan Georgiev* and Marieta Georgieva

*Address all correspondence to: kalgeorgiev@hotmail.com

Department of Pharmacology, Toxicology and Pharmacotherapy, Faculty of Pharmacy, Medical University Varna, Varna, Bulgaria

References

[1] Mizel SB. The interleukins. *FASEB J.* 1989; 3(12): 2379–88.

[2] Akdis M, Burgler S, Crameri R, Eiwegger T, Fujita H, Gomez E, Klunker S, Meyer N, O'Mahony L, Palomares O, Rhyner C, Ouaked N, Schaffartzik A, Van De Veen W, Zeller S, Zimmermann M, Akdis CA. Interleukins, from 1 to 37, and interferon-γ: receptors, functions, and roles in diseases. *J Allergy Clin Immunol.* 2011 Mar; 127(3):701–21.e1-70.

[3] Liu JK. The history of monoclonal antibody development – Progress, remaining challenges and future innovations. *Ann Med Surg (Lond)*. 2014; Sep 11; 3(4):113–6.

[4] Köhler G., Milstein C. Continuous cultures of fused cells secreting antibody of predefined specificity. *Nature*. 1975; 256(5517):495–97.

[5] Leavy O. Therapeutic antibodies: past, present and future. *Nat Rev Immunol*. 2010; 10(5):297.

[6] Sgro C. Side-effects of a monoclonal antibody, muromonab CD3/orthoclone OKT3: a bibliographic review. *Toxicology*. 1995; 105(1):23–29.

[7] Bugelski PJ, Achuthanandam R, Capocasale RJ, Treacy G, Bouman-Thio E. Monoclonal antibody-induced cytokine-release syndrome. *Expert Rev Clin Immunol*. 2009 Sep; 5(5):499–521.

[8] Dinarello CA. Interleukin-1 in the pathogenesis and treatment of inflammatory diseases. *Blood*. 2011 Apr 7; 117(14):3720–32.

[9] Pascual V, Allantaz F, Arce E, Punaro M, Banchereau J. Role of interleukin-1 (IL-1) in the pathogenesis of systemic onset juvenile idiopathic arthritis and clinical response to IL-1 blockade. *J Exp Med*. 2005; 201:1479–86.

[10] Liu C, Hart RP, Liu XJ, Clevenger W, Maki RA, De Souza EB. Cloning and characterization of an alternatively processed human type II interleukin-1 receptor mRNA. *J Biol Chem*. 1996 Aug 23; 271(34):20965–72.

[11] Dayer JM, de Rochemonteix B, Burrus B, Demczuk S, and Dinarello CA. Human recombinant interleukin 1 stimulates collagenase and prostaglandin E2 production by human synovial cells. *J Clin Invest*. 1986; 77: 645–648.

[12] Lust JA, Donovan KA. The role of interleukin-1beta in the pathogenesis of multiple myeloma. *Hematol Oncol Clin North Am*. 1999; 13:1117–25.

[13] Lust JA, Lacy MQ, Zeldenrust SR, Dispenzieri A, Gertz MA, Witzig TE, Kumar S, Hayman SR,Russell SJ, Buadi FK, et al. Induction of a chronic disease state in patients with smoldering or indolent multiple myeloma by targeting interleukin1beta-induced interleukin 6 production and the myeloma proliferative component. *Mayo Clin Proc*. 2009; 84:114–22.

[14] Mandrup-Poulsen, T, Pickersgill L, Donath MY. Blockade of interleukin 1 in type 1 diabetes mellitus. *Natur Rev Endocrinol*. 6, 158–166 (2010).

[15] Maedler K, Sergeev P, Ris F, Oberholzer J, Joller-Jemelka HI, Spinas GA, Kaiser N, Halban PA, Donath MY. Glucose-induced β cell production of IL-1β contributes to glucotoxicity in human pancreatic islets. *J Clin Invest*. 110, 851–860 (2002)

[16] Donath, M. Y. & Shoelson, S. E. Type 2 diabetes as an inflammatory disease. *Natur Rev Immunol*. 2011; 11:98–107.

[17] Stienstra R, Joosten LA, Koenen T, van Tits B, van Diepen JA,. et al. The inflammasome-mediated caspase-1 activation controls adipocyte differentiation and insulin sensitivity. *Cell Metab.* 2011; 12:593–605. doi: 10.1016/j.cmet.2010.11.011.

[18] Dinarello CA, Simon A, van der Meer JW. Treating inflammation by blocking interleukin-1 in a broad spectrum of diseases. *Nat Rev Drug Discov.* 2012 Aug; 11(8):633–52. doi: 10.1038/nrd3800.

[19] Vandanmagsar B, Youm YH, Ravussin A, Galgani JE, Stadler K, Mynatt RL, Ravussin E, Stephens JM, Dixit VD. The NLRP3 inflammasome instigates obesity-induced inflammation and insulin resistance. *Natur Med.* 2011; 17, 179–188. doi: 10.1038/nm.2279

[20] Giat E, Lidar M. Cryopyrin-associated periodic syndrome. *Isr Med Assoc J.* 2014 Oct; 16(10):659–61.

[21] Chakraborty A, Tannenbaum S, Rordorf C, Lowe PJ, Floch D, Gram H, Roy S. Pharmacokinetic and pharmacodynamic properties of canakinumab, a human anti-interleukin-1β monoclonal antibody. *Clin Pharmacokinet.* 2012 Jun 1; 51(6):e1–18. doi: 10.2165/11599820-000000000-00000.

[22] Lachmann HJ, Kone-Paut I, Kuemmerle-Deschner JB, Leslie KS, Hachulla E, Quartier P, Gitton X, Widmer A, Patel N, Hawkins PN; Canakinumab in CAPS Study Group. Use of canakinumab in the cryopyrin-associated periodic syndrome. *N Engl J Med.* 2009 Jun 4; 360(23):2416–25.

[23] Dubois EA, Rissmann R, Cohen AF. Rilonacept and canakinumab. *Br J Clin Pharmacol.* 2011 May; 71(5):639–41. doi: 10.1111/j.1365-2125.2011.03958.x.

[24] Roell MK, Issafras H, Bauer RJ, Michelson KS, Mendoza N, Vanegas SI, Gross LM, Larsen PD, Bedinger DH, Bohmann DJ, et al. Kinetic approach to pathway attenuation using XOMA 052, a regulatory therapeutic antibody that modulates interleukin-1beta activity. *J Biol Chem.* 2010; 285:20607-14.

[25] Abbate A, Van Tassell BW, Seropian IM et al. Interleukin-1beta modulation using a genetically engineered antibody prevents adverse cardiac remodelling following acute myocardial infarction in the mouse. *Eur J Heart Fail.* 2010; 12, 319–22.

[26] Bhaskar V, Yin J, Mirza AM, Phan D, Vanegas S, Issafras H, Michelson K, Hunter JJ, Kantak SS. Monoclonal antibodies targeting IL-1 beta reduce biomarkers of atherosclerosis in vitro and inhibit atherosclerotic plaque formation in Apolipoprotein E-deficient mice. *Atherosclerosis.* 2011; 216, 313–20. doi: 10.1016/j.atherosclerosis.2011.02.026.

[27] Cavelti-Weder C, Babians-Brunner A, Keller C, Stahel MA, Kurz-Levin M, Zayed H, Solinger AM, Mandrup-Poulsen T, Dinarello CA, Donath MY. Effects of gevokizumab on glycemia and inflammatory markers in type 2 diabetes. *Diab Care.* 2012; 35:1654–62. doi: 10.2337/dc11-2219.

[28] Clinicaltrials.gov www.clinicaltrials.gov

[29] Gül A, Tugal-Tutkun I, Dinarello CA, Reznikov L, Esen BA, Mirza A, Scannon P, Solinger A. Interleukin-1-regulating antibody XOMA 052 (gevokizumab) in the treatment of acute exacerbations of resistant uveitis of Behcet's disease: an open-label pilot study. *Ann Rheum Dis*. 2012; 71:563–6. doi: 10.1136/annrheumdis-2011-155143.

[30] Goh AX, Bertin-Maghit S, Ping Yeo S, Ho AW, Derks H, Mortellaro A, Wang CI. A novel human anti-interleukin-1β neutralizing monoclonal antibody showing in vivo efficacy. *MAbs*. 2014 May-Jun; 6(3):765–73. doi: 10.4161/mabs.28614.

[31] Malek TR. The main function of IL-2 is to promote the development of T regulatory cells. *J Leukocyte Biol*. 2003, 74(6): 961–5.

[32] Liao W, Lin JX, Leonard WJ. IL-2 family cytokines: new insights into the complex roles of IL-2 as a broad regulator of T helper cell differentiation. *Curr Opin Immunol*. 2011; 23:598–604. doi: 10.1016/j.coi.2011.08.003.

[33] Whittington R, Faulds D. Interleukin-2. A review of its pharmacological properties and therapeutic use in patients with cancer. *Drugs*. 1993 Sep; 46(3):446–514.

[34] Chapman TM, Keating GM. Basiliximab: a review of its use as induction therapy in renal transplantation. *Drugs*. 2003; 63(24):2803–35.

[35] Kovarik JM, Kahan BD, Rajagopalan PR, Bennett W, Mulloy LL, Gerbeau C, Hall ML. Population pharmacokinetics and exposure-response relationships for basiliximab in kidney transplantation. The U.S. Simulect Renal Transplant Study Group. *Transplantation*. 1999 Nov 15;68(9):1288–94.

[36] Lawen J, Davies E, Morad F, et al. Basiliximab (Simulect) is safe and effective in combination with triple therapy of Neoral, steroids and CellCept in renal transplant patients. *Transplantation*. 2000: 69:S260.

[37] Vincenti F, Kirkman R, Light S, Bumgardner G, Pescovitz M, Halloran P, Neylan J, Wilkinson A, Ekberg H, Gaston R, Backman L, Burdick J. Interleukin-2-receptor blockade with daclizumab to prevent acute rejection in renal transplantation. Daclizumab Triple Therapy Study Group. *N Engl J Med*. 1998 Jan 15; 338(3):161–5.

[38] Hong JC, Kahan BD. Immunosuppressive agents in organ transplantation: past, present, and future. *Semin Nephrol*. 2000 Mar; 20(2):108–25.

[39] Ding, C., Cicuttini, F., Jones, G. Targeting IL-6 in the treatment of inflammatory and autoimmune diseases. *Expert Opin Investig Drugs*. 2009; 18:1457–66.

[40] Stannus O, Jones G, Cicuttini F, Parameswaran V, Quinn S, Burgess J, Ding C. Circulating levels of IL-6 and TNF-a are associated with knee radiographic osteoarthritis and knee cartilage loss in older adults. *Osteoarthritis Cart*. 2010; 18:1441–47. doi: 10.1016/j.joca.2010.08.016.

[41] Ding C, Cicuttini F, Jones G. Targeting IL-6 in the treatment of inflammatory and autoimmune diseases. *Expert Opin Investig Drugs*. 2009; 18:1457–66.

[42] Cronstein BN. Interleukin-6–a key mediator of systemic and local symptoms in rheumatoid arthritis. *Bull NYU Hosp Jt Dis*. 2007; 65 (Suppl. 1):S11–S15.

[43] Oldfield V, Dhillon S, Plosker GL. Tocilizumab: a review of its use in the management of rheumatoid arthritis. *Drugs*. 2009; 69(5):609–32.

[44] Burmester GR, Rubbert-Roth A, Cantagrel A, Hall S, Leszczynski P, et al. A randomized, double-blind, parallel group study of the safety and efficacy of tocilizumab SC versus tocilizumab IV, in combination with traditional Dmards in patients with moderate to severe RA. *Arthritis Rheum*. 2012; 64(10):S1075. doi: 10.1136/annrheumdis-2013-203523.

[45] Mihara, M., Kasutani, K., Okazaki, M. et al. (2005) Tocilizumab inhibits signal transduction mediated by both mIL-6R and sIL-6R, but not by the receptors of other members of IL-6 cytokine family. *Int Immunopharmacol*. 5 (12): 1731–40.

[46] Kishimoto, T. Interleukin-6: discovery of a pleiotropic cytokine. Arthritis Res. Ther., (2006) 8 (Suppl. 2), S2.

[47] Zhang X, Chen YC, Fettner S, Rowell L, Gott T, Grimsey P, Unsworth A. Pharmacokinetics and pharmacodynamics of tocilizumab after subcutaneous administration in patients with rheumatoid arthritis. *Int J Clin Pharmacol Ther*. 2013 Aug; 51(8):620–30. doi: 10.5414/CP201904.

[48] Hashizume M., H. Yoshida, N. Koike, M. Suzuki, and M. Mihara. Overproduced interleukin 6 decreases blood lipid levels via upregulation of very-low-density lipoprotein receptor. *Ann Rheum Dis*. 2010; 69(4): 741–46.

[49] Genovese MC, Rubbert-Roth A, Smolen JS, Kremer J, Khraishi M, et al., Long-term safety and efficacy of tocilizumab in patients with rheumatoid arthritis: a cumulative analysis of up to 4.6 years of exposure. *J Rheumatol*. 2013; 40(6): 768–80. doi: 10.3899/jrheum.120687.

[50] Smolen JS, Beaulieu A, Rubbert-Roth A, Ramos-Remus C, Rovensky J et al. Effect of interleukin-6 receptor inhibition with tocilizumab in patients with rheumatoid arthritis (OPTION study): a doubleblind, placebo-controlled, randomised trial. *Lancet*. 2008; 371 (9617), 987–97.

[51] Genovese MC, McKay JD, Nasonov EL, Mysler EF, da Silva NA, et al. Interleukin-6 receptor inhibition with tocilizumab reduces disease activity in rheumatoid arthritis with inadequate response to diseasemodifying antirheumatic drugs: the tocilizumab in combination with traditional disease-modifying antirheumatic drug therapy study. *Arthritis Rheum*. 2008; 58 (10), 2968–80.

[52] Nishimoto N, Hashimoto J, Miyasaka N, Yamamoto K, Kawai S, et al. Study of active controlled monotherapy used for rheumatoid arthritis, an IL-6 inhibitor (SAMURAI):

evidence of clinical and radiographic benefit from an X ray reader-blinded randomised controlled trial of tocilizumab. *Ann Rheum Dis*. 2007; 66 (9), 1162–67.

[53] Rossi JF, Lu ZY, Jourdan M, Klein B. Interleukin-6 as a Therapeutic Target. *Clin Cancer Res*. 2015 Mar 15; 21(6):1248–57.

[54] Deisseroth A, Ko CW, Nie L, Zirkelbach JF, Zhao L, Bullock J, Mehrotra N, Del Valle P, Saber H, Sheth C, Gehrke B, Justice R, Farrell A, Pazdur R. FDA approval: siltuximab for the treatment of patients with multicentric Castleman disease. *Clin Cancer Res*. 2015 Mar 1; 21(5):950–4. doi: 10.1158/1078-0432.CCR-14-1678.

[55] Genovese MC, Fleischmann RM, Fiore S, et al. Sarilumab, a subcutaneously-administered, fully-human monoclonal antibody inhibitor of the IL-6 receptor: Relationship between EULAR responses and change from baseline of selected clinical parameters. *Ann Rheum Dis*. 2013; 72(Suppl 3):620.

[56] Wang L-H, Xue Y, Liu X, et al. Preclinical development of sarilumab, the first fully human monoclonal antibody (mAb) against IL-6R alpha: utilization and value of double humanized animal model. *Ann Rheum Dis*. 2013; 72(Suppl 3):375.

[57] Rafique A, Martin J, Blome M, et al. Evaluation of the binding kinetics and functional bioassay activity of sarilumab and tocilizumab to the human IL-6 receptor (IL-6R) alpha. *Ann Rheum Dis*. 2013; 72(Suppl 3):797.

[58] Radin AR, Mellis SJ, Jasson M, et al. REGN88/SAR153191, a fully-human interleukin-6 receptor monoclonal antibody, reduces acute phase reactants in patients with rheumatoid arthritis: preliminary observations from Phase 1 studies. *Arthritis Rheum*. 2010; 62(Suppl 10):S470.

[59] Radin A, Mellis S, Jasson M, et al. Safety and effects on markers of inflammation of subcutaneously administered REGN88/SAR153191, an interleukin-6 receptor inhibitor, in patients with rheumatoid arthritis: findings from Phase 1 studies. *Ann Rheum Dis*. 2010; 69(Suppl 3):99.

[60] Huizinga TW, Kivitz AJ, Rell-Bakalarska M, et al. Sarilumab for the treatment of moderate-to-severe rheumatoid arthritis: results of a phase 2, randomized, double blind, Placebo-Controlled, International Study. *Ann Rheum Dis*. 2012; 71(Suppl 3):60.

[61] Huizinga TW, Fleischmann RM, Jasson M, Radin AR, van Adelsberg J, Fiore S, Huang X, Yancopoulos GD, Stahl N, Genovese MC. Sarilumab, a fully human monoclonal antibody against IL-6Rα in patients with rheumatoid arthritis and an inadequate response to methotrexate: efficacy and safety results from the randomised SARIL-RA-MOBILITY Part A trial. *Ann Rheum Dis*. 2014 Sep; 73(9):1626–34. doi: 10.1136/annrheumdis-2013-204405.

[62] Menter A, Gottlieb A, Feldman SR et al. Guidelines of care for the management of psoriasis and psoriatic arthritis: section 1. Overview of psoriasis and guidelines of

care for the treatment of psoriasis with biologics. *J Am Acad Dermatol.* 2008; 58:826–50.

[63] Nestle FO, Kaplan DH, Barker J. Mechanisms of disease: Psoriasis. *N Engl J Med.* 2009; 2652 361:496–509.

[64] Murphy KM, Reiner SL. The lineage decisions of helper T cells. *Nat Rev Immunol.* 2002;2(12):933–44.

[65] Langrish CL, Chen Y, Blumenschein WM, et al. IL-23 drives a pathogenic T cell population that induces autoimmune inflammation. *J Exp Med.* 2005; 201(2):233–40.

[66] Zhu YW, Mendelsohn A, Pendley C, Davis HM, Zhou H. Population pharmacokinetics of ustekinumab in patients with active psoriatic arthritis. *Int J Clin Pharmacol Ther.* 2010 Dec; 48(12):830–46.

[67] Papp KA, Griffiths CE, Gordon K, Lebwohl M, Szapary PO, Wasfi Y, Chan D, Hsu MC, Ho V, Ghislain PD, Strober B, Reich K; PHOENIX 1 Investigators; PHOENIX 2 Investigators; ACCEPT Investigators. Long-term safety of ustekinumab in patients with moderate-to-severe psoriasis: final results from 5 years of follow-up. *Br J Dermatol.* 2013 Apr; 168(4):844–54.

[68] Yao Z, Painter SL, Fanslow WC, et al. Human IL-17: a novel cytokine derived from T cells. *J Immunol.* 1995; 155(12):5483–6

[69] Griffiths CE, Strober BE, van de Kerkhof P, Ho V, Fidelus-Gort R, Yeilding N, Guzzo C, Xia Y, Zhou B, Li S, Dooley LT, Goldstein NH, Menter A; ACCEPT Study Group. Comparison of ustekinumab and etanercept for moderate-to-severe psoriasis. *N Engl J Med.* 2010 Jan 14; 362(2):118–28.

[70] Gee K, Guzzo C, Che Mat NF, Ma W, Kumar A. The IL-12 family of cytokines in infection, inflammation and autoimmune disorders. Inflam *Allergy-Drug Targets.* 2009; 8:40–52.

[71] Bartlett HS and Million RP. Targeting the IL-17–TH17 pathway. *Natur Rev Drug Discov.* 2015; 14:11–12. doi:10.1038/nrd4518

[72] Langley RG, Elewski BE, Lebwohl M, Reich K, Griffiths CE, Papp K, Puig L, Nakagawa H, Spelman L, Sigurgeirsson B, Rivas E, Tsai TF, Wasel N, Tyring S, Salko T, Hampele I, Notter M, Karpov A, Helou S, Papavassilis C; ERASURE Study Group; FIXTURE Study Group. Secukinumab in plaque psoriasis-results of two phase 3 trials. *N Engl J Med.* 2014 Jul 24; 371(4):326–38. doi: 10.1056/NEJMoa1314258.

[73] Leonardi C1, Matheson R, Zachariae C, Cameron G, Li L, Edson-Heredia E, Braun D, Banerjee S. Anti-interleukin-17 monoclonal antibody ixekizumab in chronic plaque psoriasis. *N Engl J Med.* 2012; 366(13):1190-9. doi: 10.1056/NEJMoa1109997.

[74] Available from: http://www.clinicaltrials.gov/ct2/results?term=ixekizumab+AND+psoriasis&Search=Search

[75] Russell CB, Kerkof K, Bigler J, et al. Blockade of the IL-17R with AMG827 leads to rapid reversal of gene expression and histopathologic abnormalities in human psoriatic skin [abstract]. *J Invest Dermatol.* 2010; 130:S46

[76] Papp KA, Leonardi C, Menter A, Ortonne JP, Krueger JG, et al. Brodalumab, an anti-interleukin- 17-receptor antibody for psoriasis. *N Engl J Med.* 2012; 366(13):1181-9. doi: 10.1056/NEJMoa1109017.

[77] Available from: http://www.clinicaltrials.gov/ct2/results?term=brodalumab+AND+psoriasis&Search=Search

[78] Abdel-Razzak Z, Loyer P, Fautrel A, Gautier JC, Corcos L, Turlin B, et al. Cytokines down-regulate expression of major cytochrome P-450 enzymes in adult human hepatocytes in primary culture. *Mol Pharmacol.* 1993; 44(4):707–15.

[79] Huang SM, Zhao H, Lee JI, Reynolds K, Zhang L, Temple R, et al. Therapeutic protein-drug interactions and implications for drug development. *Clin Pharmacol Ther.* 2010; 87(4):497–503.

[80] Dickmann LJ, Patel SK, Wienkers LC, Slatter JG. Effects of Interleukin 1beta (IL-1beta) and IL-1beta/Interleukin 6 (IL-6) combinations on drug metabolizing enzymes in human hepatocyte culture. *Curr Drug Metab.* 2012; 13(7):930–7.

[81] Molanaei H, Stenvinkel P, Qureshi AR, Carrero JJ, Heimburger O, Lindholm B, et al. Metabolism of alprazolam (a marker of CYP3A4) in hemodialysis patients with persistent inflammation. *Eur J Clin Pharmacol.* 2012; 68(5):571–7. doi: 10.1007/s00228-011-1163-8.

[82] Yang Q, Doshi U, Li N, Li AP. Effects of culture duration on gene expression of p450 isoforms, uptake and efflux transporters in primary hepatocytes cultured in the absence and presence of interleukin-6: implications for experimental design for the evaluation of downregulatory effects of biotherapeutics. *Curr Drug Metab.* 2012; 13(7):938–46.

[83] Teng S, Piquette-Miller M. The involvement of the pregnane X receptor in hepatic gene regulation during inflammation in mice. *J Pharmacol Exp Ther.* 2005; 312(2):841–8.

[84] Beigneux AP, Moser AH, Shigenaga JK, Grunfeld C, Feingold KR. Reduction in cytochrome P-450 enzyme expression is associated with repression of CAR (constitutive androstane receptor) and PXR (pregnane X receptor) in mouse liver during the acute phase response. *Biochem Biophys Res Commun.* 2002; 293(1):145–9.

[85] Rostami-Hodjegan A, Tucker GT. Simulation and prediction of in vivo drug metabolism in human populations from in vitro data. *Nat Rev Drug Discov.* 2007; 6(2):140–8.

[86] Ufer M, Häsler R, Jacobs G, Haenisch S, Lächelt S, Faltraco F, Sina C, Rosenstiel P, Nikolaus S, Schreiber S, Cascorbi I. Decreased sigmoidal ABCB1 (P-glycoprotein) ex-

pression in ulcerative colitis is associated with disease activity. *Pharmacogenomics*, 2009; 10(12), 1941–53.

[87] Roberts DJ, Goralski KB. A critical overview of the influence of inflammation and infection on P-glycoprotein expression and activity in the brain. *Expert Opin Drug Metab Toxicol.*, 2008; 4(10), 1245–64.

[88] Miller DS, Bauer B, Hartz AM. Modulation of P-glycoprotein at the blood-brain barrier: opportunities to improve central nervous system pharmacotherapy. *Pharmacol Rev.*, 2008; 60(2), 196-209.

[89] Navarro-Millán I; Singh JA, Curtis JR. Systematic review of tocilizumab for rheumatoid arthritis: a new biologic agent targeting the interleukin-6 receptor. *Clin Ther.* 2012; 34(4), 788-802.e3. doi: 10.1016/j.clinthera.2012.02.014.

[90] Mould DR, Green B. Pharmacokinetics and pharmacodynamics of monoclonal antibodies: concepts and lessons for drug development. *BioDrugs*. 2010; 24(1):23–39.

[91] Sharpe AH, Abbas AK. T-cell costimulation–biology, therapeutic potential, and challenges. *N Engl J Med*. 2006; 355(10):973–5.

[92] Suntharalingam G, Perry MR, Ward S, Brett SJ, Castello-Cortes A, Brunner MD, et al. Cytokine storm in a phase 1 trial of the anti-CD28 monoclonal antibody TGN1412. *N Engl J Med*. 2006; 355(10):1018–28.

[93] Slamon DJ, Leyland-Jones B, Shak S, Fuchs H, Paton V, Bajamonde A, et al. Use of chemotherapy plus a monoclonal antibody against HER2 for metastatic breast cancer that overexpresses HER2. *N Engl J Med*. 2001; 344(11):783–92.

[94] Inoue K, Slaton JW, Perrotte P, Davis DW, Bruns CJ, Hicklin DJ, McConkey DJ, Sweeney P, Radinsky R, Dinney CP. Paclitaxel enhances the effects of the anti-epidermal growth factor receptor monoclonal antibody ImClone C225 in mice with metastatic human bladder transitional cell carcinoma. *Clin Cancer Res*. 2000; 6(12):4874–84.

[95] Xiong HQ, Rosenberg A, LoBuglio A, Schmidt W, Wolff RA, Deutsch J, et al. Cetuximab, a monoclonal antibody targeting the epidermal growth factor receptor, in combination with gemcitabine for advanced pancreatic cancer: a multicenter phase II trial. *JClin Oncol*. 2004; 22(13):2610–6.

[96] Dowlati A, Nethery D, Liu J. Combined inhibition of epidermal growth factor receptor (EGFR) and JAK/Stat signaling results in superior growth inhibition in A431 cell line as compared to single agent therapy [abstract]. *Proc Am Assoc Cancer Res*. 2003; 44(800):459.

[97] Finn RS, Wilson CA, Sanders J. Targeting the epidermal growth factor receptor (EGFR) and HER-2 with OSI-774 and trastuzumab, respectively, in HER-2 overexpressing human breast cancer cell lines results in a therapeutic advantage in vitro [abstract]. *Proc Am Assoc Cancer Res*. 2003; 44:235.

[98] Huang S, Armstrong EA, Benavente S, Chinnaiyan P, Harari PM. Dual-agent molecular targeting of the epidermal growth factor receptor (EGFR): combining anti-EGFR antibody with tyrosine kinase inhibitor. *Cancer Res*. 2004; 64(15):5355–62.

[99] Rose WC, Wild R. Therapeutic synergy of oral taxane BMS-275183 and cetuximab versus human tumor xenografts. *Clin Cancer Res*. 2004; 10(21):7413–7.

[100] Abuqayyas L, Balthasar JP. Investigation of the Role of Fc gamma R and FcRn in mAb distribution to the brain. *Mol Pharm*. 2012 Aug 23. doi: 10.1021/mp300214k.

[101] Suntharalingam G, Perry MR, Ward S, Brett SJ, Castello-Cortes A, Brunner MD, Panoskaltsis N. Cytokine storm in a phase 1 trial of the anti-CD28 monoclonal antibody TGN1412. *N Eng J Med*. 2006; 355:1018–28

[102] Stüve O, Gold R, Chan A, Mix E, Zettl U, Kieseier BC. Alpha4-Integrin antagonism with natalizumab: effects and adverse effects. *J Neurol*. 2008; 255 Suppl. 6: 58–65. doi: 10.1007/s00415-008-6011-0.

Chapter 13

Human Vector-Borne Transmissible Parasitic Diseases in Montenegro

Bogdanka Andric, Aleksandar Andric and Mileta Golubovic

Additional information is available at the end of the chapter

http://dx.doi.org/10.5772/61534

Abstract

Montenegro is an endemic country for a significant number of vector-borne diseases (VBD). Natural conditions and geographical position (Mediterranean area) are favorable for the existence of the disease, and its expansion (1). Current vector-borne transmissible parasitic infections that haves been registered in Montenegro includes: leishmaniasis, babesiosis, malaria, and filariasis (dirofilariasis).

The causers of leishmaniasis are the members of protozoa leishmania species (spp). The phlebotomies are the primary vectors in transmission of parasites. Documented cases of visceral leishmaniasis (VL) from 1992 to 2014 in Montenegro present 84 cases with of Kala-azar, and the 1 case of skin leishmaniasis. In 2014 the coinfection of leishmaniasis and HIV/AIDS for the first time was registered in one case.

Babesiosis is a parasitic infection similar to malaria.

In transmission of parasites, the primary vectors have different tick species, possibly the other blood meal vectors (sand flies, mosquitoes, and bugs).

Dispersion of the infection in the worldwide is enabled by a wide range of reservoirs of parasites. Examinations in Europe proved that babesia is the most frequent agent of co-infection together with *Borrelia burgdorferi*. The first diagnosed cases of human babesiosis in Montenegro were registered in 2011. By the end of 2013, 12 cases were diagnosed. The coinfection of babesia and B.burgdorferi were registered in 73% cases.

Malaria is the most known parasitic transmissible disease in the world. The causative agent is *Plasmodium*, a genus of *Apicomplexa*, which is transmitted by mosquitoes of the genus *Anopheles*. In Montenegro, the disease was officially eradicated after World War II, but we continuously register 04 cases of imported malaria per year (sailors, travelers to endemic areas). These facts are significant because of the existence of the transfers and the favorable conditions for their maintenance, and therefore the fear that the epidemiological focus can be rebuilt.

In 2014 one case of human dirofilariasis was diagnosed for the first time in Montenegro.

Keywords: Leishmaniasis, Babesiosis, Malaria, Dirofilariasis

1. Introduction

The transmissible way of spreading infection from animals to humans by different vectors is of great importance in contemporary world infectious pathology. This group includes a large number of vectors that cause different emerging diseases, the so called zoonoses. [1, 2]

Vectors play complex role in the epidemiology and pathogenesis of these diseases, with abundance of species that provide the resources for expansion into new geographic areas and direct participation in the pathogenic immunity mechanisms of infections [3]

The natural factors are adjacent to the problems of globalization and increase the importance of these diseases in the world due to: numerical magnification of human population, frequent contact between human and animal population, and behavioral changes in the human population. Also climate change is of special interest [3, 4]

Mediterranean area presents the region with frequent representations of a wide specter of vectorborne diseases (VBD). Montenegro is a Mediterranean country, geographically situated in the Balkan area. Natural conditions in Montenegro represent an ideal ecological basis for the existence of VBD [5]

New characteristics of parasitic VBD present increased frequency, severe clinical courses, and difficulties in diagnosis of nondefined way and prognosis of diseases. On the basis of this fact, they are imputed in the group of emerging zoonoses, occupying an important place [6,7,8]. Frequent multietiological (coinfective) forms of diseases represent additional problem in this group of parasitic VBD [9], based on the natural factors (coexisting of different causers in common endemic areas, natural hosts, cotransmissions of these agents with common vectors).

Based on the changes of the immunological characteristics of parasitic agents in infected humans, parasitic VBD can be provided by opportunistic action and reactivation of different and numerous intracellular microorganisms and cooperative action, with negative reflection on difficulties and uncertain prognosis of coinfections (eg: coinfection of Leishmania parasites and HIV, babesia parasites and B. burgdorferi [10,11]. In addition, coinfections represent big diagnostic problem.

Increasing multiresistance to drugs and necessary application of combined therapy represent multiple problems [12,13]. In national human pathology in Montenegro, there not enough research space has been dedicated to parasitic VBD hence they have not received attention in the light of their significance for the present or for the future.

An analysis observed four different parasitic transmissible zoonotic diseases, in different periods of the last decade, by using available diagnostic methods.

Current transmissible parasitic zoonoses that are registered in Montenegro and that should be a field for future research work include: leishmaniasis, babesiosis, and malaria. In 2014, the first registered case of autochthonous dirofilariasis in Montenegro presented a new dimension of the needs and seriousness of the disease, showing that new factors of transmissible parasitic zoonoses should be paid much more attention [14].

2. Methodology

2.1. Leishmaniasis

The number of diseased cases refers to the period 1992 to 2014. In the diagnostic procedure epidemiological, clinical, and laboratory methods were used. Diagnosis was etiologically confirmed through bone marrow biopsy analysis by direct microscoping of serial sections colored with Giemsa (stain), reticulin, and PAS method and by immune-biochemical methods (TdT, CD34, CD117, CD15, glucophorin A, CD31, CD79a, CD20, CD3, CD45RO, CD38, kappa, lambda, IgG, IgM, IgA, CD68). Serologically, with agglutination test, the diagnosis was confirmed in 56% of the cases.

Taking into consideration that in our country wild jackals and domestic dogs are the primary natural carriers of Leichmania parasites, significant for infections in humans, a screening of 1500 serum samples of both asylum dogs and stay dogs was done by using the indirect immunoefluorescence (IIF) method.

2.2. Babesiosis

The clinical characteristics of human babesiosis vary from predominantly asymptomatic (silent disease) to fulminate malignant forms, which depends on the degree of parasitemia and the strength of the immune response of the host.

Babesiosis may be suspected in cases as with tick exposure and tick exposure and history of persistent fevers and hemolytic anemia. The definitive diagnosis was confirmed by detection of intraerythrocytic ring forms of parasites in the periphery blood and by microscopic slides of bone marrow biopsy colored with Giemsa-i and Romanowsky stains. Serological testing (ELISA and Western blot (WB) and *polymerase chain reaction* (PCR) were used for detecting coinfections of babesia parasites with Borrelia burgdorferi. Microscopic slides of bone marrow biopsy colored with Giemsa-i and Romanowsky stains were also used in differentiating babesia from the malaria parasite. Detectable antibody response takes about a week s time post infection. Serologic testing may be falsely negative in an early stage of the disease progression.

2.3. Malaria

In patients with malaria malady epidemiological data play a very important role particularly with regard to residence in endemic areas and the frequent inadequate use of prevention drugs (in our sailors patients).

The golden standard for diagnosis of malaria is microscopic examination using thick and peripheral blood smears.

About 5 % of people with malaria have infections caused by several kinds of parasites therefore the analyses ought to take this into account.

2.4. Filariasis

The difficulty in making diagnosis of filariasis appears to be because of the long absence of disease symptoms in the initial stage. Therefore most people initially do not expect to have the disease. Later, symptoms are only slight and nonspecific. Eosinophilia was not observed in the blood of the patients. The serum IgE levels were normal, and signs of a specific humoral response to antigens of Dirofilaria spp. were absent, although slightly elevated antibody levels of antigens of Onhocerca volvulus could be demonstrated in all the patients.

Surgical removal of the worm and biopsy help in both diagnosis and treatment. Morphological examination of the matured adult worm has limitations in the identification of the exact species since a large number of zoonotic Dirofilaria spp. haves been described. The molecular identification is not widely available. It is also possible that there are different stain variations of Dirofilarial parasites. Molecular analysis of the highly conserved mitochondrial 12S rRNA gene of D. repens showed a 3% deviation from other filarial parasites.

3. Results

3.1. Leishmaniasis

The first cases of leishmaniasis (kala-azar) in Montenegro were registered in 1924/1925, on the Montenegrin coast (Lustica, Baosici). In period 1930 to 1932, new cases were registered in the southern coastal region, between Bar and Ulcinj. Accurate records of the number of patients with disease manifestations do not exist for the period before 1995.

Our study covers the period from 1992 to 2014, with 86 registered cases of leishmaniasis. The visceral leishmaniasis (VL) has been diagnosed in 84 cases, and 1 (1.20%) case with skin leishmaniasis. Coinfection of HIV/AIDS and leishmaniasis in one case was registered for the first time in 2014. The trend of increase in the number of patients with confirmed diagnosiswas present with 0-4 cases per year among 646000 inhabitants.

In the study sample, the child population participates approximately in 37% of the cases and adults in 48%. The diagnosis confirmation was based on microbiological-laboratory and pathohistological methods (Figure 1).

http://dx.doi.org/10.5772/61534

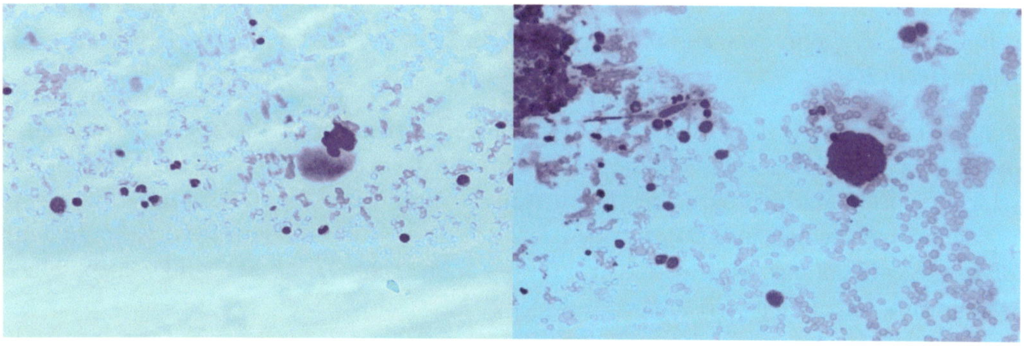

Figure 1. Bone marrow biopsy preparates colored with Romanowsky, visualizing amastigote forms of Leishmania parasites extracellular and in leukocytic cells. (Original preparates courtesy of Prof. Mileta Golubovic, Medical faculty – University of Montenegro)

According to the geographic area where VL was diagnosed, the expansion of endemic foci of the disease in Montenegro is evident. Three to four years ago, disease development was registered solely in the endemic area known between Bar and Ulcinj. According to the collected data, these areas now include the entire coastal area of Montenegro from Ulcinj to Herceg Novi, the Skaadar Lake area, including Podgorica and Cetinje, and even some northern parts of Montenegro.

In our country wild jackals and domestic dogs are the primary natural reservoirs of Leishmania parasites, significant for infections in humans. The screening of 1500 serum samples of both asylum dogs and stray dogs, from different parts of Montenegro, indicated the high infectiveness of dogs with *leishmanias,* which is 83%.

The investigation done in our country presents two types of leishmanias: L.donovani and L. infantum. The primary vectors of parasites are phlebotomi. Epidemiological studies conducted during the period 1996-1999 and in 2003 in the endemic area of VL (southern part of the Montenegrin coast) on 4770 samples of phlebotomi showed presence of five kinds: Ph. perfiliews (1%), Sergentomyia minuta (12%), Ph.papatasi (11%), and Ph.neglecticus (60%). Predominantly Ph.neglecticus is mostly found in indoor areas. It is assumed that the main vector can be found in the Bar-Ulcinj region and in the northeast Mediterranean. Evolutionary adaptability continuously allows phlebotomies to significantly expand their potential as vectors for causers of vector-borne diseases (VBD). The correlation with global changes of ecologic environment and natural base of VBD is already evident in practice and there is a tendency of further growth.

The results of clinical investigations indicate an increase in the number of clinically manifested disease syndromes of VL in humans. The clinical manifestations of Leishmaniasis are not specific and they do not make diagnosis easier. The results of complex interactions between invasiveness and tropism of parasites in relation to side and the immune response of the host. Hypothesis on long-term persistence of live leishmanias after the infection, classifies them into a group of significant opportunistic agents. Coinfective forms of disease, especially in HIV/ AIDS patients, have increased in the worldwide. In Montenegro in 2014, the first coinfection of leishmaniasis and HIV/AIDS was registered in one patient. Incidental confirmation of coinfections of L. donovani and B. burgdorferi (three cases) in a common endemic area was registered in 2003.

Pentavalent antimony drug *Glucantime,* was relatively satisfactory in therapy of leishmaniasis over a long period of time in Montenegro. Problems arose because of the increasing resistance, which has been rapidly progressing. In our study, which took place in 2008 / 2009, there were registered recurrences in 12% of patients of the total sample. Repeated treatment with *Glucantime* was not successful, neither was the use of *Miltefosine*. The best results were obtained by using liposomal *Amphotericin B.*

3.2. Babesiosis

Babesiosis (piroplasmosis) is a malaria-like vector-borne parasitic disease, the so called tick-malaria. It was first described in 1883/1884 in the Balkan (Romania) in sheep. As a cause of human infections, babesia species (spp.) were detected in 1957 in Japan.

In Montenegro the disease was first confirmed in September 2011 based on hematological and microbiological examinations. Since 2013, there have been 12 cases detected. Fourteen patients were with positive anamneses of tick bite. Six patients were with skin manifesting erythema migrans (EM) identified in examinations that were associated with Lyme borreliosis (LB). By serological methods ELISA and Western blot and PCR method, the diagnosis of coinfections of babesia parasite and B. burgdorferi was confirmed in 72% of the patients, a total of 12 patients with confirmed babesiosis.

Analyzing demographic characteristics showed all 12 cases of the diagnosed babesiosis to be between 35 and 65 years of age, with professional exposure in rural parts of Montenegro. In the clinical presentation of all patients, nonspecific symptoms are dominant. There are several dominant symptoms: prolonged febricity, feebleness, and headache and changes in the laboratory findings (anemia, indirect type of hyperbilirubinemia, and moderately increased activity of serum aminotransferases, hypoproteinemia, and hypoalbuminemia) (Table 1).

Anemia	80 %
Leukopenia	45 %
Thrombocytopenia	11 %
Increased level of serum aminotransferases	10 %
Transitory respiratory disturbances	7 %
Syndrome of infective mononucleosis	15 %
Syndrome of acute leukosis	2 %
Prolonged febricity	29 %

Table 1. Clinical Laboratory Disturbances in Manifested Babesiosis in Our Patients N-12

The confirmation of etiological diagnosis of the disease was based primarily on the fact that intraerythrocytic annular forms of the parasite have been found in the peripheral blood, stained accortding to with Giemsa, and on the basis of microscopic slides of bone marrow biopsy stained with Romanowsky in 12 cases (Figure 2).

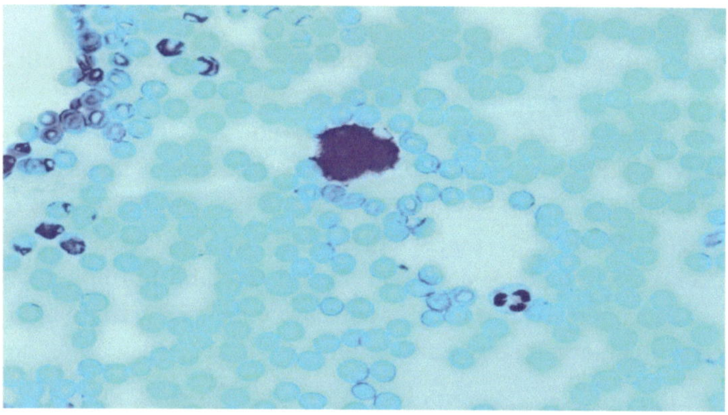

Figure 2. Ring forms of babesia parasite in intraerythrocytic position in our patient. (Courtesy of Prof Mileta Golubovic, Institute for pathology Medical faculty University of Montenegro 2011]

In endemic areas, the asymptomatic forms of babesiosis are the most frequent. Asymptomatic parasitemia can last for months, even years. This latent infection can be reactivated by stress, splenectomy, and immunosuppressive therapy. In human infections, babesia is a significant opportunistic agent.

The largest number of infected cases with babesia does not require a specific therapy treatment (silent disease). After the diagnosis was made in all cases, treatment was administered. There were two types of drugs used: *quinine* and *clindamycin* (within 7 to 10 days), which we also applied in our patients. Recent studies emphasize efficiency of *atovaquone* and *azithromycine.* Supportive and symptomatic treatment is important in severe cases.

3.3. Malaria

Malaria is the most frequent transmissible parasitic disease in the world. The causative agent Plasmodium is a genus of Apicomplexa parasites. Of the over 200 known species of Plasmodium, at least 11 species are continually competent for infection in humans. The most frequent are Pl. falciparum, Pl. vivax, Pl. ovale, and Pl. malariae. The mosquitoes of the genus Anopheles are carriers of parasites in humans. There are about 500 different species of anopheles, and 60 of them can transmit the disease. The parasite always has two hosts in its life cycle: a vector – usually a mosquito – and a vertebrate host.

Based on the historical documentation, in the period from 1923 until 1943 in Montenegro there were 28486 registered cases of malaria (data from the *Jovan Kuljaca* 1925). Most severe cases of the disease have been recorded in the vicinity of Ulcinj, Skadar Lake, Rijeka Crnojevica, and Zeta. Mild cases of disease were registered in Podgorica, Danilovgrad, Niksic, Berane, Bijelo

Polje, Andrijevica, and Plav. Extermination of mosquitoes began in 1947, so that malaria was officially eradicated after World War II in our country, but the cases of imported malaria (sailors, travelers to endemic areas), 1–4 cases per year, continued to be registered. Considering this the fear that the endemic foci can be rebuilt is justified. Fortunately some climatic factors do not favoring the anopheles species therefore malaria is very rare or even absent in the United States and Europe.

Imported malaria is a diagnostic and therapeutic problem. In the period from 2006 to 2013, we followed nonspecific laboratory analysis in 16 febrile returnees from Africa. It was found that the non-specific laboratory results were useful as an additional parameter for making diagnosis of malaria, with quick and simple diagnostic orientation. This is primarily related to thrombocytopenia, leukopenia, and hyperglycemia and increased level of serum aminotransferases activity and *lactate dehydrogenase* (LDH), urticaria, and hypocholesterinemia. It has been shown that hypocholesterinemia, severe anemia and elevated fibrinogen significantly prolonged the patient s recovery. Thrombocytopenia and increased activity of LDH were significantly associated with enlarged spleen and liver.

The most important groups of antimalarial drugs are: *Quinolone*, *Artemizin*, and *antifolates*.

New antimalarial drugs is *Atovaxon*. The big problem of treatment is resistance, particularly of Pl. falciparum. In more severe forms of the disease, in suspected resistance, combined therapy is applied. In severe forms of malaria, parenteral treatment is required.

3.4. Filariasis (Dirofilariasis)

Filariasis has systemic parasitic (worms) zoonosis from the group of VBD. Blood-feeding arthropods are those that can be transmitted. In most of cases the infective larvae (*microfilariae*) are injected through mosquito bites. A large number of mosquito species participate in transmission. Some species of fleas (*black flea*), lice, and ticks are also presumed to act as vectors. Different types of thread-like nematodes are the cause of disease in humans. The most frequent cause of filarial disease in the world is Wuchereria bancrofti. Among the many species of Dirofilaria, the most prevalent are two main filarial species (D.immitis and D.repens) that have adapted to canine, feline, and human hosts. At the same time, both the D. immitis and D. repens are themselves hosts to symbiotic bacteria of the genus Wolbachia. For the past few years, the incidence of human filariasis was increasingly reported in many parts of the world, making the disease part of the group of emerging zoonoses. The infection caused by D.repens is the most widely reported dirofilariasis with endemic foci in Eastern and Southern Europe, and Asia. In the Mediterranean area, the incidence of human dirofilariasis has increased, especially the subcutaneous and pulmonary forms of the diseases (Italy, Romania, Serbia, Germany, and France). Human dirofilariasis is typically manifested as eiter subcutaneous nodules or lung parenchyma disease, in many cases, asymptomatically [60%). Patients infected with D. repens notice a subcutaneous lump in the affected area which most commonly includes the face and conjunctiva of the eye and sometimes the chest wall, upper arms, thighs, abdominal wall and male genitalia (Figure 3). Ocular involvement is usually periorbital, orbital, subconjunctival, or subcutaneous infection. Human D.immitis infection has been associated with the human pulmonary dirofilariasis and is usually asymptomatic. Symptoms of the disease are fever, chills, malaise, cough, localized retrosternal chest pain, and pleural effusion.

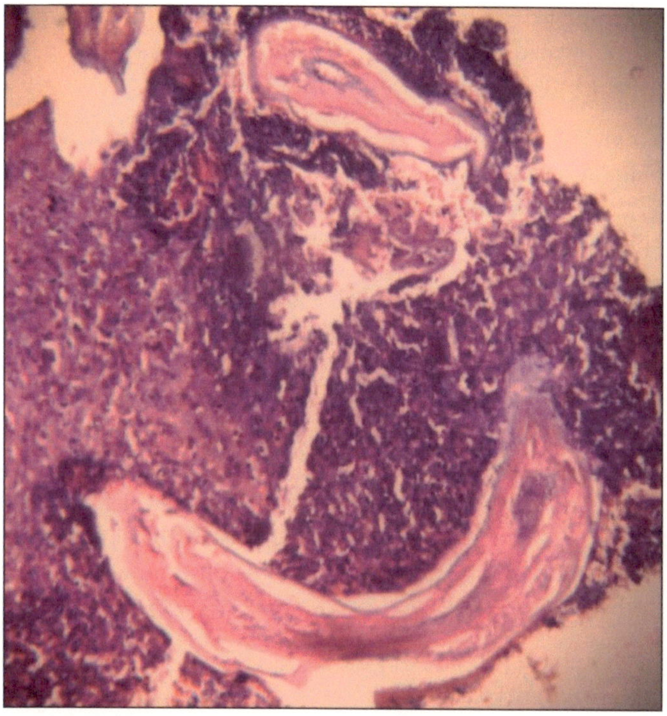

Figure 3. Human infection with D. repens are predominantly subcutaneous and most often evolved into a granuloma (Courtesy Hariish S. Permi, Department of pathology KS Haegde Medical Academy, India, 2011, (2): 199 – 201)

Our patient is a resident of Kotor and a civil servant, who has never left Montenegro. The first polymorphic symptoms occurred in January 2014 a feeling of discomfort and wriggle. Adition symptoms including the ocular disturbances that occurred later in the form of pain in short light flash, abdominal pain and dry cough that lasted for long, resulting in pneumonia. After an extensive examination was conducted, he was admitted in the surgical ward of the General Hospital of Kotor with suspected impacted epigastric hernia. On October 10, 2014, the surgeon using intraoperative method succeeded in extirpating entirely the solid fibrous granuloma, site epifascial, the midline supraumbilically. There was an indeterminate thread parasite 9.7 cm long in the excised granuloma. The pathological findings showed a granulomatous tissue with new blood vessels and giant cells of foreign body-type cells and concluded that such images can be found in filarial infections. Multipattern blood test for microfilaria was negative. Histological examination of the worms identified Diirofilaria, based on morphological exclusion of Wuchereria bancrofti, Loa-loa and Onchocerca volvulus. Serological examination of antibodies to Toxocara and Trichinella proved to be negative. After the surgical procedure the patient was treated with oral *ivermectin* (150 mg per kg) and dovicine 2 x 100 mgr. He feels good so far.

4. Discussion

Parasitic transmissible zoonoses (PTZ) in Montenegro belong to a group of emerging infections, and it is a growing public health problem. Considering the fact that enough research activity has not been devoted to this group of infectious diseases, the consequences will be reflected in the future [5,10].

Based on epidemiological studies, the extension of endemic focus of leishmaniasis in our environment is evident, based on the number of registered cases in nonendemic areas of Montenegro. Veterinary studies of domestic and stray dogs from different parts of Montenegro confirmed their high level of infection with Leishmania parasites up to 83% [16].

With filariasis (dirofilariasis), we do not have significant experience. The different types of thread-like nematodes are the cause of human diseases. Mediterranean region as to be endemic for dirofilariasis. In January 2014, the first case of human dirofilariasis in Montenegro was diagnosed. Veterinary service does not have data on the prevalence of infections in dogs in Montenegro. Numerous human cases have been reported for the European Union [16, 17, 18, 19]. In 1999, most reported cases originated from the Mediterranean area, where Dirofilaria spp. are traditionally endemic (Italy, France, Greece, Spain, Serbia), with sporadic reports of small outbreaks of subcutaneous/ocular infections caused by Dirofilaria in Germany, the Netherlands, the United Kingdom and Norway. Canine dirofilariasis was not reported earlier in Central and Northern Europe.[19, 20]

Drastic changes of ecosystem [21, 22, 23] give the basis for epidemiological changes that are characteristic for this group of infectious diseases. Agent's adaptability coverage and expansion cover the spectrum of natural hosts and vectors [24] thanks to their easy and quick transition from enzootic to zoonotic transmission cycles. This has enabled significant expansion and has given new importance to cotransmissive and coinfective forms of the diseases, with consequent difficulties in diagnosis, therapy, and prognostic assessment. [6, 10, 12, 14]

Parasitic transmissible zoonoses in our study represent a big problem due to diagnosed coinfection. Coinfection of Leishmania parasites and HIV was diagnosed for the first time in 2014 [25, 26]. Earlier studies had proven a coinfection of Leishmania parasite and the bacterial agent B. burgdorferi [27].

The latest studies in Europe have confirmed the significance of babesia parasites as the most frequent tick-borne agent in cotransmission, and participant in coinfection with B. burgdorferi. In our study common infection with babesia and B. burgdorferi is detected in 76% of cases [27, 28, 29]. Elsewhere in the world coinfections of the causative agent of malaria Pl. falciparum and the other types of Plasmodium were detected. During our investigations in 1996, Pl. falciparum and Pl. ovale were detected in the peripheral blood smear of one case, a sailor returning from Africa with a tick stroke.

Coinfective forms of diseases are not uncommon in VBD. Their occurrence highlights two possibilities. Epidemiological parth for the formation of coinfection is the consequence of cohabitation of vectors transmitted agents in common endemic areas and in the hosts and vectors. To confirm there were test results, certifying that the bacterial agent Bartonella hensellae can exchange their proteins and genetic material with B. burgdorferi and other microorganisms in a shared host or vector, which is part of their remarkable adaptability, and agent identification itself is a big problem for researchers [30].

Another possibility is the complex pathogenesis mechanisms that occurs in the infected organism caused by complex material of the agents provoking the immune response of the host, via cellular and humoral mechanisms that are able to overcome the pathogens, or contribute to the resistance against it, and against chronic infection, recrudescences, and initiation of immune and autoimmune mechanisms of infection.

The bottom line and the failures of the therapy are possible deviations. In the study it is shown that the elimination of Wolbachia induces extensive apoptosis of germ cells in adults, and somatic cells in embryos (microfilariae, larvae). The American Heartworm Society nonetheless recommends doxycycline therapy due to its beneficial effects [31].

A major practical problem is resistance or multiresistance to the therapeutic agents by which parasitic diseases have previously successfully been treated. Malaria resistance to hinolon and artemisine derivates has led to greater practical problems [32]. During our investigations, the first cases of resistance to antileishmania drugs occurred in 2008/2009. Repeated cure of treatment with *Glucantime* has not been successful, as well as the use of *Mmiltefosine*, We received good results after the introduction of *amphotericin B* in the therapy of our patients.

There is an opinion that therapy treatment for infection of B. microti for patients with good function of the spleen is not necessary and that those infections are self-confining. Therapy for infection with B. divergens is more problematic because it is more frequently found in asplenic and immunodeficient patients, with high level of parasitemia. The treatment requires combination therapy with *quinine sulphate* (600 mgr per os 3 x a day) and *clindamycin* (600 mgr per 3 x a day) for 710 days. *Pentamidine* can be an alternative drug. Examination of animal models has shown that good effects of cure can be achieved with *azithromycine*. American therapy schemes recommend curing of the heavy forms of babesiosis with combined therapy of *atovaquone + azithromycine* or *clindamycine + quinine*. In coinfections with B. burgdorferi, it is given the advantage to the cure of babesiosis and afterward it is carried on with curing borreliosis. In our study, common infection with babesia and B. burgdorferi has been detected in 73% of cases.

The much changes of natural and evolutionary factors put babesiosis in emerging human diseases. Clinical manifestations or asymptomatic infections are not always correlated with the severity of the disease. Asymptomatic parasithemia can be reactivated and take a malignant course in conditions of insufficient therapeutic treatment of coinfection and immunodeficiency. Grave manifest forms of diseases usually occur as an opportunistic infection.

Dirofilariasis has to be considered as a differential diagnosis in patients with subcutaneous or pulmonary disturbances (pneumonia). Effective therapy is possible by surgical removal of the adult worms with oral *diethylcarbamazine* (DEC) (2 mg per kg t.i.d.) over a period of 4 weeks was added to the surgical treatment in patients, only oral *ivermectine* (150 mg per kg).

5. Conclusion

In Montenegro endemic areas of leishmaniasis cover the southern part of the Montenegrin coast. More recent studies testify the extension of endemic areas in the entire coastal region and in accordance with the great expansion of the vector – Phlebotominae. Altered characteristics of leishmaniasis in Montenegro include: increase in the number of clinically manifested cases from the extended endemic area, which now includes the entire coastal areas, and increase of resistance to common therapeutic agents and drugs. The first cases of leishmaniasis resistant to *Glucantime* and *Miltefosine* were registered in 2008/2009, achieving significant results with *Amphfotericin B.*

The first cases of HIV coinfection with leishmaniasis were registered in 2014, as well as coinfection with other agents from complex VBD. Babesiosis is a parasitic disease that shares endemic areas with B. burgdorferi, which was proved in our investigations.

Dirofilariasis is a parasitic disease from the group of filariasis, which was first diagnosed in our country in 2014. There are no data in Montenegro on the experiences of veterinarians in the diagnosis of this disease among natural hosts and dogs. But it is surely present, based on data from Europe and countries in the immediate environment.

Author details

Bogdanka Andric*, Aleksandar Andric and Mileta Golubovic

*Address all correspondence to: bogdankaandric0@gmail.com

Clinic for Infectious Disease, Clinical Center of Montenegro, Medical faculty – University of Montenegro, Podgorica, Montenegro

References

[1] Fischbein DB, Dennis DT, eds.: *Tick borne diseases a growing risk.* N. Engl. J. Med., 1995; 333: 452–453.

[2] Domenico Otranto, Filipe Dantas-Torres, Emanuele Brianti, Donato Traversa, Dusan Petric, Claudio Genchi, Giola Capelli: *Vector borne helmints of dogs and humans in Europe.* Parasites and vectors, Jan. 2013

[3] Dennis DT: *Vector distribution, and evaluation of disease paterns,* 1st Congress of the European Society for Emerging Infection, Budapest, Hungary, September 13-16. 1998, Abstract3: 21.

[4] Anderson PK, Cunninghan AA, Patel NG, Morales FJ, Epstein PR, Daszak P: *Emerging Infectious Disease of patterns: pathogen, pollution, climate change and agrotehnology divers*. Trends in Ecology and Evolution, 2004 : 19 (10): 535-544 (PubMed).

[5] Gugushvil G, Sekhniashvill E, Lomtadze Z, Zerekidze L, Molashvili L: *About changes in population of transmissible disease vectors*. The collection of works of Research Institute of Medical Parasitology and Tropical Medicine, honored to Foundation (December 1999), XXXIII, 29-34: Chubaria G, Zenaishvill O, Gugushvili G, Zikarichvili L, Topuria I, et al. (eds), 2001, Tbilisi.

[6] Bogdanka Andric, Gordana Mijovic, Dragica Terzic, Brankica Dupanovic *Vector borne transmissible zoonoses* J. of IMAB-Annual proceeding (Scientific Papers), Publiesher – International Medical Association Bulgaria, 2012, Vol.18, book 1, 2012, DOI: 10.5272/j.imab. 2012181.220, p-220-225, ISSN:1312-773X, http:www.journaldatabase.org/journal/issn1312/773X, (PubMed).

[7] M. Acari, A.Badendine, CE Bennet: *A-Z Guide to Parasitology*. Vol.11. *Babesia, Tripanosomes & Leishmania*. Diasis Ltd, University Southampton, 2006.

[8] Corwin RM, Nach J: *Veterinary and Human Parasitology*. University of Missouri, College of Veterinary Medicine, USA, 1997.

[9] Berger SA, Marr JS: *Human parasitic Diseases Sourcebook*. Jones & Bartlett, Publishers,Sudbury, Massachusetts, 2006.

[10] Gray J: *Tick borne disease interaction*. 1-st Congress of the European Society for Emerging Infection, Budapest, Hungary, September 13-16 1998, Abstract.

[11] Bogdanka Andric: *Clinical features and diagnostics in associated transmissive (Ixodiae) zoonoses*. Doctoral dissertation, Medical faculty, University in Novi Sad, 2002.

[12] Krause PJ, Telford S, Pollack R, Christiansen D, Brassard P et al.: *Lyme disease and Babesiosis coinfections in Humans*. In: Cevenini et al. (eds) *Advances in Lyme borreliosis Research*. Proceeding of the 6th International Conference of Lyme borreliosis, Bologna: Societa Editrice Esculapio, 1994 : 159-162.

[13] Lucio H, Freitas-Junior, Eric Chatelain, Helena Andrade Kim, Jair L. Siguera-Neto: *Visceral leishmaniasis treatment: What do we have, what do we need and how to deliver it?* Int. J. for Parasitol.: Drugs and Drugs Resistance. 2012 (2): 11 – 19

[14] Wormser GP, Dattwyler RJ, Shapiro ED, et al.: *The clinical assessment, treatment and prevention of lyme disease, human granulocytic anaplasmosis and babesiosis – clinical practice guidelines by the Infectious Disease Society of America. Clin. Infect. Dis*, 2006 : 43 (9): 1089-1134.

[15] Bhat KG, Wilson G, Mallya S: *Human dirofilariasis*. Ind. J.Med. Microbiol. 2003: 21-65 (PubMed).

[16] Bogdanka Andric, Dragica Terzic, Brankica Dupanovic, Aleksandar Andric: *Public health aspects of visceral leishmaniasis in Montenegro.* Open J. of Clin. Diagnost. (OJDC), December 2013 (3) (Pub Med)

[17] Genchi C, Rinaldi L, Cascone C, Mortarino M, Cringoli G: *Is heatworm disease really spreading in Europe?*: Vet. Parasitol. 2005 : 24: 137-148.

[18] Pampiglione S, Rivas F, Angeli G, Baldorini R, Incensati RM, Pastormerlo M et al.: *Dirofilariasis due to Dirofilaria repens in Italy, an emergent zoonosis.* Report of 60 new cases. Histopathology, 2001 : 38 ; 344354 (PubMed).

[19] Dzamic AM, Arsic-Arsenijevic V, Radonjic I, Mitrovic S, Marty P, Kranjcic Zec IF: *Subcutaneous Dirofilaria repens infection of the eye in Serbia.* J. Helmint. 2009; 83: 129-137.

[20] Tasic S, Stoiljkovic N, Mladenovic-Tasic N, Tasic A, Mihajlovic D, Djordjevic J: *Human subcutaneous dirofilariasis in south Serbia-case report.* Second Dirofilaria days, Salamanca, Spain, 2009, p.12.

[21] Ivovic V, Depaquit J, Leger N, Urrano - A,B, PapadopulosB: *Sandflies (Diphtera, Psyhodidae) in the Bar area of Montenegro (Yugoslavia) 2. Presluce of promastigotes in Phlebotomus neglecticus and first record of Pl. kandelaki.* Ann. Trop. Med. Parasitol., 2004: 08: 425–427. Babcsiosis : Recent insigghts

[22] Oshaghi MA, Ravostan NM, Javadian EA, Mohebali M, Hajpran H et al.: *Vector incrimination of sand flies is the most important Visceral Leishmaniasis focus in Iran.* Am. J. Trop. Med. Hyg., 2009 : 81: 572-577.

[23] Corandi G, Zivicnjak T, R.Beck: *Pathogenesis of dirofilaria spp. infection.* Mappe parasitologiche 8, Cringoli G. (series ed.), Naples, 2007, p 59 - 66.

[24] Beugnet F, Clalvet Monfray K: Impact *of climate change in the epidemiology of Vector borne Diseases in domestic carnivores.* Comparat. Immunol. Microbiol. and Infect. Dis. Dec 2013, Vol 36 (6): 559 - 566.

[25] Domenico Otranto, Filipe Dantos-Torres, Emanuele Brianti, Donato Traversa, Dusan Petric, Claudio Genchi, Giola Capelli: *Vector borne Helminths of dogs and humans in Europe.* Parasites &Vectors. Jan 2013, Vol.6 (116).

[26] Alvar J. et al.: *The relationship between leishmaniasis and HIV the second 10 years.* Clin. Microbiol.Rev, 2008:21: 334-359.

[27] Rosenthal E, Marty P, Poiyot-Martin I: *Visceral leishmaniasis and HIV coinfection in southern France.* Trans. R. Soc. Trop. Med. Hyg., 1995: 89: 159 - 162.

[28] Krause PJ, Telford S, Pollack R, Christiansen D, Brassard P et al.: *Lyme Disease and Babesia coinfection in humans.* In: Cevenini et al. (eds) : *Advances in Lyme borreliosis Reschearch.* Proceeding of the 6th International Conference on Lyme borreliosis, Bologna: Societa Editrice Esculapio, 1994: 159-162.

[29] Hunfeld KP, Hildebrandt A, Gray JS: *Babesiosis: Recent insights into an ancient disease.* Int. J. Parasitol. 38: 11: 1219 - 1237, 2008.

[30] Lucio H Freitas-J, Eric Chatelain, Helena Andrade Kim, Jair L, Siquera-Neto: *Visceral leishmaniasis treatment: What do we have, what do we need and how to deliver it*? Int. J. Parasitol: Drugs and Drug Resist. 2012: (4), 11-19.

[31] Joseph E, Matthai A, Abraham LK, Thomas S: *Subcutaneous human dirofilariasis*. J. Parasit. Dis, 2011:35:140–143. [PMC free article] [PubMed]

[32] Pampiglione S, Canestri Trotti G, Rivasi F : *Human dirofilariasis due to Dirofilaria (Nochtiella) repens: A review of world literature*. Parassitologia. 1995; 37: 149–193. [PubMed]

[33] Pampiglione S, Rivasi F, Angeli G, Boldorini R, Incensati RM, Pastormerlo M, et al.: *Dirofilariasis due to Dirofilaria repens in Italy, an emergent zoonosis*: *Report of 60 new cases*. Histopathology. 2001; 38: 344–54. [PubMed]

[34] Padmaja P, Kanagalakshmi, Samuel R, Kuruvilla PJ, Mathai E: *Subcutaneous dirofilariasis in southern India: A case report*. Ann. Trop. Med. Parasitol. 2005; 99: 437–40. [PubMed]

[35] Nath R, Gogoi R, Bordoloi N, Gogoi T. : *Ocular dirofilariasis*. Ind. J. Pathol. Microbiol. 2010; 53: 157–9. [PubMed]

[36] Chopra R, Bhatti SM, Mohan S, Taneja N: *Dirofilaria in the anterior chamber: A rare occurrence*. Middle East Afr. J. Ophthalmol. 2012; 19: 349–51. [PMC free article] [PubMed]

[37] Joseph A, Thomas PG, Subramaniam KS: *Conjunctivitis by Dirofilaria conjunctivae*. Ind. J. Ophthalmol. 1977; 24: 20–2. [PubMed]

[38] Badhe BP, Sane SY: *Human pulmonary dirofilariasis in India: A case report*. J. Trop. Med. Hyg.1989; 92 : 425–426. [PubMed]

[39] Sabu L, Devada K, Subramanian H: *Dirofilariosis in dogs and humans in Kerala*. Ind. J. Med. Res. 2005; 121: 691–3. [PubMed]

[40] Poppert S, Hodapp M, Krueger A, Hegasy G, Niesen WD, Kern WV, et al.: *Dirofilaria repens infection and concomitant meningoencephalitis*. [Last accessed on 2013 Mar 19]; Emerg. Infect. Dis. 2009: 15:1844–6. Available from: http://www.cdc.gov/EID/content/15/11/1844.htm. [PMC free article][PubMed]